Second-Wave Neoliberalism

Second-Wave Neoliberalism

Gender, Race, and
Health Sector Reform in Peru

Christina Ewig

The Pennsylvania State University Press
University Park, Pennsylvania

An early version of chapter 5 was published as "Global Processes, Local Consequences: Gender Equity and Health Sector Reform in Peru," *Social Politics* 13, no. 3 (Fall 2006): 427–55. Material in chapters 3, 4, and 6 was published as "Hijacking Global Feminism: Feminists, the Catholic Church, and the Family Planning Debacle in Peru," *Feminist Studies* 32, no. 3 (Fall 2006): 632–59. Reprinted by permission of the publisher, Feminist Studies, Inc. Material from chapter 4 was published in "Piecemeal but Innovative: Health Sector Reform in Peru," in *Crucial Needs, Weak Incentives: Social Sector Reform, Democratization, and Globalization in Latin America,* edited by Robert R. Kaufman and Joan M. Nelson (Baltimore: Woodrow Wilson Center and Johns Hopkins University Press, 2004), 217–46. Reprinted with permission of The Johns Hopkins University Press.

Library of Congress Cataloging-in-Publication Data

Ewig, Christina.
    Second-wave neoliberalism : gender, race, and health sector
    reform in Peru / Christina Ewig.
        p.   cm.
Includes bibliographical references and index.
Summary: "Analyzes the politics of neoliberal health sector reform and its effects in Peru. Focuses on the intersecting dynamics of race, class, and gender in the developing world"—Provided by publisher.
ISBN 978-0-271-03711-0 (cloth : alk. paper)
1. Health care reform—Peru.
2. Neoliberalism—Peru.
I. Title.
[DNLM: 1. Health Care Reform—Peru. 2. Health Care Reform—Peru. 3. Politics—Peru. 4. Public Health—Peru. 5. Socioeconomic Factors—Peru. WA 540 DP6 E95s 2010]

RA395.P4E95 2010
362.1'04250985—dc22
2009053044

contents

tables and figures

preface and acknowledgments

When I conceived of this project in the late 1990s, I wanted to make a difference with my research. I had studied Latin American women's movements previously, and this time wanted to contribute to a movement in some way through my research. After feminists had criticized the negative effects on women of structural adjustment in the 1980s and early 1990s, it seemed that a focus on the gendered effects of the "second wave" of neoliberalism—the market-oriented restructuring of state social policies such as health, education, and pensions—was the next logical step. What impact did this latest wave of reforms have on gender equity? How did race and class interact with gender to mediate the effects of these new policies on women and men of different social strata? What were feminist activists in the region doing to address this new wave of reforms? Did gender play into the political process of social policy reform, and if so, how? Answering these questions seemed like a productive way to contribute to already established interests of feminist activists and scholars alike in gender and political economy. Latin American feminists have a long-term interest in reproductive health. In addition, health policy has historically been one of the foundational pillars of Latin American social policy systems. Therefore, I chose to focus on health policy and to do so in the racially and socioeconomically diverse country of Peru.

I began my research by tracing the formulation of Peru's health reforms, interviewing representatives of all possible interested political players, from labor unions to doctors' associations and health ministers. While Peruvian feminists, as I had expected, were keyed into debates over national reproductive health care policy, to my surprise, there was little attention paid by feminists or policy makers to the gendered effects of "mainstream" health reforms—things like privatization or decentralization of health services. This lack of attention was surprising given the rhetoric of "gender mainstreaming" at the time emanating from global forums like the United Nations Fourth World Conference on Women—forums that Peruvian feminists were actively involved in. Thus, one puzzle that this book sets out to solve is why feminists failed to intervene in the formulation of "second-wave" social policy reforms, in spite of their flurry of activity related to economic adjustment and given their strong global activism. The absence of feminists' participation in the mainstream health reform process is also one piece in understanding how the second-wave policy reform process itself was gendered.

As I researched the contemporary process of health reform, history began to draw more and more of my attention. Previous policy patterns and interest groups that had formed in response to earlier policies clearly played a role in shaping the politics of the contemporary reform process—and they did so in ways that appeared to reinforce or even create new gender, class, and racial hierarchies. I had begun to discern the importance of "policy legacies," a theoretical concept that refers to previous policy decisions that serve to shape the politics of future reform processes in important ways. Yet my research also led me to further refine the concept by demonstrating how such legacies may entrench the gender, class, and race inequalities upon which they arose. Moreover, my comparison of multiple health reforms in one country allowed me to begin to explain how and why some policy legacies were overcome in Peru's health reform process, while others remained in place. On this count, I found that transnational "epistemic communities" played an important part in determining the survival or defeat of particular policy legacies in the reform period, and also helped to shape feminists' interest in gender mainstreaming in the health sector.

But were these neoliberal reforms good or bad for women? Were they better or worse for some groups of women more than others? My second major task was to follow each of the major health reforms from formulation to implementation. I utilized mixed qualitative and quantitative methods to measure the impact of these reforms on gender equity. Market-oriented health policies tend to shift the costs of both biological and social reproduction from states and markets onto women and families—effects that are largely unanticipated in the policy-formulation stage. However, how these policies promote this shift and the extent to which they do so vary substantially according to the specific policy in question. Moreover, the same reform may have a dramatically different impact on different groups of women or men, dependent on race, class, or geographic location.

I hope that this book helps to illuminate for scholars, activists, and policy practitioners how seemingly neutral policies can have highly gendered and racialized consequences. I also hope that it provides some clues as to the political tools necessary to work toward a more equitable future.

While this book concentrates on the post–debt crisis period in Latin America, like many Latin American countries, I find myself greatly indebted today. This book entailed over fifteen months of initial research in Peru, followed by numerous follow-up trips. Many colleagues and friends in Peru were crucial in making this research fruitful. In particular, I thank Marcos Cueto, Ricardo Díaz, Ariel Frisancho, Narda Henríquez, Felipe Portocarrero, Cynthia Sanborn, and Victor Zamora for their ongoing support and assistance. For my major research stint in Peru, the Instituto de Estudios Peruanos (IEP) provided an intellectual home, with crucial library assistance at the IEP provided by Virginia García and Diana Balcazar. For their friendship and support while in Peru, I thank Cecilia Gianella, Farid Kahhat, Rocío Malpica, Caroline Mullen, and Eliana Villar.

This research depended upon the openness of policy makers, members of civil society, local community members, and health professionals in Peru who agreed to be interviewed. Those who wanted to be named are listed in the bibliography, and I thank all of those interviewed for generously sharing their time and thoughts. For help in facilitating my community studies, I thank Dr. Danilo Fernández and Antonio Moreno. I also thank my survey research assistants, Claudia Gianella, Rocío Malpica, and Madeleine Pariona Oncebay.

I am grateful to a number of institutions for their generous financial support. My major stint of fieldwork from January 1998 through April of 1999 was funded by grants from the Fulbright Foundation; from the Ford Foundation–funded exchange between the Red Para el Desarrollo de Ciencias Sociales en el Perú and the Duke/UNC Program in Latin American Studies; and from the Institute for the Study of World Politics. A Woodrow Wilson–Johnson and Johnson Dissertation Grant in Women's Health funded my expenses for interviews with representatives of international institutions in Washington, D.C. I also benefitted from a Paul Hardin Dissertation Writing Fellowship from the Royster Society of Fellows at the University of North Carolina at Chapel Hill.

This project began while I was a graduate student at the University of North Carolina at Chapel Hill. For early advice and encouragement as well as ongoing support to this day, I thank especially Evelyne Huber and Jonathan Hartlyn. Others who provided early support include John D. Stephens, Catharine Newbury, and Carol Wise. For guidance in my survey analysis I am grateful to José Sandoval. Friends and colleagues who commented on early portions of what would eventually become this book include Merike Blofield, Jenni Brier, Ethel Brooks, Sarah Brooks, Anne Marie Choup, Anne Eckman,

Maxine Eichner, Jessica Fields, Claudio Fuentes, Robin Greeley, Shuchi Kapila, Michelle Mouton, Waranee Pokapanichwong, and Carisa Showden.

The University of Wisconsin–Madison provided a stimulating and supportive environment for revising and completing the final book manuscript. I especially appreciate the generous colleagues at UW–Madison and elsewhere who read and commented on the final versions of this manuscript. Jane Collins, Joseph Harris, Yoshiko Herrera, and Rosalind Petchesky read the entire manuscript and provided detailed comments. Many others provided useful comments on one or more chapters or inspiring conversations, including Marcos Cueto, Wendy Chavkin, Paul Gootenberg, Alice Kang, Robert Kaufman, Florencia Mallon, Joan Nelson, Tricia Olsen, Joe Soss, Natasha Borges Sugiyama, Aili Tripp, and Kurt Weyland. Myra Marx Ferree helped me to get the framing right. Kerry Ratigan provided expert research assistance on the final manuscript.

Publication of early versions of some chapters allowed me to test out arguments made in this book. An early version of chapter 5 was published in *Social Politics* (Fall 2006). The story of family planning that appears in parts of chapters 3, 4, and 6 was published in *Feminist Studies* (Fall 2006). Some of the empirical material from chapter 4 appeared previously in Robert R. Kaufman and Joan M. Nelson, eds., *Crucial Needs, Weak Incentives: Social Sector Reform, Democratization, and Globalization in Latin America* (Woodrow Wilson Center and Johns Hopkins University Press, 2004).

I am especially grateful to Sandy Thatcher of Penn State Press, who agreed to take on this project and has provided helpful suggestions throughout the process. I am also grateful to Lynne Haney and another anonymous reader who reviewed the manuscript and provided constructive and useful comments, resulting in a much stronger manuscript.

My mother and father, Marianne and William Ewig, have been sources of support throughout this long process. My son, Gabriel, has been the best distraction, reminding me each day of the many beautiful things the world has to offer (beyond writing books!). Most importantly, I thank my partner, Will Jones. In addition to the critical commentary he provided on multiple versions of this book manuscript, his dedication to sharing in the tasks of social reproduction in our household, his willingness to allow me to travel for research for long periods while he cared for our family and home, as well as his unflagging intellectual and emotional support have made this book possible.

acronyms

AQV	Anticoncepción Quirúrgica Voluntaria (Voluntary Surgical Sterilization)
CGTP	Confederación General de Trabajadores del Perú (General Confederation of Peruvian Workers)
CLAS	Comité Local de Administración en Salud (Local Health Administration Committee)
EPS	Entidades Prestadoras de Salud (Health Provider Entities)
GAD	Gender and Development
GDP	Gross Domestic Product
ICPD	International Conference on Population Development
IDB	Inter-American Development Bank
IFI	International Financial Institution
IMF	International Monetary Fund
IO	International Organization
IPSS	Instituto Peruano de Seguridad Social (Peruvian Institute of Social Security)
MEF	Ministerio de Economía y Finanzas (Ministry of Economics and Finance)
MINSA	Ministerio de Salud (Health Ministry)
PAHO	Pan American Health Organization
PROMUDEH	Ministerio de Promoción de la Mujer y del Desarrollo Humano (Ministry for the Promotion of Women and Human Development)
PSBT	Programa de Salud Básica para Todos (Basic Health for All Program)
SAL	Structural Adjustment Loan
SEG	Seguro Escolar Gratuito (Free School Health Insurance)
SIS	Seguro Integral de Salud (Integral Health Insurance)
SMI	Seguro Materno Infantil (Mother-Infant Insurance)

SSE   Seguridad Social del Empleado (White Collar Social Security)
SSO   Seguridad Social del Obrero (Blue Collar Social Security)
WID   Women in Development

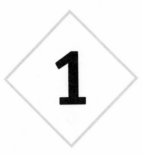

1

Intersecting Legacies of Inequality

In the early 1990s, Peruvian feminist activists and researchers were hard at work documenting the gendered effects of then president Alberto Fujimori's economic "shock therapy" and advocating for more egalitarian alternatives. They were part of a global community of feminist activists and scholars who criticized neoliberal structural adjustment programs for their negative effects on women around the world. Structural adjustment carried out by the Fujimori government in 1990, like the economic reforms promoted by major international financial institutions globally, entailed a uniform package of policies, including currency devaluation, dramatic cuts in state social services, and the opening of protected economies to global competition. Feminists argued that such policies shifted responsibility for ensuring the survival and well-being of local community members from the state to women. This critique is well known among feminist scholars and in most policy circles.

By the mid-1990s, however, a "second wave" of neoliberal reforms was well underway, the effects of which were largely overlooked. The Fujimori government, like others in Latin America, had begun to apply neoliberal tenets of privatization, decentralization, and market competition to pension, health, and education policies with the goals of making these more "equitable" and "efficient." Surprisingly, scholarship and activism on the gendered implications of these second-wave neoliberal policies—in Peru and globally—are still largely absent.

Through an examination of health sector reforms in Peru, this book demonstrates that the gendered implications of these second-wave social policy reforms are just as profound as those brought about by structural adjustment. Furthermore, the implications of these second-wave reforms cannot be simply assumed by looking at the findings from studies of the first wave of neoliberalism. Social policy reform is more complex than economic reform, involving a broader variety of policy strategies and more layers of decision making from the central government to local service providers. Second-wave reforms also took place at a different historical moment. By the mid-1990s neoliberalism had shifted from the harsh, prescriptive, one-size-fits-all recommendations of the "Washington Consensus" to a softer version. This second wave of neoliberalism was shaped by the heavy criticisms of the first wave's top-down mode of formulation and the disturbing effects of these structural adjustments on the most vulnerable members of societies. As a result, second-wave reforms not only targeted new policy arenas, but also reflected a shift in neoliberalism's own approach. This new wave of reform measures therefore requires careful scrutiny to discern their effects on equity, and gender equity in particular.

Second-Wave Neoliberalism presents both qualitative and quantitative data assessing the effects of neoliberal health sector reforms on gender equity in Peru. The analysis works intersectionally to show how reforms have different effects on distinct subgroups of women and men due to interactions among the intersecting social structures of gender, race, class, and location. Moreover, by tracing the global and national interactions that constituted the politics of the reform process, this book explains the global and local factors that led feminists *not* to carry their initial interest in economic adjustment through to analyzing the second wave of neoliberal reforms. Finally, this book takes a long-term historical view of the politics of reform, heeding how "policy legacies"—meaning the variety of interests, previous policy learning effects, and public expectations based on past policy decisions—impacted, in a gendered manner, the contemporary politics of health reform.

"Intersectionality" refers to the ways in which social positions such as gender, race, and class intersect, making the experiences, of women of color, for example, qualitatively different from either white women or men of color (Crenshaw 1994). Understanding the effects of health sector reforms requires a careful assessment of how class, race, and gender—and their intersections—interact with the new policies. Peru offers a promising venue for this study because it carried out health reforms typical of the Latin American region and because its race and class heterogeneity allows for a fruitful intersectional analysis.

Inequalities of class, race, and gender are tightly intertwined in Peru, as in much of the world. In 2001, following the economic crisis of the 1990s, 54.8 percent of Peruvians lived in poverty and 24.4 percent of Peruvians were considered extremely poor (INEI 2001). Economic recovery led to improvements in these figures by 2007, but poverty was still a major national issue: 39.3 percent of Peruvians lived in poverty and 13.7 percent were extremely poor (INEI 2007, 3). Using the poverty line method, demographers consider a household poor if the total it spends does not cover members' basic needs of food, water, and shelter. Those who face extreme poverty do not have enough resources to provide even their necessary food. Poverty and rural life are connected in Peru, especially when the extremely poor live on lands that have only limited productive capacities. Poverty is also related to race. Those who continue to eke out a living—often in mountainous terrain—are of indigenous descent and maintain their native practices. Most of Peru's extreme poor are concentrated in rural areas. In 2007 close to 64.6 percent of rural residents were poor and 32.9 percent were extremely poor (INEI 2007, 4).

Poverty does not mean the same thing to each member of a household, and this is one way that gender is crucial to our understanding of poverty. Decisions made within the household about who will receive more food and who has control over the little cash income earned through surplus agriculture will be influenced by intrahousehold gender hierarchies. Boys may be favored over girls in times of food scarcity, and most fathers will maintain greater control over the cash. National statistics show that Peruvian female children have a greater likelihood than male children to die of malnutrition (Blondet and Montero 1994, 75). Intrahousehold, gendered poverty is harder to discern as general statistics on poverty are still too often collected at the household rather than the individual level.

It is also important to point to the gendered nature of race in the Andes. Most rural indigenous men speak Spanish as well as their native Quechua, Aymara, or other indigenous language. This ability affords men access to vital information in a country where Spanish is the language of the government and the professional class. Like many rural indigenous women in other Latin American countries, those in the Peruvian Andes are more likely to speak only their indigenous tongue.[1] This tendency to be monolingual stems

---

1. This is true also, for example, in Bolivia and Guatemala.

partly from the fact that indigenous families withdraw their daughters from school after only a few years, whereas boys are encouraged to study and learn Spanish. Native-language retention is also related to the fact that women in indigenous communities are viewed as the carriers of culture, responsible for passing traditions from one generation to the next. However, certain gendered responsibilities remain constant across cultures: in Peru, as in most in the world, women are charged with primary responsibility for child rearing.

What can an intersectional analysis tell us about a specific policy like health policy? The following description and analysis of a typical research interview in rural Peru will help illustrate the connections. I conducted my survey and interviews for the rural portion of this study in the rural areas of the province of Ayacucho. I was based in the small city of Ayacucho and would travel between two and three hours from there by pickup truck or *combi* (public van service) to the rural health centers and communities for a few days at a time. On one typical trip I left at three in the morning with Madeleine, my Quechua-speaking research assistant. We piled into a pickup truck, cramped among fellow travelers and burlap bags of market wares. Public transportation to some rural areas was available only once a week, timed to coincide with market day. By the time we arrived at the end of our road trip, at the grassy plaza nestled in the mountains where the market would be held, it was about six in the morning. From there, we walked about half an hour up and over a mountain and through a valley to the first small settlement where we sought people to interview.

We arrived at a small cluster of houses and approached a home where we found our first willing interviewees of the day. The husband of this family, his breath smelling of alcohol from the carnival festivities the night before, invited us into the straw hut. We crawled through the doorway, and his wife motioned to some rocks for us to sit on. We crouched and conversed as she stoked the few thin sticks of fire that warmed the family's breakfast and stirred the thin, watery soup of a few grains of quinoa and greens and maybe a bit of *chuño* (freeze-dried potato), which gave it a grayish color. She offered me a bowl of the lukewarm soup and a large wooden serving spoon as Madeleine began our interview in Quechua. I started the tape recorder. The husband, outside the cooking hut and unseen to us, intervened in the interview with regularity, adding his commentary. The woman generally agreed with him, but sometimes gave an answer that contradicted his. By the look on her face, the questions on family planning made her uncomfortable. She appeared weathered and almost grandmotherly, yet she was the mother to the two-year old that she shooed away from the fire. Wind, sun, and hard physical labor age the faces of Andean rural women so that forty-year-olds appear seventy by the standards of wealthy nations.

The poverty in this and other villages of Ayacucho was unlike the poverty of the urban shantytowns where I also conducted fieldwork. Rice, which is the staple of meals prepared by the mother's clubs of Peru's capital city, Lima, was absent here. The few grains in the soup swam as if lost at sea. Yet this soup, which tasted mostly of salt and water, would sustain them as he worked in the fields and she tended to the grazing animals, with the toddler wrapped in her *manta* (woven cloth) on her back. In the urban shantytowns even poor families had homes of roughly constructed adobe, scrap wood, or, if they were lucky, brick. These two small huts—one for cooking, but also with a few feet for sleeping, and another about the same size, oval, and four feet in diameter—were all the indoor living space that this family had. Other than cooking and sleeping, most of their time was spent outdoors. There was no electricity for a television, common even in the shantytowns. This family may have had a communal tap for water over the next hillside, or perhaps simply used the stream. Despite the lack of amenities, they were well off compared to their neighbors because they owned a few animals, including two horses.

The poverty of this family, combined with their location in a rural sub-sistence agricultural economy, made access to and provision of health care services difficult. The majority of the population, scattered in small *comu-nidades* throughout the mountains, typically had to walk an hour to reach the local health center. Some families, like this one, faced up to a four-hour walk.[2] This family was fortunate to have a horse, which cut the travel time in half. There were no paved roads in this district, and only a path led to this particular settlement. Compared to other villages, however, this one was fairly close to the road, a half-hour walk away. If someone managed to alert the health center (there were no phones in the area, even at the health center), the ambulance could come at least to that road—if it was allotted enough gas that month, and if it was not the rainy season, when the perilous mountainside road washes out.

But access involves more than simply reaching the health center. Going there was a more daunting experience for this woman than for her husband

2. My survey of two rural districts of Ayacucho showed a range of distances to the closest health center—from a five-minute walk for those who lived near the health center, to four hours for the most distant. The average time was one hour.

because her gendered responsibility to care for children made her more socially confined in this rural setting. She was also more culturally isolated as a monolingual Quechua speaker. At the health center she would face a white or *mestizo* doctor born and educated on the urban coast who would not comprehend her language or her customs.[3] He would likely call her *mamacita* (little mama) rather than by her name. Indigenous health concepts like *pacha* (sickness from the earth) would bewilder him, which in turn would frustrate her. All of these factors would affect her access to health care, as well as the quality of care she received.

The nurse's obligatory questions about family planning, asked although the mother came seeking care for her sick child, would intimidate her, as did my own questions in the interview. At the time of this research, Peru had an aggressive family planning policy that targeted all women who visited health centers. Health workers in Peru often viewed poor women not as women, but as irresponsible baby makers. Men, on the other hand, were not expected to take responsibility for their sexual behavior. The health care workers operated within embedded gendered constructs, reinforcing these in the differentiated way in which he or she treated male and female clients.

Whereas the woman we interviewed came to the health center due to her gender-based responsibility to care for her children or for her own health, her husband never entered it.[4] Like most men I interviewed, this man believed that he did not get sick, except for an occasional work injury or alcohol-related brawl. For him, the health center was a women's place. If he had entered, however, he would have found that his status as a man and his ability to speak Spanish awarded him more respect from the health care workers. Like his wife, however, he would have been looked down upon due to his indigenous race, lack of formal education, and poverty.

Race and gender relations, combined with the poverty in which this rural family lived, have specific health consequences. Hard physical labor, poor nutrition, and less than adequate living conditions contribute to poor

---

3. Literally, *mestizo* refers to a person of mixed white and indigenous background. See further discussion of Peruvian racial distinctions below.

4. In my survey I asked respondents whether they had been sick in the past three years. Of men, 21.1 percent claimed they had not been sick, compared to 7.3 percent of women ($N = 193$). Men were also more likely than women when they were sick to either not seek health care or to simply visit the pharmacist or a market vendor to buy medicines directly. Of the men I surveyed, 9.6 percent reported that they went directly to a pharmacy when sick, compared to 3.3 of women ($N = 234$, more than the total number surveyed, as responses may have included more than one instance of sickness).

general health, rapid aging, and early mortality. The woman's health was affected by breathing the carbon monoxide from the indoor fire. She was also twice as likely as an urban woman to die in childbirth in an isolated community with no trained midwives and hours to walk, over mountains, to the health center.[5] The man's health was also affected by gender roles. From the smell of alcohol on his breath, we knew that he took part in male rituals of heavy drinking, especially at festival time. Like other poor rural men, he drank diluted rubbing alcohol, which cost only a few cents but ate away his inner organs. These are just some of the multiple ways that gender, race, and class interact in the everyday lives of poor people in Peru, and how health policy becomes intertwined in these interactions.

Legacies and Intersectional Approaches to Gender and Social Policy

The above ethnography provides a snapshot of the interactions among gender, race, and class inequalities as they relate to health, but it does not reveal the long-term processes that shaped this family's experience. For example, the family planning campaign that this woman encountered in her local health center was part of a continuum of policies in Peru dating to the nineteenth century that have viewed women's bodies as a tool of economic development. This woman's experience in the health center, faced with a *mestizo* doctor who might disparage her, also reflected a longer policy history in which the state has never viewed poor, indigenous patients as rights-bearing citizens deserving of health services. Nor was this woman's experience, and the history behind it, representative of all of Peru. Urban areas have a different policy history, one in which workers' struggles for health care benefits as a right shaped policy and ultimately resulted in a better social security health system for this group.

A "policy legacies approach" to social policy provides the historical perspective necessary to see the long-term policy trends at play for this family and others in Peru. Population policies, distinctive patterns of service

5. In the late 1990s rural Peruvian women gave birth on average five times in their lifetime (INEI 1999b). After massive sterilization and family planning campaigns discussed in later chapters, this went down to 3.7 children (ENDES 2004/5). In 1993 261 Peruvian women died in every 100,000 live births. In rural areas this number was significantly higher, 448 deaths per 100,000 live births (Blondet and Montero 1994, 74). In 2005 official figures reported an improvement of 240 maternal deaths per every 100,000 births (UN 2005), but no rural figures are available.

delivery to distinct groups of Peruvians, and interest groups such as labor unions that were emboldened by policies like social security are just some of the policy legacies that are crucial for understanding the politics of Peru's reforms at the turn of the twenty-first century. The policy legacies approach assumes that prior policies and the interests spawned in their formulation create politics that feed back into contemporary social policy reform (Pierson 1994; Hacker 2002). It is an approach that has become dominant for understanding the politics of welfare "retrenchment" in advanced industrialized countries.

I employ the policy legacies approach to understand the politics of social policy reform in Peru, but I also demonstrate that policy legacies feed back in ways that serve to entrench a particular gender, class, and race order. Thus, I develop a modified theory of policy legacies that recognizes that these have significant implications for the broader power relations of gender, race, and class. Moreover, I employ an intersectional approach in my analysis of both the politics of reform and the effects of the reformed policies. I build on the work of previous feminist scholars of welfare, who have shown that welfare regimes and the social policies they produce are gendered.[6] I add to this rich literature the additional insight that not just the policies, but the politics spawned by them (in the form of policy legacies) have critical gendered implications. But the effects of legacies are not limited to gender; they also have implications for race and class hierarchies. The intersectional approach, which I draw from feminist theorists in the United States, facilitates a focus on the interactions between gender, race, and class in the political process and helps me to better determine the impact of the resulting policies on equity. My focus on intersectionality adds a needed critical angle to existing work on gender and social policy, which has focused almost exclusively on gender. I also contribute to work on intersectionality through an empirical application of what up to now has been a largely theoretical approach. In applying the concept in Peru, I demonstrate its value to contexts outside the United States, but also caution that cross-country application requires significant care.[7]

---

6. Work on gender and social policy began as a critique of OECD welfare state scholarship. Key works include Skocpol (1992), Koven and Michel (1993), Orloff (1993), O'Connor (1996), Sainsbury (1996), and O'Connor, Orloff, and Shaver (1999). There is now an emerging literature on gender and social policy in developing countries, reviewed below.

7. Many have noted the dearth of empirical intersectional research, e.g., Hawkesworth (2003), Weldon (2006). Weldon also calls for work that considers intersectionality in comparative contexts.

Second-Wave Neoliberalism considers the four policy legacy types defined by Paul Pierson. I begin with a historical analysis of the formation of Peru's health sector that identifies the legacies resulting from this process; proceed to an analysis of the interactive effects between these legacies and the reform process; and conclude with reflections on the degree to which the reform process reshaped prior legacies and may have created its own political legacies. According to Pierson's typology, *interest group legacies* stem from policy structures that confer political assets on particular populations, including material assets and access to authority, or provide incentives for interest group formation. *Political learning legacies* are previous policies that inform the future decisions of policy makers. *Lock-in effects* give rise to widespread public expectations for policy continuity and therefore "lock in" a particular policy path. Finally, *informational policy legacies* influence the availability of information and therefore promote or deter mobilization in reaction to policy change (Pierson 1994).

I take Pierson's legacies approach a step further by demonstrating how political legacies themselves entrench the gender, class, and race inequalities upon which they arise. Interest group legacies not only have vested interests in defending existing policies that might provide them material benefits or access to power, but they often have interests based on their predominant class, gender, or racial makeup. For example, largely male unions in many countries have defended the "male-breadwinner" model of employment, arguing for higher wages in order that their wives could stay at home. Such actions uphold a social policy of breadwinner wages that confers material benefits on this group. But they also uphold male workplace dominance and traditional gender roles within households. In other words, simultaneous with defending a policy, these legacies also defend a particular gendered order. Similarly, policy learning legacies, although not as closely associated with a particular group of people, can carry with them assumptions about gender, race, or class. In the nineteenth century, when economist Thomas Malthus proposed his now disproven mathematical theorem that population growth among the poor and working classes would outstrip the earth's agricultural capacity and lead to mass deprivation, his theory reflected the fears of Malthus and other elites who felt threatened by the mass migration of peasants to British cities as a result of the enclosure movement. Population-control policies based on his ideas were aimed at the poor and working classes (viewed as responsible for their own social position) and asked nothing of elites to rectify inequality (e.g., through redistribution). Thus, these policies perpetuated the class interests of the elites that conceived of them. Current population-control policies often perpetuate these same basic elite interests. In these ways, policy legacies do not simply feed back into politics, making it more difficult to introduce new approaches; they also uphold particular hierarchies.

The legacies approach has been used to better understand the political factors, arising from past policies, that may block contemporary reform efforts. Understanding these legacies as defending particular class, gender, or race interests helps to reveal the broader interests that are at stake in policy reform periods—these are not just struggles over particular policy choices, but struggles over power and privilege. While analyses of retrenchment in advanced industrialized countries have shown that legacies successfully blocked most reform efforts, in Latin America reforms often succeeded, overcoming many old policy legacies. Thus, the reform period seemed to open the way not only for change of policies, but for configurations of gender, race, and class privilege. A puzzle that I set out to solve in the case of Peru is how and why some policy legacies were overcome while others remained in place. Related to this question, I analyze the failure of "gender mainstreaming" in the politics of health reform—why did feminists, following a flurry of activity on economic reforms and given a strong global presence and regional feminist networks, *not* successfully intervene in the formulation of second-wave social policy reforms?[8] Why—if we look from the vantage point of gendered policy legacies—did this space for reform, in which some strong "masculine" interest group legacies like unions were defeated, not open the way for the dominance of opposing "feminine" interest groups? I find that transnational "epistemic communities" (transnational networks of policy experts with a set of shared principles; Haas 1992) played an important part in determining the survival or defeat of particular policy legacies in the reform period, and also helped to shape feminists' interest in gender mainstreaming in the health sector.

---

8. "Gender mainstreaming" refers to efforts by feminists both in and out of government to assure that a "gender equality perspective is incorporated in *all policies* at *all levels* and at *all stages,* by the actors normally involved in policy-making" (Council of Europe 1998, 15). In the European Union and the United Nations gender mainstreaming is official policy. In Latin America it is rarely policy. Therefore, the focus in this book is on political factors that lead to getting gender equity onto mainstream agendas where no such policy exists. Many works on gender mainstreaming have been theoretical in nature outlining typologies of mainstreaming; see, e.g., Jahan (1995), Squires (2005), Verloo (2005). There is also a broad debate over the utility of mainstreaming as policy (see especially the essays in *Social Politics* 12, no. 3 [2005]). Others have focused on the role of state "women's machineries" and "femocrats" in incorporating gender onto policy agendas (Stetson and Mazur 1995; Franceschet 2003).

To evaluate the impacts of the resulting reformed policies on equity, I draw on the insights of scholarship on gender and development and gender and social policy in the developing world and bring to this work an explicitly intersectional approach. While the developing world is quite diverse, it is generally characterized by weak states, high degrees of informalization and casualization of labor, and reliance on family networks for well-being.[9] As a result, "welfare regime" (rather than "welfare state") more accurately captures the wide variety of practices and social supports that may or may not combine with state policies to produce well-being (Gough 2004). In "familialized" (family-dependent) regimes, the traditional concern of feminist scholars with intrahousehold distribution of resources—where gender power relations within families may result in women or children receiving fewer resources—becomes even more important (Hassim and Rasavi 2006, 12). The informalization of developing country economies also has gendered consequences because women who work tend to be concentrated in the informal sector (9). This phenomenon, in turn, has specific consequences for social policy. For example, Jasmine Gideon has shown how the concentration of women in Chile's informal sector resulted in lesser-quality health care for women than men (2007).[10]

Gender segregation in labor markets has implications for social policy when social benefits are based on paid work (Hassim and Rasavi 2006, 9). Jennifer Pribble's comparison of Uruguay and Chile demonstrated that the distinctive gendered character of each country's labor market had broad consequences for the overall "gender-friendliness" of these two social policy regimes (2006). In pension policy, scholars have shown how shifts in Latin America from state pensions to private individual retirement accounts left women with lower monthly benefits because women tend to take time out of the workforce or work part-time due to child rearing, earn less due to labor market discrimination, and live longer than men and thus stretch their funds over longer time periods (Arenas de Mesa and Montecinos 1999d; Bertranou 2001; Dion 2006).

Another recurring issue in the global north and south is the role of social reproduction. The labor that goes into social reproduction (which includes but is not exclusive to care work) is essential to the functioning of families,

9. On the informal and familial nature of developing country social policy systems, see Gough and Wood (2004), Hassim and Razavi (2006), Martínez Franzoni (2008).

10. On gender, social policy, and the informal sector, see also Benería and Floro (2006), Lund (2006).

states, and markets.[11] It is primarily carried out by women in families and in communities, and is usually undervalued, unpaid, or unrecognized.[12] Social reproduction has been a linchpin of feminist studies of advanced industrial welfare regimes, which have criticized mainstream welfare scholarship for ignoring unpaid labor and the family. Feminist scholars have also pointed to the fact that economic adjustment policies in developing countries were "male-biased" in that they did not take into account women's unpaid labor, yet relied on this labor for human survival throughout the economic crisis period (Elson 1992b).[13] Amy Lind's study of Ecuador's neoliberal reforms of the early 1990s shows that the use of women's unpaid labor became part of that country's "logic of development" (2005, 2).

Finally, scholars have focused on how social policies actively reinforce and create ideas about appropriate gender roles through their structure of benefits and through gendered policy discourses. This phenomenon has been demonstrated historically in Uruguay and Chile respectively by Christine Ehrick (2005) and Karin Rosemblatt (2000). Both authors show how the gendered discourses of political parties, state leaders, and women activists played into the formation of these countries' early health and welfare policies, resulting in different benefits for mothers and male breadwinners. The importance of gendered assumptions has also been demonstrated in analyses of more contemporary social policies that similarly reinforced women's traditional mothering roles, such as Mexico's cash-transfer poverty-alleviation program (Molyneux 2006) and Ecuador's day care and food-distribution policies (Lind 2005).

The above scholarship has focused on gender, but an intersectional analysis allows one to look at the interactions between gender and other social structures, such as race and class. The term "intersectionality" was coined by Kimberlé Crenshaw, but it emerged from previous scholarship on the relationship between gender and race largely developed by women of color in the United States and has since been refined by a number of scholars.[14]

---

11. A component of social reproduction, "care work" refers to the care-related tasks in families and communities often carried out by women. By referring to this as "work," the term emphasizes the productive aspects and signals that this work is not always out of love or devotion, as the "care" aspect of the term may lead one to believe. For a useful discussion, see UNIFEM (2000).

12. For more extensive discussions of the importance of social reproduction to political economy, see Bakker (2003), Peterson (2003), Bakker and Silvey (2008), and Hirschmann (2008).

13. See also Tinker (1990), Elson (1991), Afshar and Dennis (1992), Benería and Feldman (1992), Sparr (1994), Bakker (1994), Floro (1995), Haddad et al. (1995).

14. There is a large body of literature on the relationships between race, gender, class, sexuality, and nation that preceded Crenshaw, including, but not limited to, Moraga and

Intersectionality focuses on multiple dimensions of power and demonstrates a desire to complicate or break down essentializing categories (McCall 2005). As illustrated in the description of the rural family above, an intersectional approach is vital for understanding how social policies may impact different groups of women and men (distinguished by a combination of race, class, and location) in quite distinct ways, and how race, gender, and class interact to create these different outcomes.

Recent scholarship on intersectionality suggests an emerging methodological paradigm, one that I follow in this book. Key aspects of this paradigm include attention to more than one social position at a time (e.g., gender, race, and class); a focus on interactive effects between social positions; an assumption of dynamism or change of social structures themselves as a result of interactions between individuals and institutions; an assumption of intragroup diversity; and a commitment to multiple research methods (Weldon 2006; Hancock 2007; Nash 2008).[15] With regard to multiple research methods, I combine what Leslie McCall (2005) has termed "intracategorical" and "categorical" approaches to intersectionality. Following the intracategorical approach, I use interviews and ethnography to uncover the complexity of relations among gender, race, and class in particular locations in Peru. In the categorical tradition, I use survey data that compare "categories" of people— men, women, urban, rural, indigenous, and *mestiza/mestizo*—as a way to provide a broader understanding of the lived experiences of the variety of subgroups (and to begin to question and deconstruct these very categories).[16] An intersectional approach may focus on any number of attributes (disability, sexuality, religion). The focus of this study is on gender, race, and class, with race and class in Peru also tightly linked to location.

One cannot assume that race, class, and gender operate in the same ways across countries; thus, applying an intersectional approach developed in the United States to other contexts requires a great deal of care. "I am black, burnt by the sun," said one rural Peruvian woman to me when I inquired what race she considered herself to be (Survey 41).[17] This remark from an indigenous

---

Anzaldúa (1981), Hull, Scott, and Smith (1982), Collins (1991), Mohanty (1991), Anthias and Yuval-Davis (1992).

15. I follow Weldon in the assumption that intersectional research demands attention to interactions between social structures, not identities (Weldon 2006, 239). For an alternative view see García Bedolla (2007).

16. See methodological appendix.

17. All translations of Spanish interviews, survey responses, and sources are my own.

woman provides a small window onto the vast differences in the way that race is conceived of in Peru compared to the United States or Europe. She subtly refers to Lamarckian understandings of race, in which race is not based on biology as much as on what one does—in her case hard agricultural labor. The distinct nature of race, its close ties with class and gender, and the fluidity of racial categories in the Andes have led many to use "class" or "ethnicity" instead of "race" in Peru and other parts of Latin America. Following Marisol de la Cadena and Mary Weismantel, I use "race" to describe relations between indigenous, mixed-race, and European-descent Peruvians. The relationship between indigenous peoples, mixed-race *mestizos,* and white *criollos* (creoles) of "pure" Spanish descent is not simply one of class or occupation. Nor is it one of different "ethnic" characteristics—those things related to culture or national origin, such as ancestry, food, and language (Wade 1997). While elements related to class or ethnicity may play into the social construction of particular "races," race naturalizes economic and social hierarchies by using negative stereotypes and myths of superiority to justify inequality. Understanding indigenous-*mestizo*-white relations as racial rather than class or ethnic relations helps us to see that the encounter between the indigenous mother and *mestizo* doctor described above was as charged with racism as it was with sexism.

Peru (and the Andes more generally) has its own particularities in the way that race is understood. Persistent in Peru, as in other Latin American nations, has been a Lamarckian understanding of race in which it is thought possible to inherit acquired characteristics (Stepan 1991, chap. 3; de la Cadena 2000, 19). Lamarckism fit the Latin American reality, where elites were in fact often of mixed parentage and thus looked to education, "morality," "spirit," and other forms of cultural capital as the defining markers of race, rather than biology (Stepan 1991; de la Cadena 2000). Thus, "cultural fundamentalism" historically played at least as important a role as phenotype in defining Peruvian racial hierarchies (de la Cadena 2000, 28).

Cultural fundamentalism persists today, where education and morality are defining features of race in Peru (de la Cadena 2000; García 2005). The category *mestizo,* which literally refers to mixed indigenous and white parentage, can be reviled at one moment by a person clearly with mixed biological background but who sees oneself as a highly educated *gente decente* (person of worth) or *culto* (cultured) and thus white. Used by a person of primarily indigenous background, self-anointment as *mestizo* may imply a belief that one has, through education, attained a higher status than a lowly "primitive" Indian (de la Cadena 2000, 10, 25).

Race is also tightly linked to geography. Historically, coast and highland was not just a geographic but also a racial binary that defined the *serrano* (person of the highlands) in elite eyes as primitive while the coastal *criollo* was representative of modern Peru, and considered "white" regardless of skin color (de la Cadena 2000, 21). To elite eyes in the early twentieth century, the Amazon, by contrast, was not inhabited by primitive Indians, but by "savages" that had nothing to offer to Peru's nation-building project. Racial distinctions based on geography have softened in time (for example, *serrano* is no longer a slur, and may even be used with pride by a person from the highlands), but race and location are still tightly linked, with rural persons being predominantly "indigenous" and urban residents able to become *mestizo* regardless of their ancestral roots.

In addition to these gradations between indigenous and white, *chino* is used sometimes derogatorily and other times affectionately for all Asian-descent peoples (as in the nickname *El Chino* for former President Fujimori, of Japanese descent), while *negro, zambo,* and the more politically correct *afro-peruano* refer to the African population descended from slaves, which lives primarily on the coast. While Asians and Africans have made important social and cultural contributions to Peru, they have usually been left out of dominant Peruvian constructions of race and national identity.

Gender, race, and class are linked in a variety of ways in Peru. Bourque and Warren note that beginning in the 1960s, *mestizo* acculturation was used by men to reinforce their higher status vis-à-vis women in Andean communities (1976). In the 1990s, Marisol de la Cadena made the similar, though inverse, observation that in Andean communities women were "more indigenous" than men due to the fact that they were more likely to maintain their native indigenous language and practices (1996). In the urban areas, men also base their masculinity in part on race—poor and working-class *mestizo* men view white men as more beautiful, but also more feminine, and in this way question racial hierarchies by feminizing (Fuller 2001, 321–22). Central to racial understandings of morality is sexual control, and judgments of sexual morality fall on women, making race and gender mutually constitutive. The term *chola,* for example, often applied to indigenous-descent women market vendors who have taken on more *mestizo* ways, "racializes produce vendors, turning attention away from the women's occupation and onto their bodies, which it sexualizes in order to degrade" (Weismantel 2001, xxvii).[18]

18. For more on the term *chola,* especially in Bolivia, see also Zulawski (2007, chap. 3) and Stephenson (1999).

Despite the greater number of racial categories employed in Latin America, and the fluidity among these categories and their meanings, racism remains a powerful force. *Mestizos,* for example, according to Weismantel, "do not acknowledge partial similarity to those they stigmatize as Indians. Rather, they posit themselves as the absolute and inimical opposite of the Indian—that is, as whites" (2001, xxxii). De la Cadena takes a softer position, acknowledging that some *mestizos* posit themselves as whites, while others take pride in and recognize their indigenous roots, but not their "Indian" roots, which are associated with misery and deprivation (2000, 6). Both positions highlight that despite any number of racial categories, at discrete moments race is often reduced to "bounded pairs" such as indigenous/white or indigenous/*mestizo,* because such boundaries, as Charles Tilly affirms, "do crucial organizational work" (1998, 6). This distinct understanding of race, gender, and class and their interrelations serves as an important prelude to the intersectional analysis that follows.

Health Policy: A Sector-Specific Approach

Research on gender and social policy ranges from long- to short-term perspectives, and from sector-specific to overarching "regime type" analyses. The approach of this book is sector-specific; I analyze one sector of Latin American welfare regimes, health care policy, with special attention to the gendered political dynamics and effects of the period of neoliberal retrenchment. Health, which constitutes between one-third and one-half of all social expenditures in Latin America (Abel and Lloyd-Sherlock 2000, 1), offers a useful window onto "big questions of the state, citizenship, and struggles centered on neoliberal policies and their effects" (Briggs and Martini Briggs 2008, 17). It also offers a particularly useful site for analysis of gender inequality and its intersections with race and class within the broader framework of the Latin American welfare regime.

Because the health sector in Latin America is often composed of distinct systems (public health, social security health, and private health systems) that serve different populations, health policy captures how one social policy sector impacts the entire national population (whereas pensions, for example, only serve formal sector workers, a small slice of the population). Segmentation within the health sector reveals how welfare regimes, as Gøsta Esping-Anderson (1990) first observed, can also stratify along gender and race as well as class divides. Latin America's public health systems serve the poor, and in those countries where women or women heads of household are concentrated among the poor, these systems also serve a majority female constituency. It is also in these public systems where indigenous and Afro-descent populations are concentrated. By contrast, social security and private health systems in Latin America largely serve middle- and upper-class *mestizo* and "whiter" constituencies. Comparing these systems, their resources, and their quality (in which public health systems consistently fall to the bottom) allows one to see how the segmentation of health systems in Latin America is grounded in gender and race as well as class inequality.

A historical view of the emergence of these separate systems offers even greater depth of understanding of how gender, race, and class interact to determine access to health care. Nancy Leys Stepan has documented how Latin American public health systems were created in the late nineteenth and early twentieth centuries in a context in which the medical profession was heavily influenced by Lamarckian eugenics (1991). This form of eugenics viewed public health systems, and within these systems the molding of mothers, as central to nation building and betterment. Due in part to this history, public health systems in the region have traditionally prioritized mother-child health, and women and children have been the primary public health system clients. By contrast, social security health care, created through a process of conflict and co-optation between largely male unions and authoritarian and semiauthoritarian governments, was a masculine affair. The Colombian social security system, for example, restricted health care coverage for female dependents of male workers to obstetric coverage until 1993. In Peru, women workers in the social security system could not carry their spouses as dependents until 1992. These facts belie the gendered assumptions behind these systems—social security health systems were an essentially male privilege and the public health systems were feminized.

Gender inequalities are also evidenced in political debates during the period of neoliberal reform. For example, discussions of family planning, maternal mortality, or infant health care regularly invoked policy discourses that underlined women's contribution as mothers to the family and the nation. Feminist activists resisted these discourses, strategically invoking global conventions on women's rights to demand women's autonomy as individuals and greater reproductive rights. In these debates, women and gender were central. By contrast, in the "mainstream" health reform debates over privatization, decentralization, and targeting, policy makers told me in interviews that gender was inconsequential.[19] To them, such reforms were about reducing the role of the state, introducing the market, and promoting health care "choice" and efficiency. It was not about gender, or women. With the exception of recent reforms in Ecuador and Chile, Latin American feminists also largely stayed out of these "mainstream" health debates (Ecuador was most successful, in that "gender equity" was incorporated into the nation's general health legislation).[20] The comparison of these contrasting policies and the dynamics of gender in each reveals a lot about the politics of the health sector, and in turn, welfare regimes.

The health sector is also an ideal policy arena for a close examination of "second-wave" neoliberalism. Neoliberalism distinguishes itself from monetarism in that it is a more prevalent and looser, less ideological set of understandings on the "best way to run an economy," though both approaches fundamentally rely on the market for economic growth and equity (Fourcade-Gourinchas and Babb 2002, 571). The term "neoliberalism," rather than terms such as "openness" or "globalization" (preferred by market-oriented supporters) or "market fundamentalism" (preferred by critics of market approaches), offers a middle ground for discussing the philosophical preference for market orientation in economic and social matters (Babb 2007, 137). The pro- and antiglobalization theses are at loggerheads. This book attempts to move beyond these by outlining the changing nature of neoliberalism. Competing international discourses have forced changes in neoliberalism, while national governments have also accepted neoliberal tenets to widely varying degrees, in effect modifying neoliberalism on the ground. The range of Peruvian neoliberal health reforms covered in this book—from reforms of the early 1990s that represent "purer" forms of neoliberalism to those of the "post-Washington consensus" in the mid-2000s—illustrates these changes.

Finally, as has often been pointed out by analysts of this area (Evers and Juárez 2002; Petchesky 2003; Standing 2000), there is a dearth of empirical studies on the effects of health sector reforms on gender equity.[21] Many

---

19. I use "mainstream" here to mean those policy areas that reformers saw as central to the reform agenda; family planning policy was dramatically reformed in Peru in the 1990s, but, as I explain in later chapters, was not seen by reformers as central to overall health sector reform objectives. Thus, I place "mainstream" in quotes.

20. On feminists' role in reforms in Chile see Ewig (2008).

21. Empirical works on gender and health reform that do not focus exclusively on reproductive health are spotty. These include Hanmer (1994, 1994a) on Zimbabwe; Beall (1997) on developing nations; Gideon (2001, 2006, 2007) on Chile; Pollack (2002) on Chile; Forget et al. (2005) on Canada; Wang (2006) on China; Mackintosh and Tibandebage (2006) on Africa; Ewig (2008) on Chile; and Ewig and Hernández (2009) on Colombia. Lakshminarayanan (2003) provides an annotated bibliography, many of which are studies are based on secondary sources.

of the studies that do exist focus on the effects of reforms on reproductive health care exclusively.[22] By measuring the gendered effects of reforms to reproductive health services *and* more general health reforms, this study demonstrates how "mainstream" reforms also have important implications for gender equity, and reaffirms the need for gender mainstreaming in these more general policy areas.

Evaluating Equity: Redistribution and Recognition

In order to evaluate the effects of health sector reforms on gender equity (understood intersectionally), I draw from gender and development and welfare scholarship to create a framework for the evaluation of reforms. The crux of this framework adapts and develops Nancy Fraser's basic principles of redistribution and recognition into a rubric for conceptualizing and measuring an intersectional understanding of gender equity in the realm of health care. Equity refers fundamentally to fairness and justice; the *Oxford English Dictionary* defines "equity" as "What is fair and right." Whereas "equality" assumes sameness, the concept of equity recognizes the "differences in needs, conditions, perspectives and experiences that characterize differently situated social groups" (Petchesky 2003, 169). Moving beyond the ideal of sameness invoked by equality, equity requires "transformative change" (Reeves and Baden 2000, 10).

In many policy arenas equality of outcomes may be desired (such as equal pay for equal work or equal numbers of boys and girls attending schools), yet equal outcomes cannot be expected in the realm of health, where biological differences between men and women necessarily lead to different health outcomes. Women experience greater longevity, but also greater morbidity. Women and men also have distinct health needs, with reproductive health representing a major area, but not the only area, of health needs faced almost exclusively by women. Moreover, women and men face distinct social constraints that limit their access to health care and influence their health conditions.[23] For these reasons, as Lesley Doyal suggests, rather than focus on outputs, an evaluation of equity must focus on "the inputs that provide the basis for human flourishing" (2000, 932). Amartya Sen argues that equity

22. See, e.g., the special issue of *Reproductive Health Matters* 10 (20) (2002), Evers and Juárez (2002), Petchesky (2003), Yamin (2003).
23. For a review of the specific biological and social health needs of women compared to men, see Sen, George, and Östlin (2002).

in health is not a question of health results, nor is it solely a question of distribution of health services; equity encompasses all of the conditions that allow for the possibility to achieve good health (2002).

But how does one measure whether and how health policies are creating the conditions for the basis of equity? The link between equity and justice suggests that debates among feminist theorists over what constitutes justice offer promising ground for developing a feminist yardstick of equity. Nancy Fraser's two-ply conceptualization of justice, in which she argues that justice is composed of redistributive and recognition dimensions, brings into relief elements of equity that are often overlooked in health sector analyses— elements related to recognition, or status-based claims.[24] A focus on status-based claims helps to bring into focus those inequities related to gender and race that may not be related to distribution but have to do with respect for or valuation of differences.[25] The concept of recognition allows the analyst to work with race and gender simultaneously, thus helping to foreground intersectional inequalities. Distributive claims are clearly of consequence, and have long been a focus of analyses of equity in health service delivery. These are tied most clearly to class, but also have implications for gender and race.[26] Using the two elements together allows the researcher to cross-check the effects of policies on both forms of injustice.

According to Fraser, redistributive policies are appropriate remedies for socioeconomic forms of injustice, such as exploitation of one's labor, economic marginalization, or deprivation of an adequate standard of living (Fraser 1997, 13). The quintessential form of distributive injustice is class inequality. Examples of redistributive policies include reorganizing the division of labor,

24. For a review of gender analysis frameworks, see March, Smyth, and Mukhopadhyay (1999). For approaches to gender equity and health, see Standing (1997, 1999), PAHO (1999), Doyal (2000, 2002), Currie and Wiesenberg (2003). I am influenced by these, but prefer to modify Fraser's general theory of justice because of its parsimony. Two basic principles make Fraser's both a more flexible and powerful guide to policy analysis.

25. Fraser's conceptualization of recognition is associated with identity-based claims. In her later works she resists this association due to problems she sees in identity politics, most importantly, its oversimplification of group identities and denial of internal group heterogeneity. To distance recognition from identity, she chooses the term "status" (Fraser 2001; Fraser and Honneth 2003). Her reformulation is more consistent with an intersectional approach, but for simplicity I maintain the term "recognition."

26. In Fraser's 1997 essay she argues against an overemphasis on identity-based claims, and sets out to reemphasize material claims. Such reemphasis is not necessary in developing countries or in health policy where socioeconomic factors are considered paramount and cultural or representational aspects have been marginalized. Even in the industrialized country contexts the supposed emphasis on identity over distribution is empirically questionable (see Walby 2001).

or subjecting investment to democratic decision making (15). Recognition policies, according to Fraser, are the appropriate remedy for cultural or symbolic forms of injustice. These forms of injustice are "rooted in social patterns of representation, interpretation and communication" (14). Examples of cultural or symbolic injustice include domination by another culture that is hostile to one's own; being rendered invisible by the dominant practices of one's own culture; and being subject to disrespect or disparagement in cultural representations or everyday practices (14). Fraser suggests that policies that address recognition injustices could include positively valorizing cultural or sexual diversity (17–19). In later works she emphasizes that misrecognition is not just lack of valuation, but also subordination (2001, 25).[27]

The divide between redistributive and recognition injustices is analytical only; in practice, these two injustices often occur in tandem. Race and gender, for example, combine socioeconomic and cultural injustice, as women and people of color tend to be denied good jobs and equal wages while they are simultaneously viewed with disrespect by other members of society. This book demonstrates that health policies are not only distributive, as most would assume. They also have consequences for recognition. Fraser's dual conception of justice is a useful tool to parse out the recognition as well as distributive effects of health policies, and thus see more clearly how the two aspects intersect, just as gender, race, and class also intersect.

Applied to the health sector, distributive issues include economic and geographic access to health care as well as how policies distribute the health-related tasks essential to social reproduction. Women, due to their lower levels of paid workforce participation, lower wages, and greater levels of poverty, are more likely than men to have difficulty paying for basic needs, such as health care services. The hypothesis is similar for the culturally marginalized, who are concentrated in the lower-paid and subsistence sectors of the economy. Women and men, dependent on geographic location, may have greater or fewer health service options, with rural populations at most risk of lack of services. Moreover, geography can be gendered in that women often face greater constraints than men on mobility due to their gendered responsibilities for child care, or ideological constraints that prevent women from traveling far from family or home (Currie and Wiesenberg 2003). Finally, care work does not enter directly into Fraser's concept of distribution. However,

27. Fraser has been rightly critiqued for assuming that some social positions are entirely "recognition"-related, e.g., lesbian or gay persons. As Yuval-Davis points out, these groups also face economic or distributive injustice (2006, 200).

particularly in the case of health care, it is essential to analyze not just the distribution of medicines, clinic infrastructure, and health personnel, but also the distribution of the often unpaid burden of social reproduction. Health care, especially primary health care, is laden with gendered understandings that hinge on women's assumed responsibility for caring for the young, the elderly and the sick either unpaid or at very low wages. Reinforcing Fraser's point that the two aspects of justice often bleed together, care work also becomes a recognition issue when states fail to recognize the value of care work for social and human reproduction.

Social policy systems not only distribute labor and goods but also reinforce or change value judgments in the realm of recognition politics. On an individual level, health care workers reinforce broader cultural constructions of recognition through their everyday interactions with health care users. The attitude and approach of the health care provider can change depending on the client's gender, race, sexual preference, or class position, or some combination of these. These attitudes and interactions, in turn, can serve to open or close access to health care services. The "bedside manner" of health personnel in developing countries, for example, has been shown to be a key barrier to women's access to health care; women tend not to seek health care if they expect to be admonished or demeaned by health personnel (Mensch 1993, 242).

At an institutional level, social policies also value or demean clientele by the range and quality of services that they offer. If services essential to women's health, such as reproductive health care or breast cancer prevention and treatment, are unavailable, health services are not only neglecting to distribute essential services, they are also devaluing particular populations by denying them coverage of specific health needs. For particular cultural groups to feel that health services address their health needs, moreover, particular health practices or beliefs may need to be recognized. Stratification of health systems—for example, poorer-quality and lesser-funded services for the poor and better-quality services for the rich—are, in and of themselves, markers of recognition. Those with access to better-quality health services are recognized as "more deserving" while those denied access or with poor services are deemed lesser citizens. For justice in recognition, social policy systems must be organized in ways that recognize the "common humanity of different groups and the equal worth of each citizen" (Lister 2001, 100).

A final way in which health services can affect recognition politics is through facilitation or denial of what Ruth Lister calls "the politics of voice"

(2001, 101). Users of health care systems are recognized when they are treated not just as subjects, but as agents whose voices are heard in the processes of health policy formulation. Table 1.1 provides a summary of the distributional and recognition elements of justice as I apply them to health policy.

Peru: The Middle Road to Reform

While this is a study of one country, it is comparative because it compares the implementation of reforms in four communities and eight health centers in Peru, and it compares the political process of passing six separate health reform initiatives. The comparisons made within Peru, of comparing the effects of reforms on rural (primarily indigenous) versus urban (primarily *mestizo*) populations and of distinct health reform strategies within one country, allow for a fine-grained analysis of the interactions between gender, race, class, and health policy that could not be achieved in a multicountry study. As already stated, by examining the variety of policies within the health sector, including more traditionally feminine areas such as reproductive health as well as more strictly mainstream policies, I am able to compare how and why gender is placed on the agenda of some reforms, but not others.

In terms of its approach to health policy reform and its history of health policy, Peru can be considered a middle case in the Latin American context.

Table 1.1 Distributional and recognition elements of gender equity in health

Equitable distribution	Equitable recognition
• Wide geographic availability of services • Services economically accessible to all • Health system conscious to distribute care work equitably between men and women and state and families • Provision of health services that address the differing health needs of all citizens • Provision of health services that are of equal quality for all citizens	• Respect for and valuation of difference at the individual health provider–patient level • Equal valuation of care work and traditional paid labor tasks • Recognition of differing health needs dependent on social position and interactions among social positions • Organization of health system promotes common humanity (lack of stratification) • Voice—health care users not just subjects, but agents

Peru's health system prior to reforms was typical of Latin America: born of earlier periods of populism and authoritarianism, it was highly segmented and failed to reach a large portion of the population. Prior to reforms, Peru was considered to be in the "intermediate group" of Latin American countries in terms of the timing and development of its social policy system (Mesa Lago 1989). In the reform period Peru was considered a "moderate" case by Kaufman and Nelson in their evaluation of health reforms in six Latin American countries (2004, 43). In contrast to the more dramatic overhauls in Chile and Colombia, for example, Peru carried out its reforms in a piecemeal fashion—though the types of reforms even in these countries were strikingly similar. In terms of its degree of neoliberalism, Peru can also be considered a middle case in the Latin American context: its health reforms were neither as staunchly market-oriented as Chile's, nor as state-oriented as Colombia's. For example, while Chile and Peru both introduced private sector competition into their social security health systems, Peru attempted to promote workplace solidarity by mandating that companies as a whole (management and workers) elect one health care provider per company, rather than individual selection, to prevent private sector skimming of only the best-paid workers, as occurred in Chile.[28]

Peru lies in the lower-middle range among Latin American countries in terms of its major health indicators and health spending levels. Table 1.2 displays Peru's health indicators and spending compared to two higher-income countries (Mexico and Chile), its poor neighbor (Bolivia), as well as Costa Rica for comparison to the country with the best health indicators of the region.

Outline of Chapters

The chapters that follow are divided into analyses of the prereform health system formation period, the politics of neoliberal reform in the 1990s and early 2000s, and three chapters that analyze the effects of these reforms on gender equity. Chapter 2 traces Peru's health history from its founding moments in the late nineteenth century to the 1980s in an effort to clarify the policy patterns and policy interest groups that were formed by previous health policies. It connects the histories of public health programs and social security health care—two class-specific developments that scholars rarely

28. On Chile's "cream-skimming" health reforms see Castiglioni (2001, 43), and Titleman (2000).

Table 1.2   Basic health and health spending indicators, 2008

	Bolivia	Peru	Colombia	Mexico	Chile	Costa Rica
Life expectancy at birth[P]	65.9	71.7	73.1	76.4	78.7	78.9
Infant mortality rate, estimated (per 1,000 live births)[P]	54.0	21.0	15.9	15.7	7.6	10.1
Maternal mortality, reported (per 100,000 births)	229.0[P]	240.0[C]	73.1[P]	58.6[P]	18.1[P]	30.0[C]
Physicians per 10,000 inhabitants ratio	3.56[C]	11.5[P]	12.7[P]	14.0[P]	9.3[P]	20.0[P]
Annual national health expenditure as a percentage of GDP[C]	1.42	1.0	3.38	3.1	2.8	6.0

Sources: PAHO 2008 (denoted by "P") and CEPALSTAT 2008 (denoted by "C"). All are latest available data for each indicator ranging from 2003 to 2008.

place side by side—to make apparent the class, gender, and racial character of the health sector as a whole. The chapter puts the modified "policy legacies" approach described in this chapter to work on the Peruvian case. It contributes to theory about policy legacies by showing that "legacies" are not simply differential levels of power among interest groups or ingrained ideas of how to approach particular policy dilemmas, but power struggles that often reflect and reinforce racial and gender inequalities.

Chapter 3 is the first of two chapters that analyze the politics of neoliberal reform. Focusing on the role of global factors, the chapter asks why policy makers looked to foreign models and overcame old policy legacies in some reforms, but not in others. The answer resides in part in the strength of the competing transnational epistemic communities that advocated for dramatic policy change: the neoliberal and rights paradigms.

The global split between the rights-based and neoliberal epistemic communities also led to a gendered division of labor in Peru's national health reform process. Some reforms, like family planning, were viewed by policy makers and feminists alike as an appropriately feminist domain; others, like fees, privatization, and decentralization, were viewed as "gender-neutral" and thus not feminists' business, even though they have different effects on women and men, on different classes, and on different races. Chapter 4 traces the national political processes that led to the passage of six major health reforms: fees for services; a basic health care package; community-based decentralization;

the introduction of private sector competition into the social security health system; targeted public insurance; and increased access to family planning services. This comparison highlights the gendered nature of the reform process, and the role of policy legacies in that politics. It also helps to explain why, despite the high profile of feminists at the time globally and nationally, gender equity was not incorporated into "mainstream" health reforms.

Chapter 5 evaluates the impact on equity of key market-mimicking reforms applied to Peru's public health system for the poor: fees for services and related means testing; a basic package of guaranteed health services; and the decentralization of primary health care services to community boards. I use intersectional analysis and the conceptualization of gender equity laid out in this chapter to evaluate the effects of the reforms on different women and men, dependent on their race and class position. This chapter finds, for example, that the same decentralization reform has had dramatically different consequences for rural, indigenous poor women compared to urban poor women.

Chapter 6 analyzes the effects and politics of Peru's reformed family planning program, the only reform based on "rights-based" principles, and ironically one that abused human-rights in practice. Disturbingly, the Fujimori government in the 1990s targeted poor, indigenous women in a massive sterilization campaign that utilized feminist rhetoric to mask a neo-Malthusian and eugenicist population policy. This chapter analyzes the human effects of the policy and political fires between feminists, the state, and the Catholic Church that resulted. This chapter demonstrates that family planning policy *in practice* continued the historical policy legacy of population control in spite of its veil of rights-based rhetoric.

Chapter 7 compares the introduction of private health insurance and health provision for the middle and upper classes and the evolution of targeted state health insurance for the poor called Seguro Integral de Salud. These two reforms, despite their very different political geneses, converge on a number of counts in their denial of gender equity. In other ways, however, the targeted insurance for the poor may be setting a positive "new" policy legacy; it has set a precedent of progressively broader public health insurance that has served to ameliorate some of the long-standing race- and gender-based divisions in Peru's health system.

The conclusion summarizes the major findings regarding the effects of second-wave neoliberal reforms on gender equity and reflects on whether or not these second-wave reforms have changed the politics of Peru's health system for the long haul.

2

Colonization and Co-optation: Historical Legacies of Inequality in the State Health System

Beginning in the late nineteenth century and extending to the mid-twentieth century, organized groups in Peruvian civil society, medical doctors, and foreign interests interacted with the state in the construction of Peru's foundational state health policies. In the process, these actors and the policies themselves also actively constructed and at times contested class, race, and gender divisions. Existing inequalities shaped the formation of the health system, which in turn reinforced and perpetuated them by privileging some groups over others. But this is not to imply that the inequalities were rigid and forever maintained. Gender, race, and class continue to be immensely important in structuring Peruvian inequality, but the categories themselves have morphed and health policies have changed, leading to a reshaping of inequalities and social policies over time. This chapter explores the interaction between social policies and inequalities to understand the origins of the historical policy legacies with which future agents of change must contend. It serves as a prelude to understanding gender, race, and class in the context of the major health reforms of the 1990s and early 2000s.

Social scientists have convincingly argued that only by putting short-term events into a long-term perspective can we see the full array of factors that led to a particular outcome (Huber and Stephens 2001, 36; Pierson 2004, chap. 3). This chapter uses the concepts of redistribution and recognition introduced in chapter 1 to illustrate the ways the health system historically stratified Peruvian society. Demonstrating the multiple forms of stratification produced by Peru's health system is essential to understanding the inequities of poverty, race, and gender that had to be overcome by the reforms of the 1990s and early 2000s. Social policies such as pensions, health care, and anti-poverty programs are often conceived of as tools to ameliorate inequalities. Yet, as Gøsta Esping-Anderson (1990) first observed, social policies provide benefits *and* (intentionally or not) stratify societies along multiple cleavage lines. Scholars have offered rich analyses of how policies perpetuate gender and racial inequalities in advanced industrialized nations, but historical feminist welfare state analysis in Latin America is as yet a nascent field of inquiry.[1] James Malloy (1979) and Carmelo Mesa-Lago (1978, 1989) are often referred to as classic comparative accounts of social policy formation in Latin America, but they focus primarily on class power and state responses to class-based actions and ignore gender and race.[2] Class is indeed fundamental to understanding social policy formation in Latin America, but in this chapter I demonstrate that the formation processes were also based on gendered and racialized power relations. The resulting health system has class, racial, and gendered forms of stratification.

Policies, once implemented, can create "feedback" effects that change the dynamics of future policy debates: this is the essential lesson of the policy legacies school (Pierson 1993). Policy legacies can only be identified through historical analysis. The major proponents of this approach see legacies as neutral with regard to gender and race; this chapter demonstrates that legacies reflect and reinforce power disparities along class, race, and gender lines.[3] For feminist scholars, the legacies approach allows one not only to identify more carefully the political challenges to change that are wrought by previous policy decisions, but also to see precisely how history might influence contemporary gender dynamics of reform—obstacles to gender mainstreaming, for example. The historical perspective in this chapter informs scholars about the ways social policy legacies not only bring about

---

1. Historical comparative work on gender and social policy in advanced industrial countries includes Gordon (1990), Bock and Thane (1991), Skocpol (1992), Koven and Michel (1993), O'Connor (1996), Mettler (1998), and O'Connor, Orloff, and Shaver (1999). On race see Quadagno (1996). Initial works on Latin America include Dore and Molyneux (2000), Rosemblatt (2000), Ehrick (2005), and Pribble (2006).

2. More recent comparative historical treatments of welfare states have expanded their lens to include the roles of democracy and fiscal crisis (Haggard and Kaufman 2008) and political parties (Huber and Stephens 2001), but not gender or race.

3. Key works using the policy legacies approach include Pierson (1993, 1994), Hacker (2002), Haggard and Kaufman (2008).

stratification, but also may create political challenges to future attempts toward equity.

Stratification and legacies also conjure images of stasis, as though stratification is permanent and policy legacies will prevent any future changes. Neither phenomenon is easily budged, but particular political and economic circumstances can lead to erosion of stratification and the opportunity for agents of change to overcome previous legacies. Accordingly, this chapter also highlights change.

Policy Legacies and the Founding of Peru's Health System

As laid out in the previous chapter, policy legacies have been divided by Paul Pierson into four basic types: *interest group legacies,* which stem from policy structures and confer political assets on particular populations, including material assets and access to authority, or provide incentives for interest group formation; *political learning legacies,* essentially policies that inform the future decisions of policy makers; *"lock-in" effects,* which result in "elaborate social and economic networks that greatly increase the cost of adopting once-possible alternatives" and give rise to widespread public expectations for policy continuity; and *informational policy legacies,* which influence the availability of information and therefore promote or deter mobilization in reaction to policy change (Pierson 1994, 40–50).

The concept of policy legacies brings to the forefront the political advantage early policies offer to some groups over others, and how this advantage can be compounded over time. Like large investors who are offered a preferential interest rate, groups with greater resources and power are institutionally advantaged to have even more resources and power in future policy debates. I take this logic a step further by arguing that policy legacies afford political advantage to some races, classes, or genders over others. If policy legacies can reproduce existing power differences by explicitly affording greater power and resources to some over others, it is logical that the social policies that produce these legacies can be one of the mechanisms by which gender, class, or racial advantage can be compounded over time. Thus, social policies not only stratify, but unevenly feed back into the political dynamics of policy change, creating greater stratification or preventing change toward more equitable policy options by perpetuating or shoring up power disparities.

Interest group legacies, policy learning legacies, lock-in effects, and informational legacies all may feed back into broader societal gender, race, and class dynamics. As mentioned in chapter 1, male unions (a policy interest group legacy), for example, have often demanded the continuation of the social policy of a "breadwinner" wage, which confers specific assets on this group. At the same time, this demand also perpetuates traditional male and female roles within the household. Population control policies, similarly, evolved out of class-based interests in placing the responsibility for poverty on the sexual behavior of poor women, thus deflecting elite responsibility for distribution. When applied over and over, such policy learning legacies reinforce the class and gender bias from which they were conceived. As an example of a lock-in effect, if previous policies have invested resources or infrastructure in geographic areas where a class or racial group is dominant—but not in other areas—it may cultivate an expectation that certain areas will continue to be served well, and demands for more universal distribution may be stymied by lack of resources or initiative. Such a lock-in effect could, in turn, perpetuate class or racial distributional imbalances.

As I explore below, Peru's health sector was constructed in a two-stage process. Similar to the rest of Latin America, it began in the late nineteenth century with a public system created by internal colonialism. The concept of internal colonialism, which was first applied in Latin America in the 1960s, refers to a process by which interior portions and peoples of a single national territory are dominated both culturally and economically by a dominant elite.[4] I use the term "internal colonialism" principally because key protagonists in founding state health services characterized public health as an important tool for the state to gain control over, or internally "colonize," geographically isolated areas and improve the nation's human "stock" for economic and political ends. The state and the many doctors, nurses, and health professionals in its service saw the project of building a public health system as part of bettering Peru's people and their life conditions, even though the means used were rarely democratic or egalitarian and were tinged with racial and gender prejudice. They often bolstered their efforts with foreign cooperation, making the process in some ways more directly akin to foreign colonization, but it was primarily a nationally motivated, internal process.

4. See, e.g., Gonzáles-Casanova (1965), Stavenhagen (1965), Havens and Flinn (1970), Quayum (2002), and on Peru specifically, Cotler (1978, chap. 3). Hechter (1975) expanded the concept theoretically and applied it to the British Isles.

The term "colonialism" also highlights the interrelations between sexuality and race in contexts of economic and cultural dominance. In the vein of feminist scholars of colonialism, such as Ann Stoler and Anne McClintock, colonialism was not merely about economic and cultural conquest but equally engaged with control of "intimate" and "carnal" aspects of colonial life, a control that sought to create gender and racial hierarchies as a means of reinforcing the power of the colonizer (A. McClintock 1995; Stoler 2002). Moreover, colonial techniques of control were often reimported into metropoles with the aim of containing the actions of lower-class compatriots (A. McClintock 1995, chap. 2; Stoler 2002, chap. 4). My usage of "internal colonialism," referring to colonialism within a single nation-state, thus also hints at the complex understandings of colonialism eloquently argued by these authors, where the line between colonized and colonizer was constantly subject to construction and where not just the cultural and economic, but also sexual aspects of domination were central. Borrowing the words of Linda Gordon, I use internal colonialism as a "metaphor" to emphasize the intertwined roles of race and gender in a process of economic, cultural, and sexual domination of which the building of Peru's health system was a part. It is a metaphor meant to emphasize the complexities of processes of domination rather than flatten these into a categorical label (Gordon 2006, 428–29).[5]

Peru's process of internal colonialism depended on preconceived class, gender, and racial hierarchies. During the late nineteenth and extending through the early twentieth century, male *criollo* (meaning of Spanish descent) aristocrats from the Hispanic-influenced coast of Peru devised the public health system. They did so in part out of a desire for the betterment of the targeted populations of women, indigenous peoples (pejoratively termed *indios* and *serranos*), and the poor, but also in part out of a desire to exploit these groups so they might contribute the human resources necessary for the economic and social development of the nation as a whole. Because its designers employed hierarchal distinctions to justify their mission, the public health system that emerged had important stigmatizing aspects that further reinforced class, gender, and race inequalities. These effects were brought into greater relief in the second major phase of health policy development in Peru.

This second major period (1930s–1950s) represents an important shift in both the structure of Peruvian society and the process by which the health

---

5. Gordon (2006) provides some history of the term and applies it to the history of the United States.

system was constructed. Industrialization, migration, and urbanization led to the emergence of two new classes of workers: urban factory workers and middle-class professionals. The dominant poor/elite class division began to lose some significance as a new class category, the urban worker, emerged. These urban industrial workers and middle-class professionals represented a small new group of elites. With this shift, we also see the division between white (*criollo*) and indigenous peoples change with the advent of the idea of the *mestizo*. *Mestizo* literally meant a person of mixed white and indigenous heritage, but, as discussed in the previous chapter, it might also mean an indigenous person who took on more "European" or "educated" ways—or who simply moved from highlands to coast. An important portion of urban Peruvian society, including the new workers and professionals, began to identify as *mestizo* rather than white or indigenous. As Jorge Parodi exemplifies in his history of a metalworkers union in Lima, there were significant racial tensions between Limeño native workers and indigenous descent migrant workers from the highlands, yet in time the migrant "ceased to identify himself with his original community" (Parodi 2000, 79). This was a process of racial identity change, where migrant *serranos,* through education and movement, became *mestizo*.

The emergence of this new political class contributed in turn to health policy formation. In a context of scarce resources, white- and blue-collar workers used their newfound political power to demand better health services from the state, but they did so in an exclusive manner that layered a higher-quality social security system, serving only these workers, on top of the existing, poorly supported public health system, which it left intact. The state, in a form reminiscent of Bismarck's Germany, recognized the political advantage of separate but unequal health systems, as this form of organization limited state expenditures and served as a political tool for co-opting these new, emerging political powers.

The layering strategy reinforced class and racial hierarchies, as the resulting health system provided more and better services to *criollo* and *mestizo* workers than to the indigenous poor. Moreover, the social security health systems created for the middle and working classes served primarily male workers, with extremely limited coverage for spouses and children. The public health care system was left feminized in two senses: it was the only system free of direct cost to the majority of women and the poor, and one of its major premises was to control women's biological reproduction. A further distinction was that the social security health system came to be viewed as an exclusive right earned by its beneficiaries, while the public health system, which had never been explicitly fought for, continued to be viewed as a "welfare" benefit in the stigmatizing sense, and as a policy apparatus through which national economic objectives were prioritized over individual well-being. The next sections narrate this two-stage history of colonization and co-optation in greater detail.

Colonization: Health Care for the Poor

Peru's public health system was formed largely through internal colonialism. As discussed above, this process included exploitation of human resources in order to serve broader, instrumental national economic and political objectives. But this form of colonialism also incorporated the objective of national betterment through better health. The twin objectives of economic exploitation and human betterment may seem contradictory, but in fact they were intimately linked in the late nineteenth century as part of broader ideas of nation building and development.

The mingling of these seemingly contradictory objectives is explained in part by the ideational grounding of the early Peruvian and broader Latin American public health movements in eugenics. As discussed in detail by Nancy Stepan, eugenics gained so much traction in the region in the early twentieth century that by the 1920s "health" in Latin America had become "a matter of heredity and race" (Stepan 1991, 5, 9). Latin American eugenics thinking was based primarily on Lamarckian ideas, which asserted that acquired characteristics could be inherited, rather than the Mendelian, purely genetic, variety of eugenics that dominated in Britain, the United States, and later Germany (chapter 3). In addition, the dominance of the Catholic Church meant that Latin American eugenicists rejected negative tactics, such as sterilization, that were common in Europe and the United States.[6] Instead, along with public health initiatives, the state used prenuptial certificates, sex education, and surveillance of mothers as its primary means of promoting "Christian" eugenics (103).

Via a Lamarckian emphasis on nurture as a means to improve nature, racial improvement was a primary motivation for building early Latin American public health systems. The discourse of eugenics was as powerful in Peru as

6. Mexico's was the only eugenics movement in Latin America actually to implement sterilization, and then only briefly in one state (Stepan 1991, 128).

in the rest of the region; in 1908 conservative intellectual Francisco Graña coined the term *autogenia,* a Peruvian version of eugenics that sought to improve the "race" internally through raising health and nutritional standards (de la Cadena 2000, 17). Eugenics was also gendered in that women were seen primarily as reproducers, the vehicles through which hereditary or acquired characteristics could be cultivated (Stepan 1991, chap. 4; Zulawski 2007, chap. 4). This view of women was not unique to followers of eugenics. The notion that women were defined by their uteri, physically weak and deficient, and by extension not able to participate in political or public life was common in the medical profession in the late nineteenth century.[7] By the early twentieth century, with urbanization and the rise of the middle class, Peruvian women began to insert themselves more into public life through education and new forms of work and social organizations, but they remained idealized as mothers whose sexual honor was to be protected (Mannarelli 1999, 41–43). Doctors (overwhelmingly male) continued to view women as reproducers, akin to cows and just as dirty (46, 53). Yet, complicating a simple view, and demonstrating the importance of intersections of class and gender, middle-class and elite Peruvian women participated energetically in the hygiene campaigns of the 1910s and '20s (60–62).

While eugenics formed an important ideational basis, Peru's public health system was also spurred by economic development and the related expansion of the state in the late nineteenth and early twentieth centuries. From 1890 to 1930, Peru experienced dramatic economic growth. According to one estimate, from 1900 to 1929 the gross domestic product grew seven and a half times (Boloña 1994, cited in Contreras 2004, 177). Economic growth led to state growth. Between 1920 and 1928 the number of public servants in Lima almost tripled, from 5,329 to 14,778 (Contreras 2004, 184). Near the turn of the century, two goals in particular became major state foci that shaped the evolution of public health policy. First was increased population to meet the labor requirements of the expanding agricultural and mining sectors (Mannarelli 1999; Contreras 2004). Second was increased state control over interior territories, with the objective of exploiting their economic potential and "civilizing" the native population.

Scarcity of labor and low population levels became a point of debate in the late nineteenth century. This concern was in part economic, due to a lack of

---

7. Claudia Rosas Lauro (2004) dates the emergence of these attitudes in the Peruvian medical community to the late eighteenth century. See also Cosamalón Aguilar (2003).

labor power as a result of the abolition of slavery in 1855 and the period of dramatic growth that soon followed (Contreras 2004, 188). It was also political. Central to regional politics at the time was a pronatalist stance; "to govern is to populate," declared Argentine statesman J. B. Alberdi.[8] Debates emerged in Peru, as across the region, on the best way to increase the population. Peruvian urban elites advocated white European immigration under the premises of eugenics: Europeans would "'civilize' and populate the country, creating the basis for a robust internal market" (190). Landowners sought cheap manual labor for their plantations and were not willing to pay higher wages to compete with Chile, Brazil, or Argentina for European workers, but were content with Asian immigrants, from China and later from Japan. For a variety of reasons, immigration to Peru was minor compared to other Latin American countries. Foreigners constituted 4 percent of the population in 1876 and just 1 percent in 1940, 46 percent of them Asian and 21 percent European (194)—a defeat for those who sought to "Europeanize" the population.

With the failure of immigration as a means for population "betterment," Peruvian elites turned more squarely to public health to better the population and increase the labor force (Contreras 2004). They did this in two ways: by fighting epidemics and by initiating the first maternal-child health programs, with the aim of decreasing the extraordinary infant mortality. The government established the first national public health institutions in response to the bubonic plague, which posed a danger to coastal cities and towns between 1903 and 1930 (Cueto 1997, 27). Key among these was the Dirección de Salubridad Pública (Public Health Board), established in 1903, the precursor to today's Ministry of Health (35). The Dirección was a section of the Ministry of Development, a fitting institutional home in that it reflected the views of elite political leaders who saw state oversight of public health as essential to economic progress and development (35).

The crusades against specific diseases also became conceptually tied to poverty, and in turn to race, in large part as a result of the eugenic thinking that undergirded the process. Plague mortality rates were greater among persons of indigenous descent and Asian immigrants, because these groups were generally poorer, thus more susceptible to disease, and had less access to health care (Cueto 1997, 50). This racial and socioeconomic parallel was used by both the public and those who acted on behalf of the state to reify racial difference. Historian Marcos Cueto writes about the plague in the following

8. Quoted in Stepan (1991, 43).

terms: "the disease was associated with misery, poor living conditions and what was even worse: to be considered *chino* [Asian] or *serrano* [of the highlands], for some the scum of the earth" (51). To be targeted by public health officials was to be racially stigmatized, so much so that upper-stratum Peruvians preferred to hide illnesses altogether.

While the fight against the plague gave rise to the colonization path toward a state public health system, the system itself remained rudimentary until the 1920s. This began to change when the government of Augusto Leguía (1919–30) strengthened state public health activities with the aid of foreign counterparts, in part due to the threat of another epidemic, yellow fever. Leguía closed the Congress immediately after his election as president in 1919, and his *oncenio* (eleven-year) regime was notably authoritarian. It was also characterized by dependence on foreign support—both economic and technical—for achieving its development objectives (Cueto 1992, 9; C. McClintock 1999, 316; Klarén 2000). Leguía enhanced the state in part through spending: social spending between 1920 and 1929 increased annually at a rate of 11.6 percent (Portocarrero 1983, cited in Arroyo 2000, 190). The fight against yellow fever expanded the public health infrastructure with the help of the New York–based Rockefeller Foundation. The Foundation adopted the strategy of yellow fever eradication used by the U.S. military in Cuba and Panama at the turn of the nineteenth century, a strategy based in part on stereotypes of "the hygienic inferiority of blacks and the superiority of whites" (Stern 2006, 55).

The role of the Rockefeller Foundation in Latin American public health formation has generally been seen as motivated by U.S. economic and political interests, though recent historical works have begun to complicate this interpretation (e.g., Zulawski 2007). Marcos Cueto writes in the introduction to an important volume on the topic: "The RF's [Rockefeller Foundation's] program in yellow fever . . . can be better understood as part of a concern for the stability of the international capitalist system as a whole, and for the cultural and political role that the United States was beginning to play in it" (1994b, xi). The outbreak of yellow fever in Peru in 1919 coincided with an interest on the part of the United States and European countries in economic expansion into Latin America, Africa, and Asia. The Rockefeller Foundation was alarmed by Peru's yellow fever epidemic, which it saw as a threat to regional trade, potentially infecting ships and spreading the disease to the United States. The Leguía government, like others in Latin America at the time, invited partnership with the Foundation, as this fit its own interests of expanding state control over national territory (xiii). The Foundation provided substantial financial resources and key technical support by appointing American physicians to lead Peru's anti–yellow fever campaign. Foundation officers and doctors also brought with them substantial hubris—the conviction that the U.S. "modern" system of medicine was what was needed to address Latin America's ills (Cueto 1994c, 15–17).

Reflecting Leguía's governing style and U.S. racist attitudes toward the Latin American region, the yellow fever campaign was carried out in an authoritarian fashion.[9] The American physician who led the campaign, Henry Hanson, ignored the cultural norms and attitudes of the Peruvian people toward health care, including self-medication and reliance on native healers. Cueto writes of the episode, "The attitudes and responses of patients were treated as primitivism to be brushed aside" (1992, 21). Hanson's entourage of forty cavalry and a cruiser of sailors and marines controlled migration from affected areas, prevented public gatherings, and imposed a quarantine on the sick (15). Hanson depended on strong-arm and technical solutions to control the epidemic rather than educating the population or addressing the social factors related to the spread of the disease.[10]

Maternal-child health services formed a second strategy for increasing population and improving the national "stock." The early services in Peru demonstrate the resonance of the instrumental objective of economic development in the formation of the public health system: maternal-child health services were viewed as key to reducing infant mortality and thereby increasing the labor force and in turn economic development. These services were motivated in part by statistics from 1903–8 that showed that one-quarter of all children in Lima did not live to one year of age (Contreras 2004, 203–5). While certainly many of the professionals involved in the design and delivery of these early services held sincere desires to protect and promote human life, a parallel objective of this program, from the viewpoint of the state, was to raise population levels. Population, writes Contreras, was "viewed as a form of capital" (205n18).

Reflecting the general medical consensus in Peru at the time, the maternal-child health program was premised on the belief that infant mortality could

9. For an engaging history of the role of race in U.S.–Latin American political relations, see Schoultz (1998).

10. Similarly, Ann Zulawski writes of American doctors hired for the 1930s Rockefeller campaign against yellow fever in Bolivia adopting racist attitudes, stereotypes, and terms regularly used by the Bolivian elites to denigrate the Indian population (2007, chap. 3).

be prevented by mothers (Mannarelli 1999, 73, 78). The focus on mothers stemmed from a broader regional medical discourse, related to eugenics and again adopted from France, of "puericulture," "the scientific cultivation of the child" (Stepan 1991, 77). Central to puericulture was "a profoundly traditional view of women's role in the family and reproduction," which focused on keeping "women *in* reproduction, healthily rearing their children according to modern medical principles for the good of the country" (78, emphasis in original). Peru had officially established puericulture as a medical specialty in the San Marcos Faculty of Medicine in 1896, followed by gynecology in 1918 (Mannarelli 1999, 45). Following the U.S. example of infant mortality reduction, the new maternal-child health services were to be managed primarily by professionally trained nurse-midwives. The initial goal to appoint a nurse-midwife in each province was reached in just half the provinces by 1916. The government directed these nurse-midwives to offer free obstetric services day and night, to provide two hours daily of consultations to pregnant mothers, and to write regular reports to the central government on the number of registered births and child vaccinations. Contreras notes the authoritarian side of the program, in which infant diets were closely monitored, mothers were compelled to follow the nurses' hygienic procedures, and vaccinations were obligatory (2004).

The maternal-child health program exemplified the ways gender combined with race in the formation of the public health system. Some may quibble as to whether Peru's early maternal-child health program was any more authoritarian than the practice of the time, but the format did demand much of mothers as individuals and identified them as the cause of infant mortality. Moreover, the doctors of the emerging public health system also sought to control women's sexual conduct, which was thought to affect the health of the potential child (Mannarelli 1999, chap. 2). With their lack of political rights and greater social vulnerability, women had little ground upon which to resist (Stepan 1991, 12; Zulawski 2007, 119). Individualization of infant mortality, with responsibility falling disproportionately on women, diverted attention from the root cause: poverty. In the process, this individualization drew upon and reinforced gender inequalities. Women became intimately responsible for social reproduction, sexually controlled, and blamed for child deaths, while men had sexual freedom and little such responsibility.

While population was viewed as a form of capital for development in the early twentieth century, so were the rich untapped resources of the interior. The state, led by European-descent *criollos,* justified its closer control of distant territories within Peru partly with the belief that it was necessary to "civilize" the native populations. State public health services, based on Western biomedical practices, were viewed as an important part of this "civilizing" process.

In the late 1930s and early 1940s, an era of economic growth and urbanization, major efforts were made for an effective state presence in the Amazon jungle in eastern Peru. Similar but more limited efforts were registered in the highlands (Cueto n.d., 26). State expansion into the Amazon went hand in hand with foreign interests: American in rubber and quinine, and British in agriculture. In the 1930s the British operated a small "colony" in the Amazon that produced coffee and fruit for export (Cueto 2004b, 58). The wartime government launched the Corporación Peruana del Amazona (Peruvian Corporation of the Amazon) in 1942 and the Dirección de Asuntos Orientales, Colonización y Terrenos de Oriente (Board of Eastern Affairs, Colonization, and Eastern Land) in 1943. The former was charged with overseeing public works and rubber production; the latter authorized cattle and agricultural uses (59).

Public health services played an important role in this state colonization of interior provinces. In 1940 the Ministerio de Salud Pública, Trabajo y Previsión Social (Ministry of Public Health, Labor, and Social Prevention) established an office to oversee the public health concerns of the Amazon region. The government of Manuel Prado (1939–45), declaring that public health efforts would contribute to "colonization . . . on a scientific basis" significantly expanded the ministry's financial resources and personnel and in 1942 directed it to focus exclusively on health issues, renaming it the Ministerio de Salud Pública y Asistencia Social (Ministry of Public Health and Social Assistance) (Cueto 2004b, 66–67). This strengthened ministry contracted with Peruvian doctors such as Maxime Kuczynski-Godard and Carlos Enrique Paz Soldán to lead its efforts to colonize the Amazon. Paz Soldán himself explained in a radio address: "The modern colonizer is a hygienist. Without health, there is no lasting possession of the earth" (quoted in Cueto 2004b, 67).

Paz Soldán and Kuczynski were pioneers in social medicine, helping to establish it in Peru beginning in the 1920s (Cueto 2002, 2004b). This field, which gained significant influence in Latin America in the 1930s, is often dated to the work of Rudolf Virchow of Germany, who argued in the late nineteenth century that multiple social conditions, not unitary "scientific" factors, were significantly related to illness (Waitzkin 1998). The medical approach of Paz Soldán and Kuczynski was integral and attentive to the social dimensions of disease, such as poverty and living conditions, and thus contrasted sharply with the technical and authoritarian campaigns against single diseases discussed previously, and still dominant in other parts of Peru (Cueto 2004b, 64).

Despite the many noble objectives behind the social medicine approach of Paz Soldán and Kuczynski, the racial undertones of their hygienic colonization were also clear. Paz Soldán, a prominent physician in Peru and the Latin American region, was an active member of regional eugenics societies (Stepan 1991, 48; Cueto 2004b). Initially trained by a French medical officer who had worked in Africa as a colonial physician, he believed that public health interventions in remote areas could improve the "racial" and "moral" life of the country (Cueto 2002). Similarly, Kuczynski vaunted the positive role of the *mestizo* in the colonization effort. He argued that *mestizos* were more likely than indigenous peoples to have healthy hygiene habits and to exploit the land rationally (Cueto 2002, 190). Moreover, he saw the indigenous shamans' and *curanderos'* opposition to Western medicine as a major obstacle to colonization efforts in the Amazon (191). Similar racial undertones appear in state public health service expansion to the Andean region. Medical officials in Puno, the southernmost and highest-altitude city in the Peruvian Andes, viewed the spread of Western medicine to the indigenous-descent peasants as akin to the religious crusade of introducing Christianity (Contreras 2004b, 203).

Despite the expansion in this period, state health services still reached only a fraction of the population. Throughout the 1940s both rural and urban poor continued to rely on popular medicine and the Catholic charity hospitals in urban areas. By the end of the 1940s, the formative period of the public health system was over. Colonization attempts in the interior provinces ceased and a new focus appeared: the mobilized working and middle classes in the coastal urban cities. It was during this period, the 1930s to the 1950s, that the state, in a process described in greater detail in the second half of this chapter, created social security health care, multiple separate health systems for formal sector, mostly male workers. The process had some minor impact on the public health system. A few clinics and hospitals were built in outlying areas to serve insured workers who were far from the main hospitals in the urban centers. In some cases these could also be used by public health system patients (Mesa-Lago 1978). Along with this indirect expansion, the foreign interests continued to influence the public health system. For example, in 1957 the Pan American Health Organization and UNICEF (United Nations Children's Fund) led new efforts to eradicate malaria (Cueto

1997, 161–68). With this foreign cooperation, the public health system saw increases in personnel, training, and financial resources.

Statistics beginning in the 1950s demonstrate the scope of the public health system, so we can begin to assess its distributive character. The construction of most of the hospitals had been financed during the 1940s and 1950s by the U.S.-supported Inter-American Cooperative Public Health Service, while six were hospitals transferred to the Ministry from Catholic charities (Roemer 1964, 45, 48). In 1957 the Ministry of Health began "a basic plan of public health" to provide basic services to the population through a network of clinics, each connected to a hospital, organized in twenty geographic areas. By 1960 the Ministry of Health reported operating 32 hospitals, 71 health centers, 142 medical posts, and 177 sanitary posts.[11] Many of these, however, in practice provided very limited services. Mandated full-time posts offered services only three hours a week (39–45). Each rural post served about 17,000 people, a ratio actually far worse due to inconsistent staffing (41). In addition to these primary health facilities, the government in 1960 had 131 *botequines populares* or pharmacies that made low-cost medicines available to the population (43).

The radical, nationalist self-proclaimed "Revolutionary Government of the Armed Forces" that took power by coup in 1968 and held it until 1980 made little effort in the public health system, despite the keen interest in economic development of the first military president, Juan Alvarado Velasco. This government opted for other avenues toward economic development, such as agrarian reform, price subsidies, organizing the poor in government-created community associations, and worker participation in firm management. Although novel experiments followed in participatory development in rural areas and urban poor neighborhoods, formal sector workers were its key constituency. The government began only a handful of public health initiatives, including a basic medicine-distribution program, free medical care for birthing and newborns, and a basic health care plan that emphasized community participation (Bravo 1980). In 1975 the Ministry of Health had 103 hospitals, 344 health centers, and 994 sanitary posts. Given that the total population had grown from about ten million in 1960 to some fifteen million in 1973 (due to reduced infant mortality and increased life expectancy), the

---

11. A *sanitario* or sanitary technician who had completed primary school and another six months of weekly health-related training staffed the sanitary posts. One or two doctors staffed the medical posts, which were under the loose supervision of a health center (Roemer 1964, 40–41).

expansion of hospitals and health posts did not keep up with the population. The fraction of the population served by primary health establishments had improved little since 1960: one health center served 29,771 persons, and one health post served 14,323 (Orihuela 1980, 8–10).

While the military regime had scant interest in strengthening the public health system, population remained a core concern, as it had been since the turn of the twentieth century. The Velasco government made the long-standing state pro-natalist practices more explicit. His stance stemmed partially from a Catholic tradition, but was also a nationalist reaction to perceived imperialist interference by the United States, which was now actively promoting population control throughout Latin America.[12] In 1974 the minister of health declared that foreign powers were attempting to force Peru to adopt population-control measures and banned even private disbursement of contraceptives (United Nations 1978, 31). When Velasco resigned in 1975, ceding to more conservative generals, the centrist and free market–oriented government of General Francisco Morales Bermúdez (1975–80) reversed the pro-natalist stance and in 1976 outlined Peru's first official population policy.

Morales may have been acquiescing to United States influence, but clearly he was reacting to the rapid rise in population in Peru over the previous two decades.[13] Population growth rates for 1900–40 were 1.8 percent, for 1940–61 2.2 percent, and for 1960–72 2.9 percent (UN-DESA 1978, 3). This first official population policy reflected international currents of the time by making the "Malthusian" connection that population control was a prerequisite to sustained economic development (Varillas and Mostajo 1990, 380).[14] The new policy included access to artificial contraception and considered procreation

12. After World War II, the United States led the charge in international population-control efforts. It viewed population control as intimately linked to economic development in the Third World and thus vital to U.S. security interests (Hartmann 1995, chap. 6). See also McCoy (1974).

13. The government had shown concern over rapid population increases as early as 1964. The Belaúnde government first advocated economic development of the Amazon region as the appropriate way to manage population growth. Just prior to his overthrow in 1968, Belaúnde had signed an agreement with the Pan American Health Organization to begin a maternal-child health program that would incorporate family planning. Due to the military coup, it never was implemented (UN-DESA 1978, 6).

14. Economist Thomas Malthus argued in the late 1700s and early 1800s that population growth, stimulated by the working classes, if left unchecked, would outstrip agricultural capacity, leading to a general decline in world living standards. Historian Linda Gordon distinguishes between pure "Malthusianism," which advocated sexual restraint of the working classes, and "neo-Malthusianism," which accepts artificial birth control, something Malthus himself did not support due to its implications of separating women from their mothering role, a radical notion during his time (Gordon 1990b). In later chapters I employ the term

the decision of the couple, using the Catholic concept of "responsible parent-hood," in which couples are encouraged to use natural means to decide family size (Guzmán 2002, 190).[15] The government did not set demographic targets, resisting international pressures on this count (UN-DESA 1978, 22). It was nevertheless a dramatic reversal from traditional policies based on the idea that increased population was a pure economic gain.

By the end of the military period, the government faced a severe economic crisis that contributed to a deterioration of the public health system. In 1978 the military imposed the first in a series of economic austerity measures that severely restricted the reach of its few public health initiatives. In 1980 the Ministry of Health budget was just 3.5 percent of the overall general budget, down from 17 percent in 1968, prior to the takeover (Orihuela 1980, 7). By 1980, with few funds left for social needs, the already weak infrastructure of the public health system was in disarray. The minister of health under President Fernando Belaúnde Terry (1980–85), the first democratic govern-ment following the military government, described the state of the system when he took over: "the public hospitals—not those of the social security system—were in a state of calamity. The patients who went to be hospital-ized had to bring their own mattress and sheets" (Interview Uriel García 1998).[16] In 1980 the Ministry of Health had the responsibility of providing health care to 70 percent of the population, yet in practice it only reached half of that segment (Orihuela 1980, 7).

Public health care became even more scattershot under the new govern-ment, as part of an overall social policy trend toward "crisis" social policy interventions while letting the traditional social policy structure wither. The centrist Belaúnde government raised popular expectations as the first government elected in which the entire population had suffrage, yet it lan-guished under continuing economic recession.[17] Debt servicing and military spending to combat growing rebel movements in the provinces absorbed

---

"neo-Malthusianism" when artificial birth control in Peru supplants sexual restraint as the primary means of population control.

15. The Peruvian Church position on responsible parenthood was first outlined in the document *Familia y Población,* published by the Episcopado Peruano, March 19, 1974 (cited in Varillas and Mostajo 1990, 380).

16. This phenomenon is not unique to Peru. All over Latin America economic crises led to collapse of public health systems, and it became common for patients to provide their own sheets and basic medical supplies.

17. Not until 1980, the first presidential election after the twelve-year military govern-ment, were illiterates allowed to vote, making Peru an electoral democracy. Disenfranchis-ing illiterates had effectively suppressed the political voice of a large portion of indigenous

most of the national budget, with few resources dedicated to improving the health sector (Davidson and Stein 1988). As the state retracted its traditional social policy commitments such as health funding, it increased "emergency" social policies such as those that directed international food donations to women's groups in the poor *pueblos jovenes* (urban shantytowns), which had greatly expanded in the 1960s and '70s. As a hedge against the worsening economy, the government encouraged the communal soup kitchens run by women volunteers in poor communities, kitchens originally started by the Catholic Church. The proliferation of informal kitchens would continue after Belaúnde, and become more politicized as political parties set up their "own" kitchens in subsequent governments (Barrig 1992). With the political incorporation of illiterates, a new and substantially poor electorate became the object of clientelist politics. Social spending was siphoned off from the health system to a series of emergency aid programs that served the dual purposes of aid and politics.

The late 1980s stand out as a failed attempt to stop the downward course of the public health system. Disillusionment with the Belaúnde government resulted in a dramatic turn of the electorate toward support of the political Left. In the 1980s the Izquierda Unida (United Left) united several Left parties; in 1985, for the first time, the populist Alianza Popular Revolucionaria Americana (American Popular Revolutionary Alliance, APRA) was allowed to run a candidate in the presidential elections. Following the victory of APRA candidate Alan García Pérez (1985–90), his minister of health, David Tejada de Rivero, worked to rectify the decrepit state of Peru's public health system and shift its emphasis toward primary care. Prior to his service as minister, Tejada had worked for eleven years as assistant director of the World Health Organization. He had helped organize the 1978 WHO Alma Alta conference, which had defined the original principles of "primary health care." Primary health care shifts the emphasis away from Western hospital-based health services to basic health care services thought to address more effectively the most common health needs of the poor in developing nations (Cueto 2001, 56; 2004a).

---

peoples, poor, and women (in particular, poor indigenous women). As late as 1981, 18.1 percent of the population age fifteen years or more was illiterate, 26.1 percent of women and 9.9 percent of men. In rural areas, with a more concentrated indigenous population, 55.8 percent of women and 23.2 percent of men were illiterate (1981 census data compiled in Blondet and Montero 1994, 61). Literate women were given the vote in Peru in 1955, among the last countries in the hemisphere to grant women suffrage.

In his first year in office García passed a national population law that reiterated the Church position of responsible parenthood, but also established the right to a choice of contraceptive methods and individual freedom from manipulation or coercion in matters of family planning (Varillas and Mostajo 1990, 322–23). The government developed the National Population Program (1987–90), which outlined goals for reducing fertility rates by providing contraception coverage. Only limited economic resources were secured to carry out this plan, but it spawned the first family planning programs in Peru's social security and state-run public health systems (Guzmán 2002). Notably, the National Population Program was a component of the National Plan for Development, evidence of the continued association of population with economic development. But Tejada's efforts at introducing primary care and the launching of the first state family planning services were overshadowed by the economic and political crisis that confronted the García administration.

Legacies of Colonization

The deeper history of the public health care system in Peru left a stubborn structure of stratification that impeded full equity in the conditions to achieve good health. Its "colonization" trajectory also left some important policy legacies for the reformers of the 1990s. The stratifying effects of the public health system are evident not only in the varied distribution and quality of health services, but in the system's recognition of some groups and not others by discursively reinforcing class, racial, and gender inequalities. The urban concentration of doctors was one major distributive skew of the system. Physicians clustered in Lima and other urban areas, with little interest in serving the primarily indigenous rural or provincial populations (Cueto 1992, 10). In 1957 72 percent of all doctors were located in the capital, home to only 15 percent of the population (Roemer 1969, 165). This pattern continued with only slight improvement in the mid-1980s, with 67 percent of doctors in Lima and another 22 percent in departmental capitals (Locay 1988, 147). Doctors' preferences for urban work were somewhat offset by the rapid migration of peasants to cities in the 1970s and '80s, spurred by economic need and search for refuge from the emerging rural war with the Shining Path. By 1985, 66 percent of Peruvians lived in urban areas, but this still did not match the 89 percent concentration of doctors in the same period (INEI 2001, 39).

Moreover, the public system, although it served the majority of the population, received much less state financial support than the social security health systems created through the co-optation path explained in the next section. This centralization of resources and overall lesser financial support for public health compared to the social security system demonstrate the stratifying impact of the health system and how this stratification fell along gender, class, and racial lines. The poorest and the indigenous populations in rural areas had very limited or no access to health care. Women, stuck in the public health system because the social security system largely excluded them, also received lower-quality health services than working- and middle-class men. Few women workers had formal sector jobs; most were in the uncovered informal sector or worked as domestics, not covered by social security until the 1970s.[18] Workers' spouses had very limited coverage under social security for most of its history.

The history of the public health system also had important results for stratification based on recognition. When the state did bring health services to rural and provincial areas, it viewed the spread of Western medicine as part of a colonization and civilization process, an approach that left little room for its use along with local, popular medicinal practices. This pattern reinforced the racial differences between the urban-educated and *mestizo* doctors, who strove to bring "modernity" through Western medicine to the indigenous "backward" populations, and their patients. The racial divide between urban, white doctors and the primarily indigenous rural populations, as well as the stigmatization of Asian-descent immigrants, has left a notable rift of recognition in the public health sector between doctors and patients.

Recognition rifts related to gender also emerge from this history. State control over women's bodies and regulation of their mothering skills were essential to Peru's emerging public health system. Women, like indigenous people and the poor, were viewed as a group that had to be restrained in the name of national economic and social development. Women were viewed early on as the producers of a future labor force and bearers of the "fit" for the nation, while in later years they were viewed as threats to economic growth due to their unbridled fertility. While at one point helpers in the economic and national development project, and at another point an obstacle, women and their fertility and mothering skills became subjected to national development.

18. In 1984–93 females made up 88–99 percent of domestic workers (Gárate Urquizo and Ferrer G. 1994, 75–76), likely similar to the figures in prior decades.

This policy-formation process led to specific policy learning legacies, lock-in effects, and interest group legacies. Peru's history of medical crusades against epidemics contributed to the curative focus and vertical structure of the public health system.[19] Foreign interests tended to support efforts against a single disease, providing funding for separate offices in the Ministry of Health, a "policy learning legacy" that was repeated again and again. This process also produced lock-in effects by creating separate bureaucracies in the Ministry, dedicated to separate diseases and very often with independent budget streams. These institutions, once established, were difficult to dismantle.

Medical education in Peru was historically clinical in focus and technical in orientation, reinforced by a lack of public health programs in Peru's universities until late in the twentieth century (Cueto 1992, 10–12). This orientation encouraged the curative bias and urban focus of health policy, in that curative medicine required better facilities and equipment, which were largely located in urban areas. Medical education is slow and difficult to reorient, and helped lock in bias by encouraging state investments in hospitals and medical equipment in urban centers. While the curative focus and vertical structure were legacies not directly related to class, race, or gender, this focus and structure would become objects of reform. Urban bias would also be on the reform agenda, which, due to the relationship between geography and race in Peru, would begin to address some racial disparities.

The broader history of authoritarian approaches to medicine, especially among rural indigenous populations, and of surveillance and control of women's reproduction would also be vital to policy learning legacies. Health reforms did little to address these legacies. Health policies still see women through the lens of reproduction and motherhood, and in the countryside authoritarian sanitary campaigns, in which coercion is not out of the question, still occur.

With regard to interest group legacies, significant in this history is not the creation of interest groups or providing resources or power to a particular group, but rather their *absence*. The history of public health in Peru shows that women, the poor, and indigenous peoples—the primary public health clients—were subject to authority and control, not afforded "voice" or authority in health care decision making. This was true at the national

19. Vertical programming focuses on one disease at a time, ignoring interactions among diseases, overall health, and social dimensions of health, versus an "integral" approach, which assesses the whole.

level—policy makers in the health ministry did not ask for or listen to their concerns—as well as at the local, everyday level in doctor-patient relations.

Co-optation: The Stratified Social Security Health System

The second path to development of state health services was characterized by Bismarckian-style co-optation of the middle and working classes into the state-run health insurance programs that became known as social security.[20] Social security health care was established later than the public health system—between 1930 and 1950, a period of economic change and marked urbanization. Authoritarian rulers representing oligarchic interests promoted social security in response to pressure from interest groups, primarily the political muscle of middle- and working-class employees newly mobilized in unions and political parties. While growing in political clout, the organized middle and working classes were still a minority of the Peruvian population, the vast majority still being poor peasants and the growing segment of informal sector workers. International interests played only a minor role in the design of the social security health system. Pro-social security discourses from the International Labour Organization and the Beveridge Report, as well as experiences of neighboring countries such as Chile that had already established a social security health system, surely influenced Peru's political choices, but there were no specific foreign entities, like the Rockefeller Foundation, instrumental to this policy process (Mesa Lago 1989, 5).[21]

General Oscar Benavides, appointed president by Congress in 1933, took the first steps in Peru's co-optation path toward social security health care. He came to power soon after the political ascendancy of the APRA party, an opposition party representing the middle classes and the upper stratum of the working classes. APRA held its first national congress in 1931, which produced a number of social policy proposals, including the creation of social

20. The development of the Peruvian social security health system has much in common with the welfare state model in Germany under Bismarck. Both systems were created as largely authoritarian responses to class conflict, and both resulted in a highly stratified system. Milton Roemer's comparative work on world health systems finds that the historically stratified character of Peru's social security system is not unlike the systems of Germany and Belgium, also initially highly stratified in hundreds of autonomous sickness funds (Roemer 1969, 211).

21. The Beveridge Report, a product of an interministerial committee in Britain led by William Beveridge, was published in 1942 and recommended family allowances, free health services, and full employment. It served as the conceptual basis for the British welfare state and was internationally influential (Abel-Smith 2007).

security (Cotler 1978, 236). In an attempt to co-opt the working-class fol-lowers of APRA, the Benavides dictatorship created the Ministerio de Salud Pública, Trabajo y Previsión Social (Ministry of Health, Labor, and Social Wel-fare) in 1935 and decreed social security health insurance for blue-collar workers in 1936, called the Seguro Social del Obrero (Workers' Social Secu-rity, SSO). Benavides launched these programs to appease these class-based demands, but at the same time severely repressed their political voice in APRA. Besides co-opting demands of urban workers, he expanded existing social security health benefits for civil servants (Mesa-Lago 1978, 116).

Following Benavides' regime, restrictions loosened on working-class orga-nizing and the number of legally recognized unions rose. Thus, the civilian presidency of Manuel Prado y Ugarteche (1939–45) faced increasing pres-sures from organized class interests. Toward the end of his term, Prado legal-ized the APRA party, providing a significant opening for class-based political opposition (Cotler 1978). The escalating pressure from the working and mid-dle classes through union and APRA demands led Prado, in a manner begun by Benavides, to continue to co-opt these classes through the expansion of social policies, including health policies. Prado expanded the workers' social security health system established by Benavides, opening six SSO hospitals between 1941 and 1944 in Lima and other major cities (Mesa-Lago 1978, 117). The first of these was the Hospital Obrero de Lima (Worker's Hospital of Lima), inaugurated in 1941, the very first social security hospital in Latin America (Roemer 1964, 26).

Prior to the 1940s, the working and middle classes had organized sepa-rately, with distinct unions or associations.[22] The middle class in fact had a history of class-based strikes dating back to 1919, and achieved its first social policy victory in 1924, under the Leguía regime.[23] By the 1940s, how-ever, APRA had succeeded in blurring the lines between the working and middle classes and managed to attract the associations of both strata under its political umbrella. The middle class emerged more militantly alongside the working-class unions. This intensified militancy came from the elec-tion of APRA members to leadership positions in key white-collar worker

22. My discussion of the history of the middle class draws largely on Parker (1998). The distinction between *obreros* (workers) and *empleados* (middle-class, white-collar workers) is still important. Parker provides a history of this distinction, its underlying social (including racial) meanings, and its evolution in the first half of the twentieth century.

23. The policies gained included three months notice prior to firing, compensation for years of service, life insurance paid by the employer for employees of four or more years of service, and employer-paid disability insurance (Parker 1998, 105).

associations in the mid-1940s, including the Asociación de Empleados del Perú (Employee Association of Peru, AEP), Peru's major middle-class association (Parker 1998, 218).

While Prado represented conservative interests, his democratically elected successor, José L. Bustamente Rivero, depended on the political support of APRA.[24] The 1945 election signaled a brief interlude of influence for the allied middle and working classes. Bustamente recognized a record number of unions in 1946, and white-collar unions in particular reached unprecedented levels (Mesa-Lago 1978, 117; Parker 1998, 218). The Bustamente government acted for its constituents by raising the social security coverage initiated by the previous two administrations. Upper-echelon white-collar workers in specific industries received pensions, and he established on paper the Seguro Social del Empleado (Employees' Social Security, SSE), to serve health and pension needs of white-collar workers. Blue-collar workers also claimed new benefits, including two new workers' hospitals and insurance for occupational diseases (Mesa-Lago 1978, 117). Few of these social policy measures were carried through prior to the military takeover of General Manuel Odría Amoretti in 1948.

Tensions in the working- and middle-class alliance within APRA came to a head with the 1947 election of leaders of the middle-class AEP. Its APRA-backed leaders lost the election to opposition candidates who campaigned on issues that bolstered a distinct middle-class identity rather than solidarity with workers, such as constructing a new social security hospital exclusively for white-collar workers (Parker 1998, 221). General Odría, on taking control of the government via coup in 1948, seized on this demand as a way to co-opt middle-class interests and further divide the middle and working classes. The new hospital and Odría's expansion of the SSE succeeded as a co-optation measure, as the middle-class AEP lost strength and voice.

Odría also reinforced patterns of special benefits for specific groups that had begun in the nineteenth century. Teachers and railroad and streetcar workers won inclusion in the SSE, separate hospitals were created for the police and military, and benefits were expanded for civil servants. Blue-collar workers were not treated as well, but they did get some increased illness, maternity, and funeral aid (Mesa-Lago 1978, 117–18). Social policy provision based on occupational group continued after Odría, most notably in health

24. APRA, though legalized, was banned from running its own presidential candidate, and threw its support behind Bustamente.

policy, when President Belaúnde's government established a separate health and pension system for fishers in 1965.

The 1930s through the 1950s was the critical period for the establishment and implementation of social security health care systems, though the 1960s also saw some expansion. In addition to the separate fund for fishers, the state initiated new social security benefits for white- and blue-collar workers, some of which had been legislated but not implemented earlier (see Mesa-Lago 1978, 118–20). The Ministry of Public Health expanded in the early 1960s, building twelve new hospitals to serve insured persons who lived in areas without SSE or SSO hospitals, as well as the uninsured poor (120).

The co-optation path led to separate state health insurance systems for the middle and working classes, who each had their own health insurance programs and hospitals. The white-collar, middle-class social security health system was not only separate from the blue-collar one, it was superior. The Hospital del Empleado constructed by Odría rivaled the quality of private clinics (Parker 1998, 222). As one indicator of the lavish resources concentrated in this one hospital, in 1962 the number of employed personnel was 3.1 per hospital bed. In addition, 270 soles (about U.S. 11 dollars) per day was spent per patient at the employee hospital, compared to 150 soles at the workers' hospital. Moreover, white-collar employees who opted to use private instead of state health services were subsidized for their expenses. They opted for private services about 50 percent of the time in the 1960s (Roemer 1964, 32, 35).

These systems were financed as "pay-as-you-go" social security systems, that is, by salary contributions from the employee and the employer into a state fund. The funds also benefited from other sources of income, including fines and donations, as well as yields from investments (Mesa-Lago 1989, 187). When the systems were first initiated, employers paid the equivalent of 2 percent of an employee or worker's salary to the SSE or SSO (Mesa-Lago 1978, 139). In 1962 the SSO required a 3 percent salary contribution from the worker, 6 percent from the employer, and a 2 percent government contribution. White-collar workers in 1962 gave 3 percent of their salary, private employers 3.5 percent, public institutions 3 percent, and the government just 0.5 percent (Roemer 1964, 25, 31).[25] Unfortunately, the pay-as-you-go

---

25. Mesa-Lago (1978, 138) provides different figures for contributions. I cite Roemer's statistics because I think they are more reliable since they were recorded closer to the time. These percentages increased over time; the most recent rate, since 1996, requires the employee/worker to make the entire contribution, of 9 percent of her or his salary, deposited by the employer with ESSALUD (formerly IPSS).

health system suffered from employer evasion of payment. Workers' contributions, due to low salaries and a cap on payments at 500 soles (per a 1950 law), did not come close to covering the real costs of the services provided. Deficits were often subsidized by the state (Roemer 1964, 30; Mesa-Lago 1978, 139).

The 1968 military government was especially supportive of unions, and therefore put more resources toward social security, insuring a growing share of the population: 8.8 percent in 1969, rising to 10.1 percent in 1973 (Orihuela 1980, 10) and 17.4 percent by 1980 (Mesa-Lago 1989, 183). The resources given workers were not just material, but included authority and access to power. In 1969 administrative councils composed of representatives of the government, the insured, and employers were formed for both the SSO and the SSE, so that workers would have a role in administering their own pension and health programs.

In 1979 the worker and employee systems became partially unified when the military government, in one of its final measures, combined the SSE, SSO, and civil servants' state health insurance systems. In 1980 the pension system merged with the social security health system as a unified system renamed Instituto Peruano de Seguridad Social (Peruvian Institute of Social Security, IPSS). This consolidation only partly fulfilled the military's hopes for reform of the health sector. According to Roger Guerra García, who sat on its health reform commission, the military's "socialist vision" of a single national health system would have combined all the components, including "the social security and the armed forces health systems," with the general public health system. It faltered, in part, "because there was not support from the people" (Interview Guerra García 1998).[26] While "universal" health care was never implemented, the call for it would be often repeated in the years following the military government.

A number of factors led to a crisis in the social security health system in the 1980s and 1990s. The stratified systems originating from the co-optation path were poorly managed, especially from the 1970s on. The military government used SSO and SSE funds for other purposes without investing these wisely (Interview Uriel García 1998; Mesa-Lago 1989). According to one source, only 30 percent of the payments collected by the state for social security health care actually went to fund health services under the military government (Orihuela 1980, 8). The inflationary economy of the 1980s led

26. See also Bravo (1980).

to severe deterioration of the real value of social security deposits. The economic crisis, which mounted in the 1980s, also meant a reduction of formal sector jobs, curtailing the already small pool of contributors.[27]

Legacies of Co-optation

The historical formation of Peru's social security health system had vital consequences for inequities in distribution of health resources and recognition of particular population subgroups. The social security health system offered urban formal sector workers a "sanitized" health system of higher quality and better resources than the public health system that served the poor. The separate middle-class and military social security health systems were of even higher quality, further distinguishing these better-off groups from typical workers. Even after expansion of social security coverage under the military government between 1968 and 1980, by 1980 only 17.4 percent of the total population was insured (Mesa-Lago 1989, 183). Fifteen years later, in 1995, the state social security system insured just 26 percent of the population, the public health system served 52 percent, and a full 20 percent had no access to health care at all.[28] Despite serving only a fraction of the population, the social security health system absorbed nearly the same amount of government-directed resources as the public health system, making the distribution of health care resources highly inequitable along class lines. According to Ministry of Health estimates, based on their own and IPSS data, in 1995 spending per patient in the social security health sector was three and a quarter times that in the public health sector.

In terms of recognition, workers gained some measure of "voice" through the access to authority provided by the tripartite social security governance system set up by military government. But the effects of the co-optation path on recognition were more thoroughgoing than this fact alone. The strategy of separate systems for separate groups further stratified Peruvian society, and reinforced already existing status differentials between classes, races,

27. I do not have 1981 data on informal sector employment. However, in 1970 informal sector workers made up 31.6 percent of Lima's workforce, and household workers 9.8 percent. In 1990 that number had grown to 40.7–46.8 percent of the Lima workforce in the informal sector and 5.1 percent as domestic laborers (Sheahan 1999, 98). While these are not national figures, they give an idea of the general trend of increase in the size of the informal sector, which is related to the decline in formal sector employment.

28. Numbers provided by the Ministry of Health.

and men and women. The population insured by the social security health systems, by nature of its birth through co-optation of working-class unions and middle-class associations, was overwhelmingly male, urban, and working or middle class. Moreover, the social security health systems served a largely *mestizo* and European-descent population. Formal sector workers, even if originally of indigenous descent, had, through migration to cities, cultural adaptation to the dominant coastal culture, and economic advance in formal sector employment, become *mestizo*. The middle class furthermore differentiated itself from workers in part based on lighter skin color (Parker 1998).

The social security health system rewarded these urban-based white and *mestizo* populations. Departments with the greatest percentage of insured populations were also those with the highest index of urbanization (Mesa-Lago 1989, 182–84); 98 percent of the self-employed, who composed a significant part of the economically active population, went uncovered in 1981 (185). These included indigenous descent peoples concentrated in agriculture and female informal sector workers in "personal services." The separate and stratified social security system therefore reified not only class positions, but also racial and gender privilege.

The dichotomy between the public health system for the poor and the social security health system for workers is in and of itself highly gendered in both distribution and recognition. The workers covered by the SSO and SSE were primarily urban male breadwinners, with few women included due to their historically low levels of paid employment. Women composed just 21.7 percent of the economically active population in 1961, and 25.1 percent by 1981 (INEI 1999c). Moreover, urban women in paid employment were (and remain) largely in the informal sector or domestic workers, which were not initially covered at all by SSE or SSO. The gendered division of coverage was nominally improved in the 1970s when the military government incorporated domestic workers into the social security system (Mesa-Lago 1989, 178). However, reform was mitigated by domestic employers' evasions of payments, greater than the already high rate by employers in general. With the 1980s economic crisis, more women entered the workforce, but largely in the informal sector, which remained effectively outside social security.[29]

29. For specific numbers on the rise in informal sector work, see Gárate Urquizo and Ferrer G. (1994, 73–76). I say "effectively" excluded because informal sector workers could voluntarily join the social security health system, but the majority opted not to due to the cost. In 1987 only 12.1 percent of the nonsalaried workforce was covered by social security (Verdera 1997, 30).

Dependent wives made up just 7 percent of those insured by social security in 1961, but 23 percent by 1981.[30] The total number of adult women covered by social security was probably higher, but not dramatically so, due to the employment trends discussed previously.

For wives and common-law partners who were insured as dependents, the coverage SSE and SSO provided was extremely limited.[31] Originally, wives of insured male workers were only covered for maternity health care—all other health care for wives was either through the public health system or paid out of pocket in the private sector. In 1975 children under one year of age were added as dependents (Mesa-Lago 1989, 181; Roemer 1964). Only in March 1979 did the outgoing military government, as part of consolidating the SSE and SSO systems, expand dependent coverage to cover a worker's spouse and children under age eighteen.[32] Current legislation covers spouses, minor children, and disabled adult children who are unable to work. Dependents were, and continue to be, covered by the same contribution cap as an individual worker. The 1979 legislation also allowed self-employed (primarily informal) workers to voluntarily join the social security health system.[33] However, women workers were not able to carry a spouse or dependent on their social insurance policy until 1992, further demarcating women as less than full citizens. The extremely limited dependent coverage for most of the history of the system, and the exclusion of women workers from rights to cover dependents, effectively made social security health care a male domain and feminized the public system. While raising the status of male workers, it viewed women as actors solely in their contribution to the reproduction of the labor force.

In addition to its profound stratifying effects, this path left important political legacies that would become significant obstacles to attempts at retrenchment in the 1990s. Most important was the creation of two new powerful interest groups: workers vested with social security health care and doctors who worked in the social security health care system. Mostly male working- and middle-class workers of European or *mestizo* descent were offered superior health resources that they would later seek to defend.

30. Calculated from figures in Mesa-Lago (1989, 183).
31. Mesa-Lago (1989) points out that Peru was particularly restrictive in social security dependent coverage among Latin American countries.
32. Decreto Ley No. 22482, March 27, 1979.
33. Similar pension legislation was passed earlier, in 1974, allowing the self-employed to join and allowing coverage of dependents.

Moreover, the tripartite administration of social security provided this group with a voice in the administration of social security itself, an important means to receive vital policy information that could subsequently be transmitted through union networks, buoying their organizational advantage in responding to possible policy changes. Social security system physicians had also become a privileged group, with good salaries, working conditions, and bargaining power compared to their peers in the public health system.

A new lock-in effect also arose. The public health system was administrated by the Ministry of Health and the social security health system by the Ministry of Labor, setting up dueling ministries that "locked in" the two-tier system. The Labor Ministry in particular was loath to give up the significant resources and power afforded by oversight of the pay-as-you-go system, and would block attempts to combine the two systems.

Difficult Paths to an Equitable Future?

The historical formation of health policies in Peru was influenced by the discriminatory suppositions of doctors, policy makers, and international agencies about the relationships between gender, race, class, and disease. Discourses of inequality—such as beliefs that the poor, especially indigenous peoples and nonwhite immigrants, were carriers of disease or that mothers were responsible for high rates of infant mortality—played into the ways Peru's public health system was structured. The public system that served these groups was top-down and authoritarian, reflecting the largely disparaging attitudes of elites toward the poor, nonwhites, and women. The founding of the public system was premised not on citizens' right to health, but rather on the idea that health and population control would lead to national development—both economic and "moral." In the formative period of this colonizing path, the public health system's target populations were not even considered citizens, if suffrage is a central aspect of citizenship. These founding biases help explain the fact that Peru's public health system has remained of poorer quality and limited reach in comparison to the social security system that followed it.

But racist, classist, and gendered discourses only partially contributed to the bifurcated nature of Peru's health system. The dual system also reflected broader historical (and changing) power disparities in Peruvian society. Those groups that won political voice in the mid-twentieth century, the working and middle classes, effectively claimed for themselves a better state health system—the social security health system—via a process of co-optation by authoritarian governments. These groups effectively represented new class and race configurations in Peru (*mestizo* working and middle classes), and took advantage of the economic and political context of the time to change the nature of health policy development. They claimed a new and better health system, but it was strictly limited. They also sought to protect their newfound influence by perpetuating inequality and upholding their status differences with others. Weak Peruvian governments also knew that dividing threatening new political groups into competing camps was crucial to their own political survival, resulting in the co-optation pattern.

Disparities in power rooted in class, gender, and race became solidified and reinforced in the highly stratified health system that resulted from the combined colonization and co-optation paths to health policy. This bifurcated system also added new inequalities, most clearly new inequalities in access to and quality of health services, between the working classes, middle classes, and rich; between men and women; and between whites, *mestizos*, and immigrant and indigenous peoples. This inequitable distribution of services continues—in 2008, 43 percent of Peruvians lacked health insurance.[34] For reformers of the 1990s, who stated that they sought greater equity, ending or ameliorating this stratification should have been a fundamental objective.

Beyond producing stratification, the dual paths of colonization and co-optation left important policy legacies with which reformers in the 1990s and 2000s would have to contend. Some of these legacies became the object of reform: for example, policy makers were encouraged to "unlearn" the curative focus and vertical programming in the public health system. These legacies were not particularly related to gender, race, or class, but others more clearly were. The policy interest group legacies of material resources and authority left to working- and middle-class workers advantaged these two groups and their largely male, *mestizo* members. The privileged position of doctors in the social security health system also brought advantage to the largely male, white, *mestizo*, urban, and middle-class interest. Doctors' and unions' objectives during reform, as I outline in chapter 4, would be to defend their privilege and the stratified system that afforded it. Meanwhile, few resources and no access to authority were given to the primarily poor, female, and indigenous users of the public health system.

34. Author's calculations from ENAHO (2008).

By providing better health care and more voice in health care policy to some but not others, the dual system reinforced existing class, gender, and racial cleavages in Peruvian society. It added to the political power of white, *mestizo,* primarily male workers and offered few avenues to power for women, indigenous peoples, or the poor. These inequalities among policy interest groups foreshadow the dynamics of the reform process and the ways gender and race would play into this process. Yet, just as particular economic and political circumstances allowed for the emergence of a new class of workers and the related development of social security in the 1930s through the 1950s, subsequent chapters detail how the 1990s presented new events that would allow some of the legacies outlined in this chapter to be overcome, while others would remain in place.

Global Currents: Neoliberal and "Rights-Based"
Development Paradigms

Scholars of advanced industrialized countries have for the last decade debated the effects of globalization on these countries' well-developed welfare states. While there is still some debate, a number of studies have determined that although globalization may have narrowed the range of economic options open to policy makers, it has not actually caused significant welfare state retrenchment (Huber and Stephens 2001). These studies have pointed to policy legacies (interest group, policy learning, and informational forms) as the primary reason behind the lack of retrenchment; legacies have simply blocked reform (Pierson 1994; Huber and Stephens 2001). Many Latin American welfare states, while never as comprehensive as advanced industrialized welfare states, were founded contemporaneously with many European welfare states, and several predate the United States welfare state. One would expect, then, that the equally mature historical policy legacies of the social policy formation period described in the previous chapter—policy interest legacies such as labor and doctor's unions, learning legacies such as occupationally based benefits, and Malthusian approaches to population control—would play significant roles in protecting Latin American social policy systems from change. Yet, with the exception of Brazil, Costa Rica, and Uruguay,

most Latin American countries, including Peru, opted in the 1990s to significantly reform their existing social policies in a market-oriented direction.[1]

What explains this radical change? Why did legacies block reform in Europe
and in some Latin American countries, but not others? Did globalization play a
significant role? Or was the process of reform one of essentially domestic decisions to retrench? This chapter and the next focus on the politics of health
sector reform in Peru from 1990 to 2000 and the extent to which and why the
class-, gender-, and race-based legacies produced in the historical formation
of Peru's health care system were overcome. This chapter focuses on the transnational and global influences on Peru's major health reforms, while the next
chapter focuses more directly on the national politics at play. Both chapters
elucidate how gender did or did not play into the policy reform process.

The argument set forth in this chapter is that transnational "epistemic
communities" at key points shaped the interests of national political actors,
encouraging these in some instances to disregard previous policy legacies
(Haas 1992). The "success" of the actors that composed these epistemic communities in challenging legacies was dependent on the perceived urgency and
technical expertise required of the reform in question. In those instances
perceived as a crisis or reforms viewed as particularly complex, politicians
showed deference to the transnationally embedded professionals who offered
new ideas. However, in other instances where there was not a perceived crisis
or high degree of technicality, these same transnational ideas were ignored
in favor of previously existing policy legacies. Important to this story, and
to understanding the role of gender in the health reform process, is that
two distinct epistemic communities, neoliberal and rights-based communities, were involved in Peru's health reform.[2] In addition to crises and technical complexity, the degree to which each of these communities was able to
incorporate Peruvian policy makers and provide clear policy solutions helps
to explain the degree of influence these communities had, and in turn, why
some legacies (such as class-based union interests) were overcome in the
reform process while others (such as Malthusian policy learning legacies)
were allowed to persist.

Analysis of these two communities helps to explain a puzzling aspect of the
reform process—how was it, despite the high profile of feminists and feminist

1. On Brazil see Arretche (2004), Weyland (1996a, 2006); on Costa Rica see Martínez
Franzoni (1999), Clark (2004), Weyland (2006); on Uruguay see Castiglioni (2005).

2. As Orenstein notes, in most policy areas multiple transnational advocacy coalitions (a
term he uses synonymously with "epistemic communities") compete for influence (2008, 69).

discourses both globally and nationally in the 1990s, that the question of "gender equity" barely touched the "mainstream" health reform agenda? Accordingly, this chapter and the next answer one of the main questions posed in the introduction to the book—why feminists were *not* active in second-wave reform processes. This chapter finds that the lack of linkage between feminists and Peruvian policy makers with the broader rights-based epistemic community explains the absence of gender equity in health reform as well as the ability of President Fujimori to symbolically hijack the feminist reproductive rights discourse, rather than feel obligated to implement its principles in earnest.

Theories of Policy Diffusion

Were global factors significant to Latin American countries' move to retrench? Some scholars hypothesize that the dependent relationship of Latin American states vis-à-vis International Financial Institutions (IFIs) following the debt crisis of the 1980s allowed entities like the International Monetary Fund (IMF), through mechanisms such as conditionality, to dictate national policy (Stallings 1992; S. George 1992; Kahler 1992; Simmons 2001; Stiglitz 2002).[3] This has been a dominant argument with regard to structural adjustment, although some have questioned the effectiveness of conditionality even in the structural adjustment phase (Nelson 1990; Kahler 1992). Still others have found that conditionality has at times been requested by national policy makers as a tactic to gain the upper hand against national political forces opposed to particular policies—far from the imposition that conditionality is normally portrayed as (Nelson 1996; Teichman 2001).

In light of the unclear implications of conditionality, other scholars have argued that more diffuse forms of influence have led to policy diffusion. For example, IFIs have not conditioned policies, but rather "taught" through publications and face-to-face linkages (Finnemore 1993). Sarah Brooks finds an "indirect" process by which the economic liberalization of the 1980s and early 1990s led to a set of new incentives, namely to protect oneself from new vulnerabilities to capital. These incentives led to a greater likelihood of accepting the market-oriented pension reforms that promised diminished

---

3. Conditionality involves written requirements that specified policies be carried out in order for a government to receive loans or remain in good credit standing.

reliance on foreign capital (2004). Kurt Weyland also contends that IFIs played only a minor role in social policy reforms though "advice" and "availability" (2006, 143). Instead, he points to "bounded rationality," whereby policy makers employ "heuristic shortcuts"—when working on complex policy problems, policy makers reach for easily accessible models that appear to provide a clear, tested solution to a particular policy problem, often models from neighboring countries (2004, 2005, 2006). Weyland's argument parallels that of policy learning legacies. Whereas in the case of policy-learning legacies, policy makers reach for tried and tested policies that they have used in their own countries in the past, bounded rationality leads policy makers to opt for policy options that they see neighboring countries employ with some success.

But what leads some decision makers to look outside the boundaries of their own experience while others look to learning legacies from their own national context? And why do policy makers choose some foreign models over others? While the bounded rationality explanation is convincing in many ways, it fails to fully explain why some countries resisted neoliberal reforms. Moreover, it does not explain within countries why in some areas of the same policy sector policy legacies were cast aside in favor of foreign models, but in others they were not, as was the case of Peru. In this respect, combining a policy legacies approach with the theory of epistemic communities has a number of advantages. Peter Haas defines epistemic communities as "a network of professionals with recognized expertise and competence in a particular domain" (1992, 3). These professionals are bound by a shared set of normative and principled beliefs; shared causal beliefs regarding possible policy actions and their effects; shared notions of what constitutes valid knowledge; and a common policy enterprise (3). Epistemic communities serve to diffuse policy ideas and principles from country to country, from the international to the national and from the national to the international, through shared networks. They can help to shape the interests of political actors at critical moments.

Other studies of policy diffusion have shown the importance of networks, including in the area of social policy reform (e.g., Hall 1993; Keck and Sikkink 1998; True and Mintrom 2001; Bockman and Eyal 2002; Sugiyama 2008a, 2008b), but the theory of epistemic communities offered by Haas has a number of attractive components. The theory can accommodate the geographic clustering of diffused ideas that Weyland and also Madrid (2003) find, as in fact such communities may be stronger across adjacent national borders due to the greater opportunities to network that geographic proximity provides.[4]

But more importantly, the recognition that these communities may be transnational, and thus include members from international organizations, national bureaucracies, and civil society (Haas 1992, 17), helps to explain why so many researchers have found that national policy makers deny "influence" of IFIs over national policy matters. IFI "influence" (either in its conditional or more diffuse formulations) assumes a one-way conditioning or diffusion process, from the international to the national, or from a "model" country to another.[5] The unidirectional assumptions behind these formulations deny national-level agency in the production of new principles of reform. By contrast, the idea of a transnational epistemic community recognizes engagement of multiple actors in the creation of common "paradigm" (Haas 1992, 3). This formulation is in keeping with recent studies that have demonstrated that the line between the "national" and "international" in reform processes is quite porous (True and Mintrom 2001; Bockman and Eyal 2002; Orenstein 2008, 37). National actors may deny "influence" of IFIs because they too are engaged in the production of the common shared paradigm.

A useful feature of the epistemic communities approach to understanding health care reform is its focus on the bureaucracy. Key players in social policy reforms tend not to be presidents or political parties, but rather experts embedded in national bureaucracies (Kaufman and Nelson 2004; Weyland 2006, 12; Haggard and Kaufman 2008, 197). According to Haas, the steady increase in government and international bureaucracies since the 1970s and the growing technical nature of the problems that these try to address have led to the emergence of policy experts in and on the peripheries of bureaucracies, the individuals who form the basis of epistemic communities (1992, 9). Thus, epistemic communities are more likely to appear in areas like health reform that are embedded in bureaucracies. Another reason that epistemic communities are more likely to be influential in health sectors is that epistemic communities become more important under conditions of uncertainty. Health sectors are known for their complexity, which contributes to a significant degree

---

4. The importance of networks and clustering are classic components of the diffusion literature; see Rogers (1962, 2003).

5. Haas focuses on international and national bureaucracies, though his general definition does not preclude members of civil society. Works on similar transnational networking have emphasized the role of civil society (e.g., Keck and Sikkink 1997; True and Mintrom 2001).

of uncertainty as to which policy options are the best, a void that epistemic communities readily fill by providing "channels of advice" (12).

Moreover, it is in contexts of *crisis,* which by definition entail high levels of uncertainty, that epistemic communities become most influential, as they serve as shortcuts to solutions (Haas 1992, 14). Scholars have shown that crisis inspires a search for alternative policy solutions, often through a reliance on technocrats (Weyland 2002; 2005, 277; Haggard and Kaufman 2008, chaps. 5 and 7; Orenstein 2008, 61). Others refer to crisis as one of several possible "focusing events" that may bring visibility to a given issue and cause agents to act (Kingdon 1984; Birkland 1997). Such moments give politicians greater policy latitude than in noncrisis situations. The importance of crisis helps to explain why we see the new ideas promoted by epistemic communities prevail over preexisting policy learning legacies in some cases but not in others. In noncrisis situations, policy makers are more likely to look inward and continue with existing policy learning trends or follow the demands of policy interest group legacies rather than select a more uncertain foreign model.

Within Peru's health sector reforms of the 1990s, several policy legacies were overcome. Perhaps most importantly, the policy interest legacies of worker's and doctor's unions were pushed aside while market-oriented options of targeting, privatization, and decentralization were pursued. A transnational epistemic community rooted in both international organizations (IOs) and in Peru's government bureaucracy, with shared beliefs in the principles of neoliberalism and its causal corollaries, was instrumental in overcoming these legacies. Nevertheless, another important policy legacy outlined in the previous chapter, a Malthusian approach to population control, remained influential despite reform of Peru's family planning policy in the same period. In this case as well, there appeared to be a strong epistemic community in support of abolishing the previous Malthusian legacy, the rights-based epistemic community, which promoted a distinct vision of economic development, and, unlike neoliberalism, saw women's empowerment as central to development. In the 1990s this community had important international protagonists and adherents in Peru's civil society, yet unlike the neoliberal community, it was not sufficiently rooted in Peru's government bureaucracy nor was it called up in a moment of "crisis." Rather than buying into the principles of rights promoted by the rights-based community, the Peruvian government only symbolically and selectively used its discourse to improve its international image. As a result, the policy learning legacies of population control continued to shape national interests in this domain.

Competing Transnational Epistemic Communities

Two competing global visions of development shaped the context for Peru's health reform process: neoliberal development and the rights-based, human development paradigms, the latter rising in express opposition to the neoliberal model. Neoliberal economic theory in Latin America focused primarily on increased income; its influence was felt most directly through the Bretton Woods IFIs, such as the IMF and the World Bank, but other IOs as well as regional and national actors also played significant roles in promoting it (Orenstein 2008, chap. 2). In response, the United Nations prioritized human rights through its human development paradigm, which emphasizes not just economic but also social, cultural, and political dimensions of well-being (Haq 2003). As part of this focus, the UN also supported measures aimed at increasing gender equity and women's rights, from conventions on women's rights to the Gender-Related Development Index, which measures gender equity disparities across countries. These two epistemic communities, one promoting neoliberal principles and the other human development and rights principles, served as radically different and often "incoherent" frames from which Peruvians would develop their own national health agenda.[6] Yet only the neoliberal paradigm was sufficiently connected to the Peruvian national bureaucracy to serve as a "solution" when health care provision was at the point of crisis.

The Changing Face of Neoliberalism

The emergence of neoliberalism as an epistemic community can be traced to the late 1970s and to specific persons (such as U.S. Treasury Secretary Paul Volcker, University of Chicago economics professor Milton Friedman, President Ronald Reagan, and Prime Minister Margaret Thatcher) and institutions (such as the U.S.-based Heritage Foundation and the International Monetary Fund), all of which played a role in promoting the principle of free markets over state intervention as a solution to economic instability (Bockman and Eyal 2002; Harvey 2005; Babb 2007). In the Latin American region, neoliberalism was primarily advanced by institutions such as the IMF, the World Bank, and later the World Trade Organization that saw markets as the means for world economic growth, development, and eventually social progress.

6. On policy incoherence see Floro and Hoppe (2005).

Individual Latin Americans, however (such as the famous "Chicago Boys," who counseled Chilean General Pinochet on economic policy, and Chilean José Piñera, who advocated pension privatization worldwide), also played important roles in pushing for neoliberal reforms (Fourcade-Gourinchas and Babb 2002; Orenstein 2008, 38). These Chilean actors, among others, were important to spreading neoliberal ideas regionally.

The first wave of neoliberal policies in Latin America concentrated on economic adjustment during Latin America's economic crisis of the 1980s (Naim 1994).[7] The intents of the actors that promoted these policies were to slow hyperinflation and reorient these economies toward export production in order to repay significant debts. At that time, the dominant international policy makers agreed on the prescription for curing the region's economic ills, the so-called Washington Consensus (Williamson 1990). Removal of tariff barriers, currency protection, and interest rate controls; deregulation of enterprise; privatization of state industry; fiscal discipline; encouragement of foreign investment; and reduction of state spending were expected to rejuvenate Latin American economies. Global competition was to make these states and their economies more efficient and foster innovation.

Carried out in a form commonly referred to as "shock therapy" and designed by a technocratic elite, the reforms took place swiftly and with little political debate, despite the fact that all countries except Chile had democratic governments. The effects were shocking as well. Initially, currency devaluation led to extreme inflation, driving middle- and working-class populations into poverty. Closure of state and private industries that could not compete in the new environment led to widespread unemployment. Finally, those affected could not turn to the state for support, because state social services were also severely cut.[8] Over the medium term, neoliberal economic reforms succeeded in achieving economic stability and low inflation, though income disparities increased and long-term stability is still a matter of debate.[9]

Actors promoting the first wave of neoliberalism paid little attention to social policy, except to cut state funding for health and education services as part of an effort to shrink state spending. It was not until the early 1990s

7. Chile was a forerunner, implementing these reforms as early as 1974.
8. Publications that demonstrated the negative effects of economic reforms include Cornia, Jolly, and Stewart (1987) and Costello, Watson, and Woodward (1994).
9. See *Latin American Research Review* 39, no. 3 (2004) for articles that begin to assess the longer-term effects of neoliberal economic policy on the region.

that IFIs turned their focus to social policy. Major reforms to Latin American health systems thus took place at a different historical moment from the earlier economic reforms.[10] They were born on the cusp of the breakdown of the Washington Consensus and the shift toward "second-wave" equity-enhancing reforms. The widespread criticism of the early reforms for the toll they took on human livelihood forced proponents to rethink their prescriptions and to value stronger social policy systems. Key to the effectiveness of this criticism was the launching of several global campaigns, including "50 Years Is Enough" and "Jubilee 2000" (Edwards and Gaventa 2001).

The actors engaged in this epistemic community thus shifted their attention from bare market efficiency to a renewed interest in early twentieth-century human capital theory, which "views humans beings as a means of achieving higher levels of output or growth" (Aslanbeigui and Summerfield 2001, 7).[11] The shift to investing in human capital as a means of increasing national income allowed IFIs and other neoliberal advocates to address critics of first-wave reforms by accepting the importance of poverty reduction, social protection, and "good governance" while keeping intact the central objectives of economic development through market-based solutions and tight fiscal constraints (Hassim and Razavi 2006, 14–15; Tzannatos 2005; Razavi 2007; Bedford 2007). They followed this with reformulated solutions, such as "safety nets" to protect the poor from economic shocks, and later limited investment in and reform of mainstream state health, education, and antipoverty programs (Graham 1994). The 1987 publication *Financing Health Services in Developing Countries: An Agenda for Reform* was evidence of the World Bank's turn to an interest in human capital investment and health. Previously, the Bank had limited its interest in health to advocating population-control policies, under the belief that decreased population would be good for developing economies.[12]

Interest in social policy accelerated in the World Bank in 1995, when James Wolfensohn became president and responded to critiques of policies of the previous decade with specific measures. He started the debt-relief program for "Heavily Indebted Poor Countries," steered the Bank toward greater

10. Again, Chile is a forerunner, with major health reforms in 1979.
11. For a critical discussion of the human capital approach as essentially instrumental contrasted with the capabilities approach, see Arends-Kuenning and Amin (2001).
12. Bank president Robert McNamara (1968–81) took a keen interest in population control, marked by speeches on the topic addressed to the World Bank Board of Governors in 1968 and at the University of Notre Dame in 1969 (McCoy 1974, 66; Ruger 2006, 115). For an overview of the Bank's history in relation to health see Ruger (2006).

investment in health, and began dialogue with nongovernmental actors and the international community to combat critiques of the Bank's top-down policy dictates and lack of transparency. One Bank official in Peru noted in 1998, "New currents within neoliberalism require more participation by private organizations and civil society" (Dasso 1998).

By the mid-1990s, the World Bank and the Inter-American Development Bank (IDB) had entered vigorously into social policy matters and health policy in particular. The publication of the 1993 *World Development Report*, that year subtitled *Investing in Health*, marked the arrival of the World Bank as a major player in international health policy. Bank lending for health, nutrition, and other social services leaped from 6 percent of its overall lending in the 1980s to over 18 percent in the 1990s (Tzannatos 2006, 19).[13] By 1996, the Bank had active health projects in eighty-two countries and was the single largest source of health care funds in low- and middle-income countries (Abbasi 1999a).

The much smaller IDB historically has had a more equitable relationship with borrowers than the World Bank, and many more in-country staff members. It also has a longer history than the World Bank of supporting poverty alleviation. Like those of the World Bank, its loans to health reform escalated substantially in the 1990s. In the 1990s its goals in the health sectors of Latin America were similar to those of the World Bank: to promote efficiency, equity, and quality, especially through management reorganization (Nelson 1999, 72, 76). The IDB had supported health-related projects since 1973, but its overall spending on health between 1992 and 2001 increased dramatically, by over 250 percent (IDB 2002, 5). By 2001, 60 percent of its health-specific projects supported health reform (8). (This number excludes broader social policy–sector loans, which often also supported health-reform processes.) At the end of the 1990s the IDB had loans for reform of health systems in every Latin American and Caribbean country (Gómez Dantes 1999, 356).

The entry of these banks into health policy tied health reforms explicitly to larger processes of neoliberal state reform and displaced the World Health Organization (WHO) and its subunit for the Americas, the Pan American Health Organization (PAHO), as leaders in international health policy. The WHO and World Bank staff sizes are similar (eight thousand and ten thousand, respectively, in 2008), but WHO's budget is dwarfed by that of the

---

13. By 2008 lending for this sector was 31.4 percent of total bank lending. Calculated from World Bank lending figures available at http://go.worldbank.org/WR9THZTH00.

World Bank.[14] Its lack of major funds to lend and its traditional consultative relationship with national governments made it much weaker than the World Bank or IDB in influencing national health policies in the 1990s. These banks gain their influence primarily from the hundreds of millions of dollars they lend and donate.

The market-based principles of this new epistemic community were a stark contrast to the approach previously dominant in international health circles promoted by WHO—broad, state-facilitated access to health care. The entry of the World Bank in particular into an arena previously dominated by WHO shifted the focus of international public health from one centrally based on equity to one interested primarily in efficiency (Creese 1998; Turshen 1995). WHO had a long history of advocating for equity in health, most clearly in its core policy "Health for All by the Year 2000," a goal declared at the landmark 1978 Alma Alta international meeting on primary health care, led by WHO. "Health for All" was to be achieved through expanding "primary health care," meaning basic health care services in forms acceptable to local populations. The concept of primary care was initially rooted in the social democratic tradition, and in its most radical versions was viewed as an "adjunct to social revolution" (Cueto 2004, 1871).[15] By contrast, the World Bank does not have a mandate to work in the health arena, and legitimized its health role via economic arguments such as reducing poverty and increasing economic development. The 1993 *World Development Report,* for example, advocated investment in health not for human well-being, but as a foundation for economic growth (1993, 17). The former director of health, nutrition, and population stated in a 1999 interview, "The formation of 'human capital' is an essential prerequisite for sustained economic growth and social development" (quoted in Abbasi 1999c). Thus, while equity remained on the international health agenda, it did so based upon the more narrow human capital approach.

Coinciding with the banks' entry as major players in health policy, WHO began to shift its focus from equity to efficiency and simultaneously began

14. Koivusalo and Ollila compare WHO's budget to that of a "well-equipped university hospital" (1997, 16).

15. The more radical version of primary health care saw health as integral to development; emphasized integrated planning among distinct sectors such as economic development, education, and health; turned away from "Western" medicine and its hospital focus; turned toward attending to the basic care needs of poor people through constructing local health posts and training lay persons in basic health care services; and incorporated community members as participants in health care. Competing versions of primary care, much less utopian, emerged from other quarters shortly after Alma Alta (Cueto 2004).

to lose its international leadership capacity. This change can be traced in part to the entry of Hiroshi Nakajima as its director general in 1988. Nakajima did not carry forward the social democratic vision of equity through primary care, and his poor leadership led WHO to lose much of its international prestige (Cueto 2004; Koivusalo and Ollila 1997). WHO's turn toward efficiency is demonstrated by its collaboration with the World Bank on many levels, in particular to develop the controversial DALYs (disability-adjusted life years) (Koivusalo and Ollila 1997, 35). DALYs are a composite measure of health status and the effectiveness of particular health interventions. Introduced in the 1993 *World Development Report*, they provide a means of measuring the global burden of disease and the price of particular health interventions in terms of each intervention's ability to "buy" another year of disease-free life. The idea is for country governments to choose interventions that will cost the least and provide the greatest increase in well-being. Criticized by some as an inequitable and poorly conceived measure, DALYs highlight the emphasis of the World Bank and WHO on calculations of efficiency.[16]

While the World Bank's investment in health in itself marks a departure from "pure" neoliberalism, which would reject public investment in health, the primary strategies of health reform advocated by the World Bank, the IDB, and WHO in the 1990s continued to be guided by basic neoliberal premises. The 1993 *World Development Report* is careful to justify all state actions as contingent on the inability of markets to meet particular health needs, especially those of the poor (chap. 3). The "action plan" for health reform presented in the 1993 *Report* is also based on neoliberal principles, such as cost-benefit analysis to determine health priorities, cost containment, incentives for greater private sector participation, and more efficient state management. The 1993 action plan combined these traditional neoliberal elements with its new emphases on investing in "human capital" and increasing stakeholder participation. These elements might be considered dents in the neoliberal project, where the Bank conceded to critiques and expanded its focus to a greater interest in equity.[17]

In the late 1980s and early 1990s there had been pressure by global movements, such as the "Women's Eyes on the World Bank" and the "50 Years

16. Abbasi (1999b) reports that while WHO's official policy supported DALYs, many staff were dismayed by the change in principles that endorsement of the DALY represented. For more on the DALYs see Murray and Lopez (1996), Petchesky (2003, 164–72). For a gender critique see Hanson (2002).

17. I thank Rosalind Petchesky for this insight.

Is Enough" campaigns, for the World Bank and IMF to make their policies more gender-sensitive. The Bank had been relatively slow in incorporating gender into its development policies, but by the early 1990s, when arguments that structural adjustment affected women more negatively than men were well known, overall criticism of the Bank was at its height, and the UN Fourth World Conference on Women was on the horizon, the Bank began to pay greater heed to gender issues. President Wolfensohn attended the Fourth World Conference, where he committed himself to work with women's NGOs to develop a gender and development focus within the Bank (Barker and Kuiper 2006, 1). Shortly afterward, "Women's Eyes on the World Bank" succeeded in making the Bank agree to integrate the principles established at the Conference into Bank policy (Women's International Network News 1997). In 1996 an External Gender Consultative Group composed of fourteen gender specialists from around the world met to advise the Bank on gender policy (Long 2006). Finally, in 2001, the Bank published *Engendering Development: Through Gender Equality in Rights, Resources, and Voice*, its most comprehensive treatment to date on gender and development issues.[18]

Despite all this activity on gender and development in the 1990s, there was still little connection with the health reforms the World Bank and the IDB were promoting at the time. The Bank's External Gender Consultative Group met only once a year and had limited funds and no real power over bank policy (Long 2006, 49). Both the Bank and the IDB had divisions dedicated to gender and development, but my interviews with officials (in and outside the gender divisions) indicate that neither bank systematically took gender into account in the health reform process.[19] The major health reforms recommended by the banks changed over time toward greater attention to human capital investment, but gender equity was not directly considered in any of these reforms.

After the initial recommendations in the 1993 *World Development Report*, the policy experts of the IFIs, WHO, and others engaged in this epistemic community developed a series of specific health reforms as new solutions to long-term human capital deficits. Not all were implemented in every country, but surprisingly similar reforms were implemented in regions as disparate as South Asia, Africa, and Latin America. These reforms can be loosely divided into three periods. The first period, the late 1980s and early 1990s, included *financing reforms*, which sought a greater role for private financing

18. For more detailed history of gender in the Bank see contributions in Kuiper and Barker (2006).

19. Interview Anon. 14 (2000), Interview Anon. 16 (2000), Interview Anon. 17 (1999).

of health care to control costs and encourage cost recovery. Under this rubric are user fees, prepayment schemes, and insurance. In addition, *reforms of human resource management* were proposed, which used market mechanisms to leverage greater worker accountability and productivity. Through *targeting,* state health resources were focused on populations most in need, whom the market could not reach. Targeting referred to both particular populations and particular health interventions, bundled in a "basic package" whose elements were selected based on their ability to increase DALYs at lowest cost. *Decentralization* was advocated, on the premise that local actors would be more responsive to user needs and that smaller, competing units would be more efficient. For example, the World Bank's action plan emphasized success of community control in covering 38–49 percent of the operating costs of community-run local health centers (1993, 165). *Private sector provision of health services* (by for-profit or nonprofit entities) was encouraged based on the belief that the private sector should play a role wherever possible and that market competition would lead to greater efficiency as public and private providers competed for clients and market share. Finally, initiated by African nations in the Bamako Initiative but later advocated by the World Bank, *community financing and administration schemes* were proposed, where community members take responsibility for self-administrating and self-financing basic health services.[20]

The second period, from the mid- to late 1990s, focused on sector-wide approaches called SWAPs. SWAPs sought to overcome tepid national commitment to reforms and lack of discernible improvements in health indicators in the first phase of reform by bringing together stakeholders from state, society, and international spheres, and by building institutional capacity and sustainability in the health sector. In an effort to coordinate donor demands and ease state management of reform, lending for SWAPs was coordinated in a common pool of funds from various donors and also often included state funds (Evers and Juárez 2002; Petchesky 2003, 158; Standing 1999).

At the beginning of the 2000s, when former World Bank chief economic advisor Joseph Stiglitz began to critique both Bank and IMF policies publicly, we see a renewed appreciation of the role of state regulation of health service provision.[21] This further loosening of the Bank's position vis-à-vis

20. Elements of the first phase are modified from Standing (2002).

21. Stiglitz criticized first-generation neoliberal policies as theoretically and historically inaccurate (1998). He also denounced the lack of transparency in the policy process itself. See Stiglitz (1998, 2002, 2004).

state involvement was combined with other factors such as the rise of the UN human development model, along with regional factors such as the election of more leftist leaders and economic expansion in Latin America. Together these factors allowed for greater state leeway. As a result, several countries introduced broad state insurance programs such as Seguro Popular (Popular Insurance) in Mexico in 2001, Seguro Integral de Salud (Integral Health Insurance) in Peru in 2001, and Plan AUGE in Chile in 2003. These latest reforms might not be considered neoliberal at all, given that they incorporate greater numbers of the poor into social policy systems. Yet, like the reforms that preceded them, these insurance programs still mimicked markets by separating financing and delivery elements of health coverage, as well as offering narrowly defined packages of health care services selected on a cost-efficiency basis.[22]

Even while recognizing their evolution over time toward a greater role for the state, these three phases of health reforms still reflected a neoliberal affinity to market mechanisms. A central point of this overview is that "neoliberalism" is far from a static economic theory; rather, it is a set of policy solutions actively constructed by members of an epistemic community that have changed over time. The underlying principles of a preference for market-based solutions as the best route to development and measurement of development by economic growth have remained constant, while other factors have been added in that have served to soften the neoliberal paradigm.[23]

Rights-Based Development and Feminist Affinities

The human development discourse promoted principally by the United Nations offered an alternative to the neoliberal paradigm that dominated the 1980s (McNeill 2007). The roots of this paradigm within the UN can be traced

22. For example in Chile, neoliberal opponents accepted the AUGE law that was ultimately passed only when the most equity-promoting elements of the proposal (a compensatory solidarity fund) was eliminated, leaving a reform that ultimately did not radically alter the previous neoliberal health system (see Ewig and Kay 2008). In Mexico the Seguro Popular was boycotted by the leftist-led Mexico City government due to its imposition of fees for health services on the poor. Moreover, its primary architect, Julio Frenk, has been a regional proponent of the "structured pluralism" model of health reform (on which the Seguro Popular builds), which includes a significant degree of market participation (Londoño and Frenk 1997).

23. Even the 2001 Bank publication *Engendering Development*, although it begins to incorporate talk of "rights" and "resources," still defines development as economic growth (Schoenpflug 2006, 119).

to the institution's founding. Promotion of development was one of the four main ideas on which the UN was based (along with peace, independence, and human rights; Emmerij 2005). As early as 1962, the UN warned that over-emphasis on the "material aspects of growth" may lead to "human beings seen only as instruments of production rather than as free entities."[24] In the 1970s the UN was at the center of new ideas for promoting development; for example, the International Labour Organization (ILO) pushed for measuring development not just by economic growth, but by employment as well (Emmerij 2005; Jolly 2005, 53). Also in the 1970s and 1980s, the women and development movement within the United Nations Development Programme (UNDP), in particular its subunit, the United Nations Development Fund for Women (UNIFEM), advocated for the inclusion of women in the development process, and for individual development rights for women (Murphy 2006, 200–211; Snyder 2006). The basic needs approach, another precursor, emphasized poverty reduction and was developed in the 1970s in both the UN and the World Bank, in a period before the Bank became ideologically tied to market-based solutions.[25] In 1986 the UN formalized its position that human rights and development were fundamentally related with its Declaration of the Right to Development (Hansen and Sano 2006, 38).[26]

It was only in the 1990s, however, that "human development" was consolidated and recognized as a development paradigm with its own epistemic community. It began with the launching of the first *Human Development Report* in 1990 by the UNDP. Reacting to structural adjustment policies had been tried, with dire human consequences; human development took on resonance especially among those opposed to such policies. The paradigm was the brainchild of economist Mahbub ul Haq, who collaborated closely with Nobel laureate economist Amartya Sen and Paul Streeten, an economist who worked on the basic needs approach at the World Bank in the late 1970s.

Human development as a paradigm draws heavily on the economic and philosophical writings of Amartya Sen, which emphasize the importance of human capabilities and political freedoms, in addition to economic growth, for development.[27] Capabilities refer to the degree to which economic and social policies contribute to people's abilities to live a fulfilling life, such as

24. Quote in UN (1962), cited in Jolly (2005).
25. In the 1970s the Bank, under Robert McNamara, was focused primarily on poverty reduction. This changed in the late 1970s and 1980s when A. W. Clausen became Bank president and Ronald Reagan and Margaret Thatcher took office (Tzannatos 2006).
26. For more on development as a human right, see Andreassen and Marks (2006).
27. See, e.g., Sen (1989, 2001).

nourishment, education, and good health (Fukuda-Parr 2003).[28] As described by its innovator, Haq, human development involves five key aspects. First, it places people at the center of the development process. The objective of development is "the betterment of people's lives, not just the expansion of production processes." Second, it emphasizes the formation of human capabilities (such as health, knowledge, and skills) that can then be used toward productive, political, or leisure ends. Third, economic growth and production are included, but are evaluated on the extent to which they improve people's lives. Fourth, economic, social, and cultural factors are incorporated. Finally, people are both the means and ends of development, "but people are not regarded as mere instruments for producing commodities—through an augmentation of 'human capital'" (Haq 2003, 18–19).

Key to the popularity of the human development paradigm was the development of the Human Development Index (HDI), a composite statistical measure. Deliberately simple, the HDI is composed of average measures of life expectancy, literacy, educational attainment, and GDP per capita. Although criticized for its simplicity, it has gained popularity for precisely this reason. The index graphically demonstrates that countries with the highest GDPs do not necessarily come out on top by this broader indicator. The indicator is also more sensitive to within-country inequalities, in contrast to simple GDP measures, which mask these. Reflecting the UN dedication to gender and development issues, shortly after the creation of the HDI, two other gender-specific measures were developed, the Gender Development Index (GDI) and the Gender Empowerment Measure (GEM).

The United Nations has been criticized for not fully including gender in its projects and programming, yet it has gone farther than any other international organization in incorporating and promoting gender analysis. The UN first incorporated gender at its founding through its human rights framework and the creation of the UN Commission on the Status of Women, established in 1946. The first major UN convention to support women's rights and equality was the Convention on the Elimination of All Forms of Discrimination Against Women (CEDAW), first adopted by the General Assembly in 1979. CEDAW promotes women's equality in political, social, and economic realms and is the only human rights convention that affirms women's reproductive

---

28. Martha Nussbaum has applied the capabilities approach with a central focus on gender. Sen's approach is open-ended; Nussbaum has sought to pin down a set of "fundamental entitlements" that constitute capabilities (see, e.g., Nussbaum 2000, 2003). The UN opted to expand on Sen's more open-ended version for the HDI (Fukuda-Parr 2003).

rights. Following the UN declaration of 1975 as International Women's Year, and the subsequent declaration of the International Decade for Women (1975–85), the UN hosted a series of world conferences on women. Over time, these conferences became an important node for feminist transnational networking and international visibility for the feminist movement (Zinsser 2002; Friedman 2003). Feminists were also able to gain significant international visibility at other UN conferences. For example, at the 1993 UN Conference on Human Rights in Vienna and the 1995 Copenhagen World Summit for Social Development, feminist activists were successful in placing women's rights on the international human rights agenda and women's poverty on the development agenda (Bunch 2001; Snyder 2006).

Women's movement activists were also influential at the 1994 International Conference on Population and Development (ICPD) in Cairo. The ICPD produced a significant change in the global discourse on population. From the view of population control as a means to security and economic development, the discussion shifted to an approach that valued women's reproductive rights and gender equity (Lane 1994; Petchesky 1995; Smyth 1998; Presser and Sen 2000). Access to reproductive health services for all men and women was one objective of the accords, and reproductive rights were explicitly linked with human rights. Participants agreed on a comprehensive definition of reproductive health that included "a state of complete physical, mental and social well-being and not merely the absence of disease or infirmity, in all matters relating to the reproductive system." This definition included but was not limited to "the capability to reproduce and the freedom to decide if, when and how often to do so." Furthermore, the definition encompassed not only family planning but infertility treatment and quality health care for pregnant women and newborns (ICPD 1994).

The crowning moment for international feminism in the 1990s was the Fourth World Conference on Women, held in 1995 in Beijing, China, in which participants agreed to a declaration and platform of action that reached beyond any previous international agreements to promote gender equality.

In addition to the significance of the Cairo accords, the life expectancy measure in the HDI put health squarely in the human development paradigm. Some have argued that the attention given to the HDI in the early 1990s may have been part of the impetus for the World Bank to begin to invest in health (McNeill 2007). In the early 2000s the UN went further and developed a set of policies that built on the human development paradigm by linking poverty reduction to human rights. This link was built by outlining fourteen human rights (such as health, education, work, housing, and political freedom) that clearly reflect the human development approach (UN 2002).[29]

The declaration that resulted from the Fourth World Conference also referred to health care in three separate points:

1. By supporting women's reproductive rights: "The explicit recognition and reaffirmation of the right of all women to control all aspects of their health, in particular their own fertility, is basic to their empowerment."
2. By supporting women's right to primary health care: "Promote people-centered sustainable development . . . through provision of . . . primary health care for girls and women."
3. By supporting equity in access to health care: "Ensure equal access to and equal treatment of women and men in education and health care and enhance women's sexual and reproductive health as well as education."

In addition, the declaration pointed to the related issue of prevention and elimination of violence against women.[30]

Few concrete health policy proposals emanated from this rights-based epistemic community. Unlike the banks, the UN did not have teams of health policy consultants, and its health arm, the World Health Organization, as described above, had been severely weakened in its level of influence vis-à-vis the banks. It was only in the 2000s that the UN devised specific policy recommendations—the Millennium Development Goals, which have several health components—to carry forward its rights-based vision of development. Notably, these goals were arrived at through a consensus-building process with the World Bank and IMF, and were criticized for their minimalist approach as well as concessions made to global capital (Soederberg 2005).

Thus, the rights-based epistemic community had distinct principles from those of the neoliberal community, but also showed some degree of convergence with the neoliberal community over time. Its lack of power and resources made it less influential, as will be detailed below, but it also lacked clear and specific policy proposals that could be tapped by policy makers looking for alternative solutions. This lack of clear proposals helps to explain its lesser influence in health reform, as does its timing. This epistemic

29. For a useful discussion of international human rights agreements that support the social right to health, see Yamin (2003), 65–78.
30. Fourth World Conference on Women: Beijing Declaration, http://www.un.org/womenwatch/daw/beijing/platform/declar.htm.

community gained global and national recognition for its applicability to general health policies outside reproductive health only *after* the perceived crisis of health care in Peru was over.

While little came from the rights-based community in terms of health reform proposals, proposals related to gender and health did emerge from the Cairo and Beijing declarations, as outlined above. This fact, coupled with the increased appearance of women's issues on the global agenda leading up to the Beijing conference, including the sharp spike in transnational organizing among feminists in the 1990s, seemed to make for a propitious time to push for mainstreaming *gender equity* into health sector reform processes. (The concept of gender mainstreaming, meaning systematically integrating gender into all government policies and programs, was first introduced at the 1985 Women's Conference in Nairobi. The goal of gender mainstreaming was reiterated in the Beijing declaration.) Yet, as the next section will show, in the 1990s and even in the 2000s, feminists made few inroads in Peru.

Global Influences and Peruvian Policy Making

The two transnational epistemic communities influenced Peruvian health policy unevenly. The neoliberal community held greater overall sway during the most active period of Peruvian reform. The broader UN human development paradigm had only limited influence, but one aspect of the model had significant resonance in Peru: the call for greater gender equity, especially through the 1995 Fourth World Conference on Women in Beijing, China. The reason for the uneven impact of each paradigm was the differing perceptions of "crisis" in the separate health policy domains that the communities were able to influence (the neoliberal paradigm held most influence over general health reforms and the rights-based paradigm over reproductive health) and the differing degree to which each epistemic community hooked into the Peruvian policy bureaucracy at the time, a factor related to the financial influence of each community. As a result of these factors, actors engaged in the neoliberal community (both in and outside Peru) were best positioned to set the agenda for reforms that took place, especially those of the 1990s.

The Neoliberal Paradigm and Peruvian Policy Making

Deference to the neoliberal epistemic community as opposed to previous policy legacies or alternative epistemic communities was substantially aided by a perceived "crisis" in the public health system. This crisis created uncertainty and thus a need for quick recourse to expert knowledge. In Costa Rica the existing health model was working well and thus Costa Rican leaders preferred to follow their own policy learning legacies rather than adopt outside models (Weyland 2006, 150). But in Peru the severe economic crisis, combined with civil war in the 1980s and 1990s, had wreaked havoc on the health system, drawing into question the validity and sustainability of previous policies.[31] Moreover, the close connection between the economic crisis and the health crisis led to a confluence of policy solutions, due in part to an overlap between the main government institutions, such as the Ministry of Economy and Finance and the prime minister's office, that were responsible for addressing both issues.

Peruvian health spending peaked in the 1970s and early 1980s, then dropped severely due to economic crisis and was further slashed in 1990–91 with adjustment. The poor were hit hardest by the cuts, as they relied on a public health system that saw its budget slashed to only 15 percent of what it received in 1980 (MINSA 1996, 26). The human effects of economic crisis and shock therapies were compounded by Maoist guerrillas, who targeted government health clinics. One Ministry of Health administrator reported that health establishments were open only six hours a day due to lack of funds to pay employees, and that 32 percent of state health centers were closed due to loss of state control in regions dominated by the Shining Path guerrillas. Medicines and supplies were practically nonexistent (Interview Vera 1998).

A health minister in Fujimori's early administration recalled that in reaction to the crisis the president insisted "that there be health care," but left the minister to worry about the "details" (Interview Freundt-Thurne 1998). The crisis context predisposed Fujimori, at least in the initial stages of health reform, to support dramatic steps to rectify problems, overcoming the incentive barriers that often stymie reform in health sectors (Kaufman and Nelson 2004). But he left the details to the policy experts in the Peruvian bureaucracy, effectively deferring to technocrats, many of whom were engaged in the then-dominant neoliberal epistemic community.

Alberto Fujimori ran on a platform that stressed the ineffectiveness of traditional political parties and a desire to avoid economic shock. Yet in August 1990, less than a month after taking office, Fujimori reversed position and

---

31. Weyland does not use a legacies argument, but rather attributes Costa Rican reticence to change to Costa Rican "values" (2006, 150). Costa Rica's resistance may be better understood by policy learning legacies, as reformers insisted that the policies in place were working.

implemented a draconian economic stabilization program that stabilized the economy but nearly eliminated Peru's social safety net. His position was in direct opposition to the heterodox economic approach of his predecessor, Alan García, whose policies had thrown Peru into great economic trouble and bad standing with international creditors. Fujimori's shift also entailed a sudden change in government personnel. By 1991, conservative national economists with links to the IMF and World Bank took over the president's economic team. (Even in this phase, the two-way street of neoliberal ideas was evident; for example, the blueprint for Peru's stabilization was coauthored by Peruvian economist Carlos Paredes and American economist Jeffrey Sachs; [Conaghan 1998].) Thus, in the early 1990s, when Peru's economy was beginning to stabilize and second-wave social policy reforms emerged on the political agenda, key officials in the Peruvian government were largely neoliberal in their economic outlooks but looked to the IFIs for spending approval in the interest of avoiding the economic instability to which their previous bad credit standing had contributed.

But Peruvian policy makers did not wait for IFI "influence" to take action on health reform. In 1993 the prime minister's office outlined a plan for targeted spending in the areas of health, education, justice, and emergency food aid as a means to address the crisis in the health and other social policy sectors. In October the minister of economy and finance took this conceptual document to a meeting with the Paris Club creditors, who were enthusiastic about the plan (Interview Manrique 1998).[32] Paris Club approval was a signal to Peru of the changing winds of IFIs, which were moving toward a softer neoliberal approach that saw some place for investment in human capital. In its letters of intent addressed to the IMF in the 1990s, Peru outlined its economic and social policy plans, which followed the general shape of the softened neoliberal consensus of the period. For example, in its 1996 letter of intent Peru promised to promote private investment in health and education sectors and increased, targeted social spending aimed at the poor.[33]

The letter of intent set much of the basis of Peru's subsequent health reforms (Interview Anon. 4 1998; Interview Guerra García 1998), but the ideas that fleshed out the reform agenda were produced by actors in the neoliberal

32. The Paris Club is a group of financial officials from nineteen of the world's wealthiest countries. They offer debt restructuring and debt relief to countries when other alternatives have failed.

33. *El Peruano* (1996). See also the letters of intent of May 1998, http://www.imf.org/external/np/loi/050598.htm, and June 1999, http://www.imf.org/external/np/loi/1999/060799.htm.

transnational epistemic community, which included Peruvian policy makers and a variety of IOs. A Peruvian technocrat summed up the process of building a shared set of principles: "We are in a process of internationalization of the politics of health. Like in economics, you see that there are a series of economic policies that have an international level of consensus. Health is in a process of that kind" (Interview Anon. 5, 1998). Some of the key components of this consensus and the channels through which they were generated were clear in remarks by Peruvian policy makers and local IO officials. For example, the public remarks in 1996 by the World Bank representative in Peru, Fred Levy, revealed the centrality of the human capital approach to health reform, and the role of local Bank representatives in indirectly promoting this emphasis. Criticizing the slow pace at which the reforms were being implemented, Levy announced: "These sectors [health and education] have not yet carried out the structural changes necessary to establish the human capital base that the country needs to develop over the long term."[34] A policy maker in the health ministry remarked that the strategy of targeting (which was carried out with solely Peruvian national funds) came to be accepted due to the experience of pilot projects carried out in Peru by bilateral agencies, as part of Peru's mandate to fulfill its letter of intentionality with the IMF, and as a strategy that would "complement efforts underway by the World Bank, IDB and USAID" (Interview Anon. 4, 1998). These comments point to the ways in which Peruvian experience (e.g., pilot projects) combined with international influences to make targeting what this interviewee termed "a Latin American tendency."

One indicator of the density of the network between IOs and Peruvian policy makers was that the distinction between these two "sides" was not clear at all. For example, the head of the World Bank's health reform unit in Washington, D.C., at the time of reform was Peruvian Daniel Cotlear, who maintained close personal ties to Peruvian policy makers. Most Peruvian policy makers, moreover, had at some point served as World Bank or IDB consultants, either in Peru or in Washington, D.C. These individuals regularly moved between job opportunities in government and job opportunities with international organizations.

The network between these international and national actors was not based on shared principles or career paths alone. Several international financial institutions and agencies directly financed national health reform efforts,

34. Quoted in *Diario Gestión*, September 24, 1996.

and such financing allowed the proponents of the neoliberal epistemic community to gain a greater foothold in the Peruvian bureaucracy. The most significant was the IDB, which cooperated with Japan and the Peruvian government to finance the Programa de Fortalecimiento de los Servicios de Salud (Program to Strengthen Health Services), a sector-wide approach (SWAP). During the 1990s this SWAP funded the teams of Health Ministry consultants that spearheaded health reform from within the ministry. These teams were financed by loans of sixty-eight million dollars from the Inter-American Development Bank, twenty million dollars from the Overseas Economic Cooperation Fund of Japan, and ten million dollars from the Peruvian national treasury.

The World Bank, the United States Agency for International Development (USAID), and the British Department for International Development (DFID) also supported the reform effort. The World Bank funded a major targeting project, the Programa de Salud y Nutrición Básica (Basic Health and Nutrition Program), supported by 44.4 million dollars in 1994–2000 (Yamin 2003, 117). USAID personnel led workshops on health reform for ministry members, began pilot reform initiatives, and funded short studies on particular aspects of the health sector. Most of these were activities of USAID's Proyecto 2000 (Project 2000), financed by 30 million dollars each from the U.S. and Peruvian governments (Yamin 2003, 117). DFID worked to build the technical capacity of Peruvians engaged in designing reforms (Interview Anon. 12 1998; Interview Lewis 1998).

In addition, the major health-related reform projects financed by the agencies described above were located in the Ministry of Health itself. The Program to Strengthen Health Services, for example, had its own offices in the ministry, in which Peruvian consultants were hired to work on behalf of the IDB and Japan. Project 2000, financed by USAID, and the Basic Health and Nutrition program, financed by the World Bank, were also run by Peruvians in the ministry. Essentially, international organizations became embedded within the Health Ministry itself, blurring the line between "Peruvian" and "global" actors but also further cementing the shared ideational basis of this epistemic community.

International organizations and Peruvian actors contributed ideas to this network via publications, conferences, training workshops, and person-to-person contact. For example, IOs disseminated their U.S.-produced publications to Peruvian policy makers, such as the World Bank's 1993 *World Development Report* and *Financing Health Services in Developing Countries*, both of which were cited by Peruvian policy makers in interviews. But they also financed the Peruvian studies of reforms, which in turn informed these agencies' opinions on the effectiveness of particular reform approaches; USAID, in particular, funded numerous Peruvian studies published by its Proyecto 2000. These organizations would also regularly hold workshops on health reform (often led by Peruvian representatives of these institutions) for government policy makers and representatives of other IOs. Finally, the Washington offices of the IDB and World Bank would regularly send missions to Peru to evaluate the progress of reform, thus facilitating greater Washington-Lima interactions.

This epistemic community was not just in IOs and in Peru's bureaucracy; it also reached across national borders. Peru's neighbors, such as Bolivia, Chile, and Colombia, were similarly engaged with neoliberal health reforms. As a result, regional sharing of expertise and experience also proliferated within this epistemic community. Peru was influenced, for example, by the Chilean and Colombian examples of social security health reforms, and hosted experts from each of these countries to explain their mechanics, though it ultimately opted to modify Chile's reform (Interview Torres 1998). Peru was also influenced by the Bolivian maternal-child health program when designing its maternal-infant health insurance. The main innovator of the Bolivian program was Peruvian David Tejada, who later returned to Peru to head Peru's similar reform. In recent years, as Peru seeks to refine its own public insurance program, the Seguro Integral de Salud, the Health Ministry has also hosted visits from Mexican experts on that country's Seguro Popular and Chilean experts on the Plan AUGE (see chapter 7).

Peruvians were never coerced into accepting neoliberal premises or policies. IFI representatives I interviewed claimed a supportive role only, without intent to influence or condition health reform, while Peruvian informants claimed significant autonomy from international influence.[35] "Through a costly learning process," as one Peruvian policy maker put it, Peru had developed ways to maintain national autonomy. For example, by seeking multiple sponsors for a project or reform, they could say to a demanding foreign donor that they were not the principal financier and thus would have to compromise (Interview Anon. 12, 1998). However, while national bureaucrats successfully created wiggle room to innovate outside the desires of IFIs, through

---

35. This was the position of interviewees such as Anon. 15 (1999), a World Bank Lima representative, and Anon. 16 (2000) of the Inter-American Development Bank, 2000.

their tight networks with these organizations, they were more than just accepting of neoliberal principles, but active participants in their creation. As one informant who was central to the reform process put it, at no point in the reform process was there conditionality; rather, there was a certain "ideologization" of the process itself (Interview Anon. 5, 1998).

Because of epistemic communities' shared ideas of cause and effect, these can redefine interests in a given policy realm (Haas 1992, 15). The new discursive primacy of neoliberalism and the leadership of IFIs and bilateral agencies rather than WHO in the health field led to new understandings of the primary political challenges to health sector reform. Specifically, the IFIs framed certain interest groups as "obstacles" to reform, namely, organized labor and doctors' associations (IDB 1996)—precisely the groups that had historically fought for health benefits as a right (labor) and that had built their livelihood on providing health care in state systems (doctors). Market interests were seen as troublingly absent from health systems, and reformers believed that their entry would lead to greater efficiency through competition. This new causal understanding reshaped the interests of policy makers to see political and material benefits in confronting these policy interest group legacies head-on.

In addition to redefining interests, an epistemic community can also "agenda set" by effectively limiting the range of issues under consideration (Haas 1992, 16).[36] Gender equity, for example, was not part of the neoliberal reform agenda in Peru. Nor were women, organized feminists, or indigenous peoples part of the political calculations as interest groups that might block reform. The lack of attention to organized women and organized ethnic groups was not surprising, as they did not have historical legacies of power in the health system or vested interests to defend. The absence of gender equity on the health reform agenda, however, was surprising given the high profile of gender issues in international and national spheres at the time due to preparations for the Fourth World Conference on Women.

This epistemic community did not dominate in every policy area, however. One reform that emerged later and outside the crisis context, Seguro Escolar Gratuito (Free School Health Insurance, SEG), defied neoliberal principles in a number of ways, as is detailed in chapter 4. Moreover, the family planning policy, as detailed below, was seemingly influenced by the alternative

---

36. Agenda setting is a process whereby certain issues or approaches are placed on the political agenda and others are effectively closed out (Bachrach and Baratz 1962; Schattschneider 1960; Lukes 1974; Livingston 1992).

rights-based community, but was ultimately shaped more by previous policy legacies than by epistemic communities.

The Rights-Based Paradigm and Peru's Health Reform

The rights-based human development paradigm and its related UN projects did not influence Peru's health reform agenda significantly; instead, policy legacies in the area of population policy prevailed. The lack of influence of this epistemic community had to do with its weaker global position in the early and mid-1990s relative to the neoliberal community, the lack of financial resources of UN agencies, and the related relatively weak network relations between national policy makers and international proponents of the paradigm. Moreover, in the one area in which the rights-based community was stronger and did have strong links to the Peruvian bureaucracy—family planning—the same "crisis" conditions did not exist as they did for basic health care services. Due to these factors, rather than turning to this community for solutions, President Fujimori's administration simply hijacked the rights-based discourse in order to improve its international reputation, while duplicitously maintaining the same basic Malthusian population policies that had previously guided Peru's population policy.

The influence of the rights-based paradigm was particularly weak in the health sector in the 1990s because, as described previously, the UN agency with the greatest clout in the health sector, WHO, was itself weak and had begun to defer to the World Bank's efficiency approach. Moreover, WHO, PAHO, and other UN agencies such as UNICEF or UNIFEM had little money to dedicate to in-country policy plans in comparison to the major banks and bilateral agencies. In my process tracing of the formulation of Peru's six major health reforms of the 1990s (see chapter 4), UN-related agencies played a role in only two instances, both of these quite peripheral. Policy makers involved in one reform, the CLAS, emphasized the influence of the World Bank's 1993 *World Development Report* and UNICEF's 1990 book on the experience of community participation in health administration in Africa, *The Bamako Initiative,* for the ideas behind the CLAS (Interview Bendezú 1998).[37] In this case we see the discursive influence of UN publications that are also endorsed by the World Bank. The Seguro Escolar Gratuito was endorsed by UNICEF, but only after the program was established; UNICEF did not play a role in its formulation.

37. For more on Bamako, see McPake, Hanson, and Mills (1993).

It was only in the 2000s that the UN human development/human rights paradigm began to gain some attention from Peruvian health policy makers outside of reproductive health circles. In 2002 the UN appointed Paul Hunt Special Rapporteur of the Commission on Human Rights, charged with defending the right to the enjoyment of the highest attainable standard of physical and mental health. Hunt visited Peru in 2004 and 2006. He urged Peru to consider the rights-based approach to health, including the ramifications for health of signing the Free Trade Agreement of the Americas (UN News Service 2004). Such attention came well after Peru's major health reforms had already been enacted.

While the broader human development paradigm had little currency in Peru at the time of Peru's major reforms, the Beijing platform and its promotion of reproductive rights were highly visible to Peruvian policy makers and of special interest to President Alberto Fujimori. Moreover, feminists were well positioned to influence national policy at the time. Peruvian feminists were active participants in the preparations for Beijing and at the conference itself. With their roots dating back to the 1970s in Peru's political Left and based in a number of autonomous feminist organizations founded in the 1970s, Peru's feminists were among the most organized and active on the South American continent.[38] Preparations for Beijing served as an additional spur to bring disparate feminist organizations together behind a single focus. A grant from USAID allowed feminist NGOs in Peru to elaborate a nationwide consultative process to formulate a national agenda on women (Rousseau 2006, 127). The state led a similar process of consultation in developing its own agenda for Beijing. Peruvian feminists also had substantial regional visibility, as evidenced by the fact that the NGO representative for the Latin American region at Beijing was Peruvian feminist leader Virginia Vargas. Other feminists, such as the umbrella group Grupo Mujer y Ajuste Estructural: Debate y Propuesta (Women and Structural Adjustment Group: Debate and Proposals), were linked to other global feminist networks such as Women's Eyes on the World Bank, which criticized Bank economic policies for their negative effects on women.

Despite this actively engaged and globally linked women's movement and the sound position the Beijing Declaration provided to advocate for gender

---

38. Peru's major feminist organizations are Manuela Ramos and Flora Tristán, both founded in 1978–79. These were preceded by a number of earlier feminist organizations and women's sections of political parties. Today there are several other smaller feminist organizations as well. For more see Vargas (1989, 2006, 2008); Cevasco (2004); Rousseau (2006).

equity in the health reform process, a feminist influence was barely felt in the general health reform process. My interviews with feminist activists at the primary feminist NGOs in Peru revealed that feminists were not particularly interested in health sector reforms other than those related to family planning. Feminist attention to reproductive health was driven by a long-standing interest in reproductive rights and by experience in global feminist advocacy at both the ICPD and Beijing. As a result of the ICPD conference, feminists in Peru were successful in the creation of a tripartite commission, composed of representatives of the state, civil society, and international agencies charged with overseeing state follow-through on the Cairo population accords to which Peru was a signatory. This significant gain would allow them access to the state on matters of reproductive policy (see chapter 4).

Like that of Peruvian policy makers engaged in the neoliberal epistemic community, Peruvian feminists' interest in reproductive health was also shaped by global funding patterns. As feminists in Latin America became professionalized in the 1990s in NGOs with greater financial needs, their foci and influence became increasingly shaped by international funds (Alvarez 1999; Ewig 1999). The Ford Foundation had a long history in the region of funding feminist work on reproductive health (Shepard 2006). In 1995 one of Peru's largest feminist NGOs, Manuela Ramos, in coordination with another NGO, the Centro de Investigación y Educación Popular Alternativa (Center for Alternative Research and Popular Education), was granted the largest sum ever awarded to an NGO in Peru for Reprosalud, a project financed by USAID that investigated the reproductive health needs of poor Peruvian women. There were few feminist health projects outside reproductive health. In these, feminists collaborated with the World Bank. For example, the Bank contracted feminist NGOs to interface between the Bank and the local health promoter volunteers in the participatory component of the Bank's Basic Health and Nutrition Project.[39] Thus, global funders saw feminists as well positioned to work on reproductive health issues, and their funding served to reinforce this focus. They also saw women's NGOs as ideal for carrying out the World Bank's objective of incorporating civil society into its projects.

The great irony was that, despite their significant visibility and strength, feminist goals, even in the narrower realm of reproductive health, were co-opted and transformed to serve the interests of the state and international institutions. Peruvian feminists and a good segment of the international

39. Incafam was one of the NGOs to whom the Bank contracted out.

population establishment were engaged in the reproductive rights epistemic community, but this community did not adequately incorporate Peruvian policy makers. Instead, the Fujimori administration seized on the political opportunity of the Beijing forum, Peruvian feminists' high profile, and the values of "modernity" and "democracy" implicit in the reproductive rights discourse to further his international and domestic political agendas.

Seen through the theoretical lens of sociological institutionalism or political science constructivism (both of which emphasize the role of global norms and culture in influencing national political decisions), reproductive rights discourse had come to represent an emerging new global norm, one of modernity and democracy through the practice of reproductive freedom.[40] While among some economists and environmentalists a Malthusian approach to population control is still viewed as legitimate, the sea change that took place at the 1994 Cairo accords led to the dominance of the reproductive rights frame at the global level (Petchesky 1995; Halfon 2007).

The symbolic association between reproductive rights and modernity and democracy made the discourse an attractive vehicle through which President Fujimori could appear more democratic amid growing criticism of his authoritarian tendencies. Less than a year after the Cairo Population and Development accords, during his second inauguration speech in 1995, Fujimori announced a major change in population policy. He proclaimed a concerted "struggle against poverty," and promised that family planning would play a critical role in this new initiative. Fujimori's political power at this point was strong. Congress was newly reconstituted following Fujimori's closure of that body and a brief rule by decree in 1992. Nationally, the president was lauded for taking a forceful position against the worst economic crisis in Peru's history and against guerrilla insurgencies, but his 1992 self-coup was viewed poorly by international observers. His 1995 inauguration announcement was followed by an international commitment in September, when he was the only male head of state to address the United Nations Fourth World Conference on Women in Beijing: "as part of its policy on social development and the fight against poverty, my government has decided to carry out an integral strategy of family planning that confronts openly, for the first time

---

40. On sociological institutionalism, see, e.g., Boli and Thomas (1997) and Meyer et al. (1997). For these approaches in comparison to constructivism see Finnemore (1996). A number of studies document the symbolic relationship established between women's rights, reproductive rights, and modernity and democracy. See, e.g., Berkovitch and Bradley (1999), Barrett and Tsui (1999), Bergeron (2003), and Htun (2003).

in the history of our country, the serious lack of information and services available on the matter."[41]

These announcements of expanded family planning courted both global and national audiences. The Beijing speech garnered Fujimori badly needed kudos from the international community. Outspoken support of women's reproductive rights appeared to be a democratic gesture, assuaging countries that looked unfavorably on Fujimori's closing of the Congress. After his 1992 self-coup, USAID had pulled funding for its two major health programs, one of them family planning (Interview Anon. 6, 1998). Fujimori's new policy served to shore up international alliances and win tacit approval, and eventually financial backing, from important bi- and multilateral agencies such as USAID.[42]

Nationally, the announcements were an attempt to win the favor of Peruvian feminists, while continuing an ongoing dispute with the Catholic Church. In these ways, rights discourse served as a symbolic tool that aligned with Fujimori's domestic political objectives. Peruvian feminists had substantial national visibility in 1995 due to the Conference and its preparatory meetings. Fujimori arrived at the Beijing conference at a critical moment, when conservative actors like the Catholic Church were attempting to roll back some of the rights established in the Cairo accords. His announcement at the conference led to what some observers have called "an implicit alliance" between Fujimori and some feminists in civil society, though others remained wary of the Fujimori agenda, which was indeed mixed on women's issues (Alfaro 1996).[43]

At Beijing, Fujimori, dressed in jeans and tennis shoes, not only shed the traditional formal attire of presidents and UN delegates, but also shed Peru's traditional alliance with the Catholic hierarchy on issues of artificial contraception. This significant expansion of family planning services in Peru was made possible by a long-standing conflict between the Fujimori government and the Peruvian Catholic hierarchy. Church-state conflict in Peru began in 1990 when Cardinal Augusto Vargas Alzamora of Lima openly supported the candidacy of Fujimori's political opponent, Mario Vargas Llosa. Lacking Catholic Church support, Fujimori was elected with the strong support of

41. From speech by President Fujimori (in Spanish) to United Nations Fourth World Conference on Women, September 15, 1995, Beijing, China, translation by author. My thanks to UN staff for a fax of the original speech, and to Heather Roff for her assistance in obtaining it from the UN.

42. In a quantitative study of 114 countries, Barrett and Tsui (1999) show that democratic countries with clear population policies are more likely to receive aid from USAID.

43. Other cabinet members supported conservative positions, and Peru signed the Beijing Platform for Action with reservations.

Protestant sectors. According to some observers, the distance between the Catholic Church and the state progressed to "open war" in 1995 when Fujimori took an active stance on family planning (Interview Wicht 1998).

Though the Catholic hierarchy is opposed to artificial contraception in general, it particularly opposes surgical forms of contraception, which it views as mutilation of the body. Surgical sterilization had been illegal in Peru, except in cases where pregnancy was considered a mortal risk, until September 1995. Just days before the Beijing Conference, after lively debate, the Fujimori-dominated Congress passed legislation that legalized "voluntary surgical contraception," creating more dissent between the church and the government.[44] Fujimori's Beijing announcement targeted the church, accusing "the Catholic hierarchy" of trying at all costs "to prevent the Peruvian State from carrying out a modern and rational policy of family planning" that would help "the poorest sectors of our population."[45]

This speech, portraying his government as modern and the Church as irrational and backward, heightened tensions between the two and led the Peruvian bishops to proclaim the government family planning initiative a "satanic" proposal that would turn "the entire country into a whorehouse."[46] Despite this vehement opposition, the government expanded access to state-provided contraceptive services, including "voluntary" vasectomies and tubal ligations.

It is evident from Fujimori's placement of family planning within his broader "struggle against poverty" that he viewed family planning as a means to reduce poverty, rather than to promote women's rights; a policy learning legacy from previous political periods. However, his courting of feminists at global forums such as Beijing and his citation of feminist-influenced development accords created the impression that the policy would balance poverty-reduction objectives with reproductive rights, especially since Fujimori explicitly cited the Cairo accords in legal documents pertaining to population policy in Peru.[47] A lack of "crisis" of reproductive health and only a

44. Voluntary surgical contraception was legalized through modification of the National Population Policy (Law 346), passed September 7, 1995, days before the Beijing Conference. Congressional debate on the law included conflict with the Catholic Church and discussion of poverty-alleviation objectives (congressional debates in *Diario de Debates,* Primera Legislatura Ordinaria de 1995, Thursday, September 7, 1995, 463–535).

45. Fujimori, speech to UN Fourth World Conference on Women.

46. Quotes by bishops in "Peru's Family Planning Fight Forgets the Poor," *National Catholic Reporter,* October 6, 1995, 11.

47. See, e.g., Decreto Supremo No. 055-97-PCM, the law that created COORDIPLAN, as well as follow-up legislation, D.S. 011-98-PROMUDEH.

tepid movement of Peruvian bureaucrats toward the relatively new reproductive rights discourse and its principles meant that this epistemic community was too weak to serve as an incentive for Peru's government to redefine its interests toward reproductive rights over the old legacies of Malthusianism in a full-fledged manner.[48]

Conclusion

An alternative explanation for why neoliberal reforms prevailed in some areas, populist reforms in others (such as the SEG discussed in the following chapter), and policy legacies in still others would be that politicians are simply following their political "interests." This chapter does not deny the importance of interests, but rather lays out two important mechanisms that shape interests: epistemic communities and policy legacies. In so doing, it helps to explain when and why some policy legacies are overcome, while others continue to shape future policies. In times of crisis and great technical complexity, epistemic communities that are sufficiently rooted within national bureaucracies can serve to shape politicians' interests in new directions and away from preexisting legacies; they provide clear solutions to impending political problems. Absent a crisis, policy learning legacies are more likely to prevail due to their familiarity among policy makers, their lock-in effects via either institutions or acceptability among the broader public, and the political clout of interest group legacies seeking to defend these policies. For example, in Costa Rica and Uruguay existing health policies were working well and were supported by a broad sector of the population; thus, politicians' interests were shaped by these policy legacies rather than by members of epistemic communities, despite efforts of World Bank officials and others to move these health systems into a more market-oriented direction (Clark 2004; Castiglioni 2005).

In Peru there was a severe crisis of the general health care system—fiscal and physical deterioration of the public health system, which lacked a strong track record or an organized constituency to defend it. Crisis led policy

---

48. While feminists certainly considered the lack of family planning services a crisis, this was not a new situation and thus not viewed as a crisis by general policy makers. Most importantly, however, the traditional mode of family planning delivery through Malthusian means was seen as unproblematic by these policy makers. See, e.g., Smyth (1998) on global population organizations also only accepting the new reproductive rights discourse discursively.

makers to rely on the advice of Peruvian and transnational actors engaged in the neoliberal epistemic community as a source of solutions. In the narrower realm of family planning, it was unclear to policy makers that previous legacies were necessarily unworkable (in fact, policy documents showed a preference for these legacies), and these old policy learning legacies provided clear, simple solutions of population control, while the alternative "solution" of reproductive rights had failed to be absorbed fully by Peruvian policy makers and was a more complex idea to implement. These contrasting contexts of crisis, as well as the lack of embeddedness of the rights-based community in the Peruvian bureaucracy, explain why in several general health reforms Peruvian policy makers opted for new ideas that forced them to challenge and overcome policy legacies, whereas in other cases policy legacies like Malthusianism were allowed to persist. These distinct conditions in each sector led to the ability of an epistemic community, in the one case, and legacies, in the other, to dominate the shaping of politicians' interests.

The argument outlined in this chapter is consistent with that found by other scholars of health reform in Latin America, who also highlight the importance of crisis for policy change, but it looks at the issue from a meso- rather than macro- or microlevels. Stephen Haggard and Robert Kaufman, for example, emphasize the importance of legacies in shaping policy in the region, except in cases of fiscal crisis, which served to spur a shift toward neoliberal solutions (2008). Their multiregional study is macro in its focus and, due to its broad sweep, does not dwell on policy differences within given countries. Kurt Weyland (2005) also cites the importance of crisis leading policy makers to look to foreign models for solutions. But his analysis focuses on the individual, psychological level: what psychological factors lead policy makers to look to foreign solutions. This chapter adds to these analyses by looking at the meso-level: the role of networks in shaping policy decisions within one country.

Finally, the weakness of the rights-based epistemic community at the time of Peru's major health reforms helps to solve the puzzle of why gender equity did not enter into the "mainstream" health reform agenda, and only superficially influenced the more specific reproductive health care policy area, despite a particularly vibrant and high-profile feminist movement at the time. Despite the uneven effects of these two epistemic communities, each helped shape a gender division of labor in the national policy-making process. This division is explored in the next chapter.

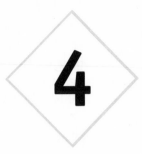

Gendered Divisions: The National Politics of Health Reform

Within the neoliberal epistemic community, international organizations defined working and middle-class labor unions and doctors' associations as the key obstacles to health reform. Given that these groups defended the existing occupationally stratified health system, their defeat in the reform period might have signaled an opportunity to alter the health system radically and create access to health care based on universal citizenship, rather than continue the existing system, where different classes, races, and genders were subject to health care of differing quality. Moreover, as explained in the previous chapter, global and national conditions seemed especially propitious for feminists to argue for "gender mainstreaming" in the health sector, which might have included eliminating stratification and paying attention to women's and men's specific biological and social health needs. Yet ultimately neither of these possibilities came to fruition.

The principles of those who led the reform efforts were part of the reason for this failure; a single-system, universal citizens' rights health system was never on the limited "human capital" agenda of those engaged in the neoliberal epistemic community. But given the fact that the IFIs at the time were pressured to consider gender equity and local level input, and that gender mainstreaming was being actively promoted globally, the absence of any gender mainstreaming effort is curious.[1] The absence may have been due to the factors outlined in the previous chapter—gender equity was not well incorporated into the principles of the neoliberal epistemic community, and the rights-based epistemic community, which did incorporate gender equity into its principles, was not well incorporated into the Peruvian bureaucracy at the time. These were surely factors, but the absence of interest in gender equity is still curious when one considers the national political context of the 1990s, where, according to Peruvian feminist leader Virginia Vargas, "The Fujimori government, more than any other in [Peruvian] history, advanced women's rights in institutional terms and in terms of placing women in visible positions" (2008, 112). Among its accomplishments, the government established the first women's ministry in the region and passed a quota law for women's representation in politics.[2] So why was gender equity not considered in the "mainstream" health reform process?

This chapter answers this question by connecting the global currents discussed in chapter 3 to the national politics of health reform through comparison of the policy processes of six major Peruvian health reforms between 1990 and 2000.[3] Part of the reason behind the lack of gender mainstreaming lies in the manner by which the neoliberal and rights-based transnational epistemic communities shaped the politics of reform along a distinctly gendered division of labor. The neoliberal community influenced the "mainstream" elements of the reform agenda, which were viewed as gender-neutral and largely outside the interests of women or feminists.[4] Family planning, on the other hand, was viewed as a women's and feminists' interest and shaped

1. See discussion of IFIs and gender equity, previous chapter. In contrast to Latin America, in the late 1990s in Malawi, Mozambique, Uganda, and Ghana gender advocates had significant success in mainstreaming gender onto health agendas in those countries (Theobald et al. 2005, 144).

2. The proceedings of the 1975 UN International Women's Year Conference was the first international call for the establishment of "women's machineries," or institutions within state structures specifically designed to monitor and advocate for improvements in women's status. This demand was reinforced at the 1995 Beijing Conference (True and Mintrom 2001, 30). Following on these recommendations, Peru was the first country in Latin America to establish a women's ministry. Executive-level women's institutions, however, existed prior to this in a number of Latin American countries, including Chile and Nicaragua.

3. I do not discuss two minor reforms in the period: autonomous hospital management and a plan to organize health clinics into networks. I also do not discuss the passage of the general health law, which served as a legal framework for the sector.

4. As stated previously, by "mainstream" I refer to those policies such as targeting, privatization, and decentralization that were deemed by policy makers as central to the reform process; other policy reforms such as family planning were viewed as outside of this agenda, as explained below.

by the rights-based community. This division of labor went unquestioned, surprisingly, even by Peruvian feminists, and it helps to explain why gender mainstreaming did not occur except in the policy area of family planning.

But there were also other factors at play, including the growing authoritarian nature of the Fujimori regime, the characteristically neoliberal form of the policy-making process, and policy legacies. Policy legacies helped to shift the attention of actors in civil society toward some reforms, but not others. Analyzing the noise and silences of policy interest group legacies in particular, such as labor unions and doctors' associations, in addition to other groups in civil society vis-à-vis the proposed reforms helps to explain the absence of gender mainstreaming. It is also revealing of the underlying class, gender, and racialized nature of the legacies themselves.

Six National Policy Reforms

The neoliberal epistemic community, composed of international organizations, consultants from neighboring countries, and Peruvian technocrats themselves, eschewed a gender analysis and instead saw health reform as a highly technical, managerial exercise that did not need to take social relations into account. As a result, gender was simply not on the "mainstream" reform agenda in Peru in the 1990s. Nor, at the time, was gender equity on the reform agenda elsewhere in the region; only in the early 2000s did some attention begin to be paid to gender equity and health reform. The policy makers involved in Peru's health reforms were mostly male, and most came from traditionally male professions such as medicine, economics, and engineering. As Elsa Baca, leader of the FENUPSA health workers union (the only female union leader to reach a national union leadership position at the time), commented with regard to women's political representation in the health sector, "I imagine that in the United States as well, and in all the world, there is machismo which [as is the case in Peru] excludes women from the most important positions in the health sector, even though we are the majority of workers in the sector" (Interview Baca 1998). Figures provided by the Ministerio de Promoción de la Mujer y del Desarrollo Humano (Ministry for the Promotion of Women and Human Development, PROMUDEH) for 1998 showed only minuscule percentages of women in each major state agency. The women's ministry itself employed only 2.78 percent women. Surprisingly, these figures showed the Ministry of Health had the greatest percentage of women among its ranks, 21.38 percent (PROMUDEH 1998). Yet, in my research experience during the same year, only two of about fifty top health reform decision makers were women.

But more important than the sex and education of the policy makers was the fact that these policy makers did not believe gender equity needed to be central to their thinking. Similar to what Diane Elson (1991, 1992b) found for economic reforms, health reforms were largely "male-biased" in that policy makers viewed them as gender-neutral, and thus reflection on their implications for gender equity was deemed unnecessary. In over thirty interviews with national policy makers in Peru's health sector, only one subject indicated a concern for gender issues. The interview instrument was tailored to the position and expertise of the interviewee, but each contained questions regarding gender and women. These probed (1) whether women beneficiaries of policies were considered in the formulation of reforms; (2) whether groups in civil society, including women's groups, were consulted in the policy process; and (3) whether gender equity was a policy objective. Most of the time responses to these questions were a simple "no." Some dismissed gender as irrelevant, while a few noted that at the implementation stage in some cases gender issues became more apparent. In one interview a former health reform team member stated, "We never even thought that the issue [of gender] existed; if it does exist, it must be very tangential" (Interview Anon. 41, 1998).

Surprisingly, Peruvian feminist activists accepted the supposed gender-neutrality of these reforms and the assumption that the reforms were not their business. This is despite the existence of a coalition of women's NGOs, bound together in an umbrella organization called Grupo Mujer y Ajuste Estructural: Debate y Propuesta (Women and Structural Adjustment Group: Debate and Proposals) that had formed to confront the deleterious consequences economic adjustment had had on women. This group, composed of smaller NGOs, had not yet identified "second-wave reforms" as an issue. Meanwhile, Peru's larger women's NGOs were heavily engaged with reproductive rights, not other aspects of health care. Feminist activists' greater engagement with reproductive rights issues, as discussed in chapter 3, stemmed not only from a long history of work on this topic, but also from the global epistemic community on reproductive rights that they had helped to develop, which included significant global funding that further directed their interests toward reproductive health and rights. These larger feminist organizations did gain an important foothold in the health reform process— but only in the narrower domain of family planning policy.

Part of the reason for feminists' successful participation in family planning was that technocrats in the Ministry of Health viewed reproductive health as a female and feminist domain separate from general health reform. At a 1998 academic conference on social policy reforms in Lima, a consultant for the Lima office of the Pan American Health Organization proclaimed that "family planning is not part of the health reform process." However, changes in family planning policy clearly fit the definition of health sector reform as "sustained purposeful change to improve the efficiency, equity and effectiveness of the health sector" (Berman 1995, 15). In fact, the overhaul of family planning policy in Peru in the 1990s was a radical reform in that previous policies were not just changed, but reversed altogether (though, as explained in the previous chapter, basic Malthusian policy legacies were maintained).

Racial equity in health care access was also notably absent on the reform agenda. One top policy maker defended the state's failure to address the needs of indigenous populations on the grounds that to take into account all of Peru's diversity was simply too complex (Interview Anon. 2, 1998). Race, like gender, did not fit the technical reform agenda. Peru is notable among Latin American countries with large indigenous populations for its lack of an indigenous movement (Yashar 1998; García 2005). Yet race was clearly a factor in Fujimori's and Toledo's elections: in both cases the majority of Peruvians opted for nonwhite presidents. And they both regularly dressed in typical highland indigenous clothing during their campaigns and presidencies. Yet, despite his blatant use of race in his campaigns, Fujimori did not seek to change the system of racial privilege that is an organizing principle of Peruvian political life, and its health system.

Preexisting policy legacies and the competing transnational epistemic communities instead helped to foster a gender division of labor that kept gender equity off the "mainstream" health reform agenda, and feminists were only able to influence the more "feminine" family planning agenda, as the following comparison of the political processes of six major reforms in Peru's health sector in the 1990s demonstrates.

Public Sector Reforms: Fees, Means Testing, Targeting, and Decentralized Administration

The four major reforms to Peru's public health system in the 1990s—fees, means testing, targeting a basic package of services, and community-based decentralization—sought to expand health services. Yet these also were formulated with fiscal and efficiency concerns at the forefront and in insulated political processes. What is surprising about these reforms is the degree to which they did not provoke the attention of civil society; they passed with relatively little difficulty despite the important degree to which they employed market-mimicking mechanisms. In part, the lack of dissent is related to the fact that the programs expanded state health care services. But another reason for the lack of attention is the fact that the reforms took place in the historically ignored public health sector, which served the needs of the poor, indigenous peoples and, traditionally, women—groups that had never been emboldened into interest group legacies that would defend the public health system, unlike workers and doctors in the social security health system. As illustrated in chapter 2, public health for subordinate groups was traditionally carried out in a top-down manner, and the way reform in these sectors was carried out in the 1990s did not stray far from this legacy. The policies themselves, however, were dramatically different from previous policies in their emulation of market models.

Fees and the measure of means testing to determine who would be exempt from these fees constituted Peru's earliest health reforms of the decade and reflected the "purer" form of neoliberalism of the late 1980s and early 1990s, which focused on cutbacks in state services. There was little domestic opposition to fees and means testing, in part because the Ministry of Health declared these reforms directly and they required no outside approval by Congress or the president. The public appeared to accept them due to the crisis context, which demanded action in the public health system to avert its collapse. In a system that was previously officially free of charge, user fees were the government's response to the devastating economic situation at the time. More a survival strategy than a carefully conceived reform, the central ministry simply allowed hospitals and clinics to officially begin charging fees to maintain themselves in the face of a deep economic crisis.

But the practice of charging fees lasted beyond the crisis period, under the neoliberal premise that they would deter "free riders"—those who had the ability to pay for private health care but used the public system anyway. In addition, in theory, fees would enable significant cost recovery and encourage public institutions to operate more like private entities. In 1999 fees for services accounted for 19.7 percent of the Ministry of Health budget (MEF 2000); by 2002 it reached 22.7 percent, and dropped only with the implementation of public insurance schemes discussed later in this chapter, to 16.1 percent in 2005 (MINSA 2008, 52). The above arguments constituted the neoliberal basis for fees, but policy proponents also made other arguments. The World Bank (1993) suggested that relatively low fees would expand coverage and increase the quality of services. An IDB official asserted that fees would lead to greater valuation of health care services by users (Interview Anon. 16, 2000).

Simultaneous with the introduction of fees, Peru's public health system implemented means testing, in which patients' incomes and familial resources were scrutinized to determine whether they would receive reduced fees or fee waivers. There were no official criteria for means testing, but the practice was promoted by the Ministry of Health and carried out in most health establishments. A top ministry official described the policies of fees and means testing in Peru in the 1990s in this way: "The majority of [public health] establishments charge fees . . . but without an explicit, discriminate policy, rather with criteria that they develop within each of these places, including whom to charge, who not to charge and the amount of the fee" (Interview Anon. 5, 1998).[5] In addition to the concern with free riders, pressure on health establishments to generate income through fees was an added incentive to practice means testing to maximize income. The turn toward means testing followed the neoliberal premise of reducing state benefits as much as possible. Only those most in need ought to benefit from free public services; all others ought to pay or utilize private providers.

By the mid-1990s Peru sought to step up its investment in human capital through providing targeted, primary health care. Following the Paris Club approval for social spending in 1993, which reflected the changing currents of neoliberal discourse toward greater investment in human capital, Peru implemented the Programa de Salud Básica para Todos (Basic Health for All Program, PSBT) in 1994. This program paralleled other efforts to expand primary care across the region at about the same time—for example, the Equipos Básicos de Atención Integral de Salud (Basic Health Teams, EBAIS) in Costa Rica and the Programa de Ampliación de Cobertura (Expanded Coverage Program, PAC) in Mexico. The Mexican program was the most similar to Peru's in that it also only offered a very basic menu of primary health services.[6] The health sector was still facing crisis when this reform was passed in December 1993 as one article of the extensive 1994 budget law, so there was some urgency behind it. The article allowed the release of funds for

5. See also Remenyi (1999), 45.
6. On Costa Rica see Clark (2004); on Mexico see Pérez and Medina (n.d.).

a number of targeting initiatives, health being just one. No other legislation was required, and Basic Health for All was developed from that point on within the Ministry of Health by a team of five appointed by Minister of Health Jaime Freundt-Thurne. The program was financed entirely by the national treasury.

The reform targeted a basic package of primary health care services to the poorest Peruvian communities. It involved an inflow of resources to these communities, in terms of clinic construction, personnel who were attracted to poor and remote areas by competitive salaries, and medicines and medical supplies. The basic health package approach sought to expand the reach of public health services in remote rural and urban poor areas at minimal cost. While the principal intent was to increase equity in access to care, cost-efficiency was also a concern of targeted programs (Haggard and Kaufman 2008, 217). The basic health care concept came from the World Bank, which advocated low-cost primary care interventions as the most cost-effective manner to increase disability-adjusted life years, or DALYs. The basic package of services involved necessary but minimalist government intervention to boost human capital (World Bank 1993). While targeting the poor is an important remedy for an otherwise class- and geographically inequitable health system, the risk is that these programs are more vulnerable to fiscal cutbacks than programs that serve broader, and more organized, constituencies (Nelson 1992).

The Basic Health for All program also borrowed from neoliberal tenets by introducing private sector models into public systems. Specifically, health professionals were hired under a private sector labor regimen. Unlike traditional state health workers, who held "named" positions and were virtually immune to job loss (but also paid poorly), these health professionals were hired on short-term contracts, which would be renewed based upon productivity levels.[7] Though these workers were paid competitive salaries, they forfeited job stability and benefits—they received no health, pension, vacation, or even sick-day benefits. The new employment regimen directly challenged the existing policy interest group legacies of doctors and other health professionals. In Basic Health for All, contracts were extremely short (three to six months with no benefits) and productivity expectations were high. For example, persons working in rural areas with low population density had the

---

7. The 1991 Ley de Fomento de Empleo allowed the use of temporary contracts for up to three years per employee, and in 1995 this was extended to a five-year period.

same productivity requirements as those in densely populated high-demand urban areas (leading to high incentives for rural workers to lie about productivity, as was professed to me by some health care workers). With quotas to meet and jobs on the line, efficiency was successfully promoted, but there were no incentives to provide high-quality care.

This radical change in employment practices was possible due to significant reforms in labor policy. Important for health sector unions, bargaining shifted from sector-level to firm-level (Saavedra 2000). This meant that the union of health professionals working for the Ministry of Health, the Federación de Trabajadores del Ministerio de Salud (Federation of Ministry of Health Workers), had to bargain with each regional health director, not the ministry as a whole. The union of health professionals thus became ineffective and nearly dissolved. In addition, labor law reforms made strike days unpaid days, thus reducing the incentive to strike or to maintain a strike.

Throughout the 1990s, Peru had an overabundance of young health professionals seeking work. These unemployed professionals welcomed the well-paid work opportunity that the Basic Health for All Program presented. The program effectively opened an alternative health labor market to the scarce "named" positions in the social security health system and the Ministry of Health. These workers, however, could not unionize. While the Ministry of Health at one time had had a very strong nurses' union, it disappeared due to these changes in labor practices and hostility against its leaders. This left only the nurses' union of the social security health system. As a leader of Peru's social security system nurses' unions explained, "The contracted nurses do not join unions out of fear of being fired, because the current laws give all the rights to the employer to determine the contract" (Interview Bottger 1998).

The impact of Basic Health for All on primary level public health care in Peru was notable when measured by its level of coverage—by the end of 1998, the program covered 89 percent of all primary level public health establishments. The percentage of centers covered later dropped, to 79 percent in 2001, because some of these centers converted to the CLAS model, discussed below.[8] By 2007 the program had disappeared as a program in name, though many of its elements remained, such as contracting most health professionals. Moreover, the idea of a "basic package" would continue in future programs, such as Integral Health Insurance (Seguro Integral de Salud), discussed later.

8.   Data provided by former CLAS program director Ricardo Díaz Romero, February 19, 2001.

At about the same time that the Basic Health for All Program was developed in the Ministry of Health, another small team was working on a policy called the Programa de Administración Compartida (Shared Administration Program). This program came to be known simply as CLAS, after the local health administration committees (Comités Locales de Administración en Salud) it created. In 2007 35 percent of Ministry of Health establishments were CLAS (MINSA 2007, 109). The concept of administrative decentralization comes in part from the idea of subcontracting. The neoliberal premise behind subcontracting is to have smaller entities take over components of administration or service provision, to create minimarkets within a larger market. In theory, these small markets will be more efficient and responsive to client needs. Applying this concept to state health sectors, reformers reasoned that smaller administrative units, which were closer to their clients, would more efficiently manage health resources than a centralized national health ministry. For example, local administrators would be able to target scarce resources more effectively to those who really needed them. With the right incentives, these smaller units would compete to produce better services at lower cost. Better services, in turn, were thought to generate greater disposition on the part of users to pay for services.

While Argentina, Brazil, Colombia, and Chile all carried out major decentralization initiatives as part of their health reforms of the 1990s or earlier, these countries decentralized fiscal and administrative responsibility for health services to states or municipalities. Peru also engaged in some fiscal decentralization to regional health authorities in the 1990s, but policy makers looked to community participation as a unique means of administrative decentralization. Colombia, Brazil, and Costa Rica all call for some form of participatory oversight in their health systems; only in Peru was a participatory model effectively implemented (Nelson 2004, 60–61).

The participatory component of the CLAS draws from an intersection of philosophies that seek to promote empowerment and democratization through participation, and the move by IFIs in the mid-1990s from top-down prescriptions to more local approaches that saw the "organizational capacity of the poor" as key to poverty reduction (Narayan 1999, 2). This curious combination of neoliberal and more democratic ideals perhaps lies in the global entities whose publications inspired it: the World Bank and UNICEF (as discussed in the previous chapter). The CLAS reform team members were funded through the Inter-American Development Bank/Japan SWAP loan, as well as a small amount of international funding from USAID that allowed the team to hire a foreign consultant in the development of the policy.[9] But fund-ing for the implementation of CLAS, as for Basic Health for All, came entirely from the public treasury, with no bi- or multilateral financial support.

The CLAS program decentralized local health clinic administration to a board composed of six community members and the clinic head doctor. The community elected three board members, and the head doctor selected the other three from local community health–related groups such as mothers' clubs.[10] These boards had significant responsibilities, including hiring and fir-ing personnel, deciding how money raised through fees for services would be spent, and approving an annual community health plan each year. The inde-pendent nature of CLAS health centers created minimarkets where each com-peted with other nearby health clinics to attain more patients who might be attracted by the particular services a CLAS center might offer. The CLAS would benefit from more clientele by earning more user fees, which, in contrast to non-CLAS health centers, it was allowed to keep and spend on improvements.

Each health center that converted to the CLAS model legally became a private nongovernmental organization (termed *personería jurídica*). Yet each was dependent on the Health Ministry (in the case of the Lima CLAS) or its regional health authority (in the provinces) for its main budget, primarily salaries. The CLAS health center infrastructure also remained state prop-erty. The ability to spend their own fees led many CLAS centers to improve their infrastructure and hire additional staff members. CLAS members were required to approve a local community health plan each year, a component that urged greater responsiveness of health services to community circum-stances. Finally, the health workers in the CLAS centers were hired directly by the CLAS members, who evaluated these workers on at least an annual basis. This oversight provision in the policy increased worker productivity (Altobelli 1998a). Like Basic Health for All workers, CLAS professionals were contracted, but generally for a year rather than a few months at a time, and, unlike Basic Health for All workers, CLAS workers received regular benefits such as vacation and pension contributions—though their salary scale was lower than that of their Basic Health for All counterparts.

9. This consultant, Dr. Carl Taylor of Johns Hopkins University, has since supported a number of similar initiatives in other countries.

10. Mothers' clubs are a common grassroots organization in poor Peruvian communities. They are groups of mothers that originally organized to volunteer in distributing daily gov-ernment milk rations to children and the elderly. Some clubs expanded to other community services activities.

The CLAS policy was developed entirely within the Ministry of Health by a small reform team appointed by Minister Freundt-Thurne. The team at first consisted of eight people and was eventually reduced to three. This core team wrote the Supreme Decree that created CLAS. Freundt-Thurne supported the project within the ministry, and successfully sought the support of the president, whose signature was required on the Supreme Decree to make the reform legal (Interview Anon. 11, 1998; Interview Bendezú 1998; Interview Vera 1998; Interview Freundt-Thurne 1998). President Fujimori's interest in the policy was only improvement in health services; whether it "was CLAS or not CLAS was not important" (Interview Freundt-Thurne 1998). CLAS was tied financially to Basic Health for All, receiving its funds from the same budget line approved by Congress for targeting, as part of the same health sector–restoration effort. As a result, it did not need to go to Congress for inclusion in the budget, and key state institutions, such as Congress and the Ministry of the Economy and Finance, played no role.

The expansion of CLAS depended on the will of the autonomous regional health authorities. Some of these were enthusiastic and implemented the program widely, while others saw decentralization, especially to community members, as a political threat to their authority and refused to implement it well, or at all. By 1997, three years into the program, CLAS covered only 10 percent of all primary level health establishments connected to the Ministry of Health—a far cry from the 72 percent coverage of Basic Health for All, which started at about the same time (MINSA 1996b).

The CLAS would stall and then spurt depending on government support through the Fujimori and Toledo administrations. In 1999 it was salvaged only through the support of coordinated parallel loans from the World Bank and IDB, who viewed the program positively. The government of Alan García (2006–) has once again supported the CLAS, declaring it to be an efficient and effective form of health delivery that ought to be expanded.[11] As of this writing, the program has survived for thirteen years, despite political resistance. Notably, despite its legal origin as an easily reversed "supreme decree," in October 2007, after regular lobbying by a small but well-positioned handful of CLAS supporters in Lima's civil society, the Congress passed Law 29124, which officially made the CLAS model part of Peru's permanent health structure.

Policy legacies shaped the attention of actors in civil society so that most of these public health reforms were ignored by organized sectors. Continuing

11. Personal communication with Laura Altobelli, May 30, 2007, Lima.

organized labor's historic focus on the social security health system, the health care unions at the time—the most powerful being the Federation of Ministry Workers and the Asociación Nacional de Médicos del Ministerio de Salud (National Association of Doctors of the Ministry of Health, ANMMS)— did nothing to challenge the changes in labor regimen that primarily affected the public health sector. The ANMMS formed part of the national doctors' guild, the Federación Médica (Medical Federation), which opposed reforms in the social security health system but ignored the new hiring regimen in the ministry and did not attempt to organize the workers hired under that system. The lack of protest against the reform—either its basic package approach or the labor regimen—is revealing of the degree to which the public health sector was not viewed as an important domain for political contestation. It was only in 2005, ten years after the initial reform, that the Medical Federation mobilized against the contracts, and for a short period of time doctors regained the right to named positions.[12]

In response to the CLAS reform, there was some resistance from medical associations, as this reform was initially viewed as "privatization." The Colegio Médico (Peru's equivalent to the American Medical Association) issued a statement in opposition to CLAS after the Supreme Decree was first passed. The Medical Federation also opposed the reform. A member of the Medical Federation explained, "We were not in agreement with giving the community the responsibility to finance health services, in other words the possible privatization of health services or self-administration" (Interview Díaz 1998). In addition, the Federation of Ministry Workers, fearing the negative impact of further decentralization on the unity and viability of their union, vocally opposed the measure (Interview Vera 1998). The protests went unheeded by policy makers, however, who, with the support of the president, viewed new ideas as the only way out of a crisis situation and, like the IFI representatives they interacted with, viewed labor and doctors' associations as obstacles to reform rather than interests to court. By simply avoiding public discussion, the formulators of the CLAS policy did not allow the opposition to stop or slow the reform. One of the three reform team members stated: "We never responded. We simply took a very low profile" (Interview Bendezú 1998).[13]

12. In 2005 many doctors, but no other health professionals, were shifted from contracted to named positions. Naming has once again stopped since that time, but previously named doctors continue in named positions. Naming grants not only protection from termination, but also fewer work hours in a day.

13. Vera (1998; Vera was also a member of the team) and Freundt-Thurne (1998) made similar comments.

Reform of the Social Security Health Sector: Health Provider Entities

Whereas the health sector reforms that served largely the poor and the indigenous population aroused little dissent from civil society despite their generally neoliberal contours, the reform of the social security health system, serving the white and *mestizo* middle and working classes, provoked massive opposition. This reform took aim at the most entrenched interest group legacies: both organized labor, which had fought for the institution of social security health in the first place, and organized doctors in the social security health system, who benefited from much better salaries and benefits than their public sector peers. Ardent opposition from these interest groups and others helps to explain the roughshod manner in which the Fujimori administration attempted to pass this reform.

Social security reform allowed private health care companies to offer health insurance to workers previously only covered by the state social security system. Drawing on principles offered by professionals engaged in the neoliberal epistemic community, Peruvian policy makers expected that market competition between the state and private providers would improve the quality of social security health care and reduce costs (Johnson 1998). Policy makers also expected the reform to provide an incentive for expansion of the tiny private sector insurance market (Interview Torres 1998). Finally, they hoped that the introduction of private sector providers would reduce congestion in the social security health system (Carbajal and Francke 2003, 517; Johnson 1998). As was the case for Peru's pension reform, Chile was looked to by policy elites as a model (Interview Freundt-Thurne 1998; Interview Manrique July 15, 1998; Interview Torres 1998). The original proposed reform was in fact very similar to the Chilean health social security reform, though the law that was finally implemented, as explained below, involved a number of important modifications.

In the early 1990s, health ministers Freundt-Thurne and Eduardo Yong Motta made unsuccessful bids to create the legal framework for Organizaciones de Servicios de Salud (Health Service Organizations, OSS) on the heels of pension reform. This reform would have allowed private insurers to compete directly with the state social security health system. The OSS reform was passed by legislative decree in 1991, but it was never implemented due to strong opposition from organized labor, retired persons, and health care professionals. The plan lay dormant until Marino Costa Bauer—a former insurance executive explicitly appointed to see the reform's passage—was appointed minister of health. In 1996 the president passed a second legislative decree, based on a modified version of the OSS policy developed by Costa Bauer's team, titled Entidades Prestadoras de Salud (Health Provider Entities, EPS) rather than OSS. This time opposition members of Congress protested that the decree was unconstitutional because it extended beyond the decree-making powers Congress had granted the president. It had authorized decrees related to privatization but not to social security system reform.

Ultimately, the proposal passed Congress in May 1997 as the Modernization of Health Social Security Law (Ley de Modernización de Seguridad Social en Salud). Peru's weak party system and presidential control of Congress at the time made passage of the law relatively trouble-free, and Congress made few changes to the 1996 decree. Neither the passage of the OSS bill by legislative decree nor the EPS bill, despite the fact that the latter finally passed Congress, allowed for more than a few hours of public debate. The Congress made only minor modifications to six of the final law's nineteen articles. Congressional debate was acrimonious, and a significant contingent of congressional members from opposition parties walked out and refused to participate in the final vote.[14]

Similar to the Basic Health for All and CLAS reforms, the failed OSS and successful EPS proposals were devised by small reform teams appointed by the minister. The Health Provider Entities team, furthermore, was funded through the generous IDB/Japan SWAP loan mentioned above (Interview Torres 1998; Interview Anon. 12, 1998). As a result of resistance to all-out privatization (the route taken with pensions), the initial reform simply introduced private competition to the state system. Second, in contrast to the Chilean model, it allowed for "solidarity" among workers, in that workers as a whole in each company voted on which provider would obtain a company health insurance contract. Company-by-company rather than individual selection avoided potentially different plans for different types of workers—management and labor, for example. In addition, as a cost-containment measure, Health Provider Entities provided only primary and secondary care, while more expensive complex care was reserved for the state system. As a result of this final measure, of the total paycheck contribution (9 percent of a worker's pay), 25 percent went to private health providers and 75 percent to the state system. For that 25 percent contribution, an EPS had to offer a minimal package of

14. *Diario de los debates,* Segunda Legislatura Ordinaria de 1996, Tomo II, 17.4.97–16.5.97, 17a sesión, Thursday, May 8, 1997.

services, a *plan mínimo,* whose contents were determined by the state. (The *plan mínimo* also distinguished this reform from Chile, which initially had virtually no regulation over its private providers.) Any services beyond the basic package could be purchased individually from the health provider. Once a company opted for a Health Provider Entity, individual workers could also opt to maintain affiliation with the state social security system.

One of the leaders of the health sector reform effort noted that, of all the health reforms during the Fujimori administration, Modernization of Health Social Security was the "most jealously guarded" (Interview Anon. 5, 1998). Guarding was necessary to overcome strident opposition, especially from policy legacies both in government and civil society. Opposition stemmed in part from the Peruvian Institute of Social Security, which would not only lose funds and prestige, but would have to bow to the less prestigious Ministry of Health that was envisioned in these reforms as the overseer of general health policy, across Peru's segmented health system. It also stemmed from organizations of health professionals and retired persons, organized labor— and even feminist organizations—who joined together in protest just after the passage of the final Health Provider Entity law. In May 1997 the National Front in Defense of Health and Social Security (Frente Nacional de Defensa de la Salud y la Seguridad Social, FRENDS) was formed. FRENDS, composed of sixty-four different organizations from civil society opposed to the Health Provider Entity reform, vowed to stop its implementation (Interview Sánchez Moreno 1998).

Social security health system reform faced much greater resistance than the Basic Health for All and CLAS reforms for a number of reasons. Although the state social security health system covered a smaller portion of the population (23 percent, compared with the 74 percent covered by the Ministry of Health), it affected the most powerful interest group legacies, including organized formal sector workers and social security health system workers, who remained better organized than public health sector workers. Second, because this reform initially mirrored the previous privatization of the pension system, the opposition was primed to oppose a reform of this type. Finally, whereas the Basic Health for All and CLAS reforms brought an increase in state health resources, the reform of the social security sector implied job and resource loss for the state system. The opposition failed to stop it, in part because many white-collar workers wanted a choice in health care options and the improved care quality that Health Provider Entity reform promised. Another reason was that organized labor was especially weak at this juncture

due to the economic crisis, which had led to significant job loss and low salaries, and the Fujimori government's drastic antiunion measures, discussed
below. The reform also progressed to implementation because the Fujimori
administration used every political tactic possible to overcome interest group
and previous policy learning legacies to impose what it viewed as the "solution" to the crisis of social security health care: neoliberal-inspired private
sector competition.

Family Planning: A Rights-Based Reform?

The reform of the family planning program contrasts with the public sector
and social security sector neoliberal reforms in two primary ways. First, at
least in its official documents and public statements, it followed the international human and gender-rights principles established at the Cairo and
Beijing conferences. Second, feminists played a central role, whereas they
were absent in the other reforms. This contrast points to a gendered division of labor in which the above neoliberal public health and social security
health reforms were viewed by policy makers and feminists alike as "gender-
neutral," whereas reproductive health was viewed as a feminine and feminist
domain.

Rights-based rhetoric and feminist engagement in the policy process led
to quite admirable official family planning policies. But other government
documents related to poverty reduction and analysis of the implementation
process reveal that government leaders deceptively employed rights-based
and feminist discourses while maintaining old policy learning legacies of
using the public health system to promote economic development via the
control of poor, primarily indigenous, women's bodies. Ironically, in the one
policy area where feminists and rights rhetoric seemed to have influence, a
policy outcome antithetical to both feminists and the broader rights-based
epistemic community prevailed: the mass sterilization of primarily indigenous, poor women.

Following Fujimori's national and international pronouncements that family planning in Peru would be central to his war on poverty, the program
was thoroughly overhauled. The revised program, outlined in the document
"Reproductive Health and Family Planning Program 1996–2000," was largely
in line with the Cairo Programme of Action and revised the earlier Peruvian
Family Planning Program, the mismanagement, corruption, and disarray of
which had led to the threat of termination by international aid agencies

(Interview Anon. 6, 1998). The revised plan followed Cairo in defining reproductive health as "the condition of complete physical, mental and social well-being that men and women require in order to develop reproductive functions with security during all periods of life." This plan considered family planning a priority in overall reproductive health and modified the Cairo approach only in the reference to the Catholic concept of "responsible parenthood" and the inclusion of "modern and secure" forms of contraception (MINSA 1996c, 5).

This plan also echoed Cairo in naming gender equity as a goal to be achieved through equal rights for both sexes and "health services that will diminish the barriers that limit women's access to quality care." The plan attempted to ensure warm interactions between caregivers and clients, high-quality attention, and respect for clients' self-determination within their cultural values (MINSA 1996c, 30, 28–29). Finally, for the first time, this family planning program included the option of sterilization as a contraceptive choice. While largely reflective of the Cairo agreements, the document did contain some important flaws, which were later identified by Peru's Defensoría del Pueblo (human rights ombuds office). The Defensoría decided that program documents set goals that ran counter to full reproductive rights and did not allocate adequate resources. Among fifteen goals for service provision, the Defensoría required a change in three in March 1998 after an investigation by the Defensoría, the Congress, and a special commission named by the Ministry of Health. The goal of "reaching" 50 percent contraceptive coverage of all women in their fertile years and 70 percent of women in their fertile years in union was edited to "making the effort to reach" these numbers. The goal of making contraception available to 60 percent of adolescent women in union was changed to the simpler goal of "avoiding unwanted adolescent pregnancies." The goal of ensuring that every woman who gives birth in a health establishment leaves the establishment using some form of birth control was changed to individually counseling postpartum women on the family planning options available.[15]

In addition to the president's rhetoric about women's rights and the echo of the Cairo language, advertising for the family planning program appeared feminist in emphasizing the rights of women and couples to choose the number of children. A newspaper ad for the program read: "There are those

---

15. See Ministerio de Salud 1996c, 26–27, for original wording and Ministerial Resolutions 089-98-SA/DM and 076-98-SA/DM for the changes.

that still do not understand that Peruvian women, or the couples in Peru, have the right to choose."[16] These factors produced an image of a progressive government program that favored individual liberties and reproductive well-being for women and men.

Coupled with this rhetoric was the direct involvement of feminists themselves in overseeing implementation of the policy. In the 1990s, several feminist NGOs successfully forged a significant access point to the state in the area of family planning: a tripartite monitoring committee (the "Mesa Tripartita") devised as a mechanism to ensure fulfillment of the population accords agreed on in Cairo. The brainchild of the broader women's health network in the Latin American region, the Peruvian committee was composed of representatives of the state, civil society, and international agencies, with three feminist NGOs serving as the primary representatives from civil society.

Despite the rights-based rhetoric and involvement of feminists in the oversight of its implementation, other government documents reveal that the upper echelons of the Fujimori government—the presidency and the prime minister's office—viewed family planning principally as a tool for economic development, with little regard for reproductive health or rights. An influential document entitled "Basic Social Policy Guidelines," developed in 1993 by the prime minister's staff, projected dramatic population growth and argued that this increase, if left unchecked, would outstrip the economy's ability to provide adequate employment and basic social services. While this document does not offer a specific population-control strategy, it does provide justification for such a policy based on economic and demographic trends.[17]

Another document, "Social Policy: Situation and Perspectives," discusses family planning services more explicitly as one of a number of goods to be distributed to the neediest communities. This approach had the potential to expand access to family planning methods to the poor, who had not previously been served. But the document also demonstrates the executive branch's clear preference for sterilization over other methods of family planning: one of the thirteen indicators for success of social policies was the number of "people who opt for a permanent method of family planning."[18] No

16. From a full-page ad in *El Sol,* January 21, 1998, 3A. Ads like this ran frequently in 1998.
17. "Lineamientos básicos de la política social," Primer Ministro, Lima, November 1993.
18. Comisión Interministerial de Asuntos Sociales internal report, "Política Social: Situación y Perspectiva a Agosto 1997," Documento de Trabajo 21-08-97, App. E, unnumbered page titled "Comisión interministerial de asuntos sociales: Indicadores de seguimiento." Neither tubal ligation nor vasectomy is technically irreversible, but the surgery is essentially unavailable to the poor in Peru.

indicator for any other form of contraception was included. Thus, the number of surgical sterilizations performed became one of only thirteen criteria for evaluating the Fujimori administration's struggle against poverty. The motivation for the emphasis on sterilization appeared to be at least in part the cost-effectiveness of a one-time intervention and the assurance that this would lead to fewer births (Interview Anon. 6 1998).[19] The fact that these high-level authorities privileged sterilization over other forms of contraception was not only contrary to the norms of reproductive health agreed upon at Cairo, which required a choice of contraceptive methods, but also exposed their orientation toward population control.

Despite the official policy language, which was in line with the rights-based approach, and the overt attempts to win feminists as allies to family planning reform, the primary goals of the program became economic growth and poverty reduction. The logic of the executive branch was that a reduction in population would lead to an increase in GDP per capita. Elite, primarily white male, policy makers sought control of women's bodies as a means to meet their goals of economic growth. They continued a policy learning legacy of Malthusianism established in the late nineteenth century, but disguised it with rights-oriented rhetoric. Thus, although the policy reform process in the case of family planning reflected a rights-based approach, the implementation of the program was quite the opposite. How this mass sterilization campaign was allowed to transpire under the noses of activist feminists and in a seemingly new, more rights-oriented climate is explored in chapter 6.

Neopopulist Reform: Free School Health Insurance

In July 1997 Seguro Escolar Gratuito (Free School Health Insurance, SEG) was introduced. Like the neoliberal reforms, it was devised entirely by a small team designated by the executive. Some proponents also used the argument that it would improve Peru's human capital. However, free school health insurance reflected important changes in the Peruvian context by 1997: a weaker, and changing, neoliberal epistemic community; and a lack of crisis in the health sector at this time. While neoliberal principles were clearly relied on in the Fees, Means Testing, Basic Health for All, CLAS, and Health Provider Entities reforms, in the SEG populist politics trumped the neoliberal principles on which the other policies were based. School health insurance

19. Barrig (1999) also found this connection.

thus demonstrates the limits of the influence of the neoliberal epistemic community when confronted by a president without a need for the "short-cuts" provided by policy experts. Moreover, in this case there were no policy legacies to block this reform; instead the reform fit a long-standing pattern of populist politics (see, e.g., Roberts 1995; Weyland 1996b).

School health insurance reform provided free health care coverage through the public health system to all children preschool through age seventeen enrolled in the public schools. The insurance promised to increase access to health care. It was also targeted to the extent that primarily poor people and the lower classes attend Peru's public schools. Some national health figures, like the regional health director in the province of San Martín, Victor Zamora, argued that the reform fit with the broader neoliberal focus of the time on investment in human capital: "We are thinking of free school health insurance as a collective measure of human capital investment; an essential conceptual element of the social reforms."[20] For the president, however, it simply made political sense: free school health insurance would cover a broad population at low cost, since this population was relatively healthy (Jaramillo and Parodi 2004, 16). It was an ideal tool for cultivating support for his government.

The president, at this time more distant from the debt crisis and health sector crisis of the early 1990s, saw little need to rely on the technocratic advice of policy makers in the neoliberal epistemic community. From a public health perspective, targeting an age group that has a low incidence of infirmity compared with other age groups made little sense. According to the IFI representatives I interviewed, if better health outcomes were the goal, the money aimed at the SEG would have been better spent on children in the age range from birth to five years, who faced the greatest health risks. International consultants from the IFIs bristled at the idea of broad insurance for a group that did not warrant it based on their cost-effectiveness calculations.

Fujimori announced the free insurance in his July 1997 Independence Day address to the nation. Free school health insurance was an extension of his ongoing interest in education. (He had been using school construction in poor communities as a populist tool for some time.) His consultants on education policy conceived of the concept, and his address was the first notice of the reform to Ministry of Health officials (Interview Jorge 1999; Interview Zamora 2002). The health ministry, charged with developing the specifics of

20. *Diario Expreso,* September 2, 1997.

the reform and launching it in the space of a month, assembled a small team of consultants led by Ulises Jorge Aguilar, former head of a regional health authority.

According to Jorge, the process of formulating the free school health insurance program "surged from his strong authority," where he "ordered things." Not only was input not invited from civil society, but the advice of other reform teams and program administrators within the ministry was rejected (Interview Jorge 1999). As a result of the president's strong support for the reform and this authoritatively led reform team, the reform proceeded from announcement to implementation in less than a month, with no time for either support or opposition (though in this case there were no clear "losers" to protest). Nor did legal institutions pose barriers, as the program proceeded without any legal basis for the first two years of its existence.

Free school health insurance was also independent of international influence. The program's formulation and implementation were funded entirely through the national treasury. Only after over a year of implementation did one international agency, UNICEF, begin to take an interest in the program and support it in small ways (Interview Jorge 1999). And over time it came to serve a significant population—in 2001 the combined Seguro Escolar and Seguro Materno-Infantil covered 4,602,000 individuals.[21]

Perhaps unwittingly, with the populist free school insurance, Fujimori set a template for expansion of health care to the poor, which was built on at the end of his administration and by the subsequent administrations of Alejandro Toledo and Alan García. Broadening the free school health insurance concept began at the behest of IFIs, which sought to focus government health spending on greater epidemiological threats, such as Peru's disturbingly high maternal mortality. Specifically, in 1998 the World Bank and IDB (through the same parallel loan that supported the CLAS program) asked Peru to develop a similar free social insurance plan for infants and mothers, Seguro Materno-Infantil (Mother-Infant Insurance, SMI). This was implemented by the outgoing Fujimori administration. But because many ministry officials resisted a program that they felt was pushed on them by the IFIs, it was implemented poorly. Mother-Infant Insurance was subsequently folded into the Seguro Escolar program by the transitional Paniagua government, thus diluting much of its original focus. When Toledo took over the presidency in

---

21. "SIS Necesita S/.127 milliones más para brindar mayor cobertura," *Gestión Médica*, February 2003.

2001, both Free School Health Insurance and Mother-Infant Insurance were replaced by yet another, but more encompassing free insurance program, Seguro Integral de Salud (Integral Health Insurance, SIS), aimed at adults in poverty. Like Fujimori, Toledo used the free insurance as a populist political tool to gain the political support of the poor, and his approach was continued by President Alan García. Following the political approach of populism rather than neoliberalism or human rights, the SEG, followed by the SIS, has potentially spawned a new policy legacy—broad public support for the policy has created a "lock-in" effect whereby it is now difficult to reverse.

Explaining a Lack of Gender Mainstreaming

The above comparison of these six policy processes demonstrates how transnational epistemic communities and policy legacies shaped what were considered "feminine" and "masculine" policy areas, with gender equity not entering the health reform agenda except in the area of family planning. Feminists themselves accepted this division and did not attempt to influence "mainstream" reforms, even those in the public health sector that would affect poor women the most. The critical importance of the transnational epistemic communities for shaping feminists' interests is proved by later events. In the early 2000s a few feminist activists began to shift their attention to gender mainstreaming in the health sector. But this only came about after the Pan American Health Organization, with funds from the Ford Foundation, pressed Peruvians to consider this as an important area, and funded a gender and health sector reform project based in the Ministry of Health.[22] The efforts of the PAHO-supported Ministry of Health program ultimately succeeded in gaining the passage of a norm, supported by Minister of Health Pilar Mazzetti in 2006, which required gender mainstreaming in the health sector, and the project within the ministry also continued beyond the PAHO/ Ford initial funding period.[23] In addition, there was the broad interest by the Peruvian government (like others in the Latin American region) in reaching the UN's Millennium Development Goals, a set of eight development goals to be reached by the year 2015. The goals gave a central place for gender equity,

22. The Pan American Health Organization promoted gender mainstreaming projects in both Chile and Peru in the early 2000s. For the Chilean case see Ewig (2008).

23. Resolución Ministerial 638-2006/MINSA, "Norma técnica de salud para la transversalización de los enfoques: Derechos humanos, equidad de género e interculturalidad en salud."

and may be part of the reason why the concept of gender equity was incorporated, for the first time, in the health ministry's 2007 National Health Plan (MINSA 2007). In the late 2000s, in other words, the global currents seemed to have shifted significantly toward the rights-based epistemic community, which gained currency, at least in rhetoric, within the Peruvian bureaucracy. Whether its goals of gender equity will be carried out in practice remains an open question.

Observing the reactions from organized groups in civil society to these six processes of reform also reveals the gender, race, and class contours of the policy legacies at play in this process and how these shifted attention to some reforms, while ignoring others. The reform of the social security health system was the most bitterly contested. Largely male-led unions and doctors' associations aggressively fought against the reforms of the social security sector, which represented one of the hard-won historic political gains of these interest groups. These unions also kept gender equity off the political agenda. As union leader Elsa Baca explained, despite the fact that women union members were on the front lines of protests against health reforms that would affect their salaries and working conditions, the "union movement did not recognize this as an opportunity to develop work related to gender" (Interview Baca 1998).

Other major reforms were achieved in the public health system, yet in these reform processes what is most notable are the silences, the relative lack of contestation over reforms that would affect the majority of the population: the poor, the indigenous peoples, and the majority of women. The noise, contrasted with the silences, of civil society in the reform process reveals the underlying gender, race, and class assumptions of the organized sectors. The one reform apparently worth fighting against—social security—was that which served the middle- and working-class *mestizos* and a constituency that historically has been male.

While policy legacies and epistemic communities provide the broadest explanations for the gendered character of Peru's health reform politics and the lack of feminist interest in mainstream health reforms, other factors also played a role. These included the authoritarianism of the Fujimori regime, the closed character of the neoliberal policy process, the weakness of the Ministry of Women that Fujimori had established, and the class position of feminists themselves.

As the Fujimori regime became gradually more authoritarian during the 1990s, it was exceedingly difficult for any groups in Peru's civil society to influence the government. Early in his tenure Fujimori had significant political support for the twin achievements of controlling the economic crisis and the Shining Path. However, a stable but stagnant economy and a lack of a clear constituency demanded steps to ensure continued support. His rule became increasingly authoritarian. In 1992 he staged a military-backed self-coup and closed the Congress until international pressures forced him to restore formal democracy. Fujimori weakened Peruvian political parties with an antiparty discourse and by constitutional changes that reduced veto points in the policy process, where parties could previously intervene. Fujimori also sought to weaken opponents in civil society, in particular organized labor, which vocally opposed his market-oriented reforms. Beginning in 1991, the government radically revised labor laws from the most protective in the hemisphere to among the most flexible. The reforms eased restrictions on terminating employees, eliminated tripartite bargaining, and, as noted previously, liberalized the use of temporary contracts (Saavedra 2000). As the regime grew more authoritarian, key union leaders were assassinated, such as CGTP leader Pedro Huilca. The government laid blame on Sendero Luminoso for the murder of Huilca, but union leaders were convinced it was the work of the government.[24] Regardless of the perpetrator, these acts chilled union protests substantially. Specific to the health sector, leaders of health worker and doctors' unions that questioned health reforms were sometimes fired from their jobs and intimidated by the government (Interview Vidal 1998, Interview Baca 1998). Feminists were not immune to the regime's authoritarian tactics. When one feminist investigator began to reveal the administration's sterilization campaigns in the Peruvian countryside, her house was broken into and key evidence taken.

The government's characteristically neoliberal mode of policy making also made advancing reforms over opposition possible and gender mainstreaming more difficult. I call this "characteristically" neoliberal because the closed process was similar to neoliberal economic reform in Peru and elsewhere in Latin America, and to neoliberal health reform in Mexico and Colombia, where small teams made the key reform decisions (González Rossetti 2004; Ramírez 2004).[25] In particular, policy making was characterized by lateral loading

24. The case of Pedro Huilca is still not resolved. For a review of the evidence see the report of the Peruvian Truth and Reconciliation Commission: http://www.cverdad.org.pe/ifinal/pdf/TOMO%20VII/Casos%20Ilustrativos-UIE/2.58.%20PEDRO%20HUILCA.pdf.

25. On the insulated character of the economic reform process in Latin America, see, e.g., Bresser Pereira, Maraval, and Przeworski (1992); Nelson (1994); Haggard and Kaufman (1992, 1995); Smith, Acuña, and Gamarra (1994).

and executive decrees. "Lateral loading" refers to decision making that is pushed out of elected spheres to courts, quasigovernmental institutions, or executive-level agencies (Banaszak, Beckwith, and Roudt 2003, 5). By avoiding elected spheres, lateral-loading and executive decrees make it easier to overcome vested interest-group legacies because many reforms never become subject to public debate.

As demonstrated in the six processes outlined above, in a lateral-loading fashion, health policy reforms in Peru were formulated by small, insulated teams of technocrats in executive ministries prior to being passed into formal policy by presidential decree, ministerial resolution, or Congress. As one health sector reform leader explained, "We are talking fundamentally about a small reform team that tries to push forward health sector reform ideas" (Interview Anon. 3, 1998). Not only were these insulated teams, but they were also fluid in their composition, making it difficult to gauge the changing plans of the ministry. As one feminist active in health issues said, "in 1994 we calculated that the average permanence of a head of a program was seven months. You coordinate, and arrive at an agreement with one, and the next one arrives, and it is as if none of that coordination existed" (Interview Güezmes 1998). Of the six major reforms discussed in this chapter, only two passed through the Congress; the rest were passed by ministerial resolution, presidential decree, or simple implementation without any formal legal status (table 4.1). The lack of democratic debate on health policy fit an ongoing pattern that began during the 1980s economic crisis and intensified under President Fujimori: half of all laws in Peru in the 1990s were passed by executive decree (Levitt 2000).

A final factor contributing to the lack of gender mainstreaming was the weakness of PROMUDEH. In October of 1996 President Fujimori created this women's ministry by legislative decree; it was one of only a handful of ministries worldwide at the time dedicated to the promotion of women's issues. Yet unlike some similar institutions in the region (such as SERNAM in Chile), PROMUDEH did not play the mainstreaming role that these organizations were envisioned as carrying out when first proposed by global feminist activists.[26] Divorced from the major reforms underway in the line ministries, PROMUDEH did not review health policies for their gender implications. This institution, supposedly symbolic of the Fujimori government's dedication to

---

26. On SERNAM see Franceschet (2003); on SERNAM and health sector mainstreaming see Ewig (2008); on women's ministries elsewhere around the globe see Stetson and Mazur (1995).

Table 4.1 Legal basis of major health reforms, 1990–1999

	Fees and means testing	PSBT (basic health program)	CLAS (local health administration committees)	EPS (private health providers)	Family planning	SEG (student health insurance)
Ley Law Passed by Congress		Articles 29–32 of *Ley 26268* (1994 Budget Law), December 1993		*Ley 26790* May 1997		
Decreto legislativo Law decreed by president with powers authorized by Congress				*D.L. 887* 1996 * *D.L. 718* 1991**		
Decreto supremo Law decreed by president without need for Congressional authorization			*D.S. 01-94-SA* April 1994			
No law Created through ministerial resolution, norm, or other means					*Resolución Ministerial* 071-96-SA/DM February 1996	No legal basis; president's project, 1997
No law No legal basis; implemented around 1990	No legal basis; implemented around 1990					

*Disputed by Congress as unconstitutional.
** Never implemented.

women's issues, was relegated to the role of creating and administering isolated women's assistance programs, such as craft production and food distribution. The ministry's mission was also diluted—it served not only women
but also the elderly, the disabled, and the poor. It oversaw adoptions and
even housed the national institute of sports. PROMUDEH also had no formal
mechanisms for dialogue with its stakeholders in society. An activist with the
feminist organization Manuela Ramos noted about PROMUDEH, "There are no
mechanisms installed, so, yes, there is contact and there is dialogue, if you
take the initiative. But my concern is that there is no formal space" (Interview Carrasco 1998). Another activist from the feminist NGO Flora Tristán
reinforced this view (Interview Cambria 1998). Without formalized dialogue
with organized women in society, feminists could not link into the state
through this institution.

It appears that Fujimori's efforts to promote women and women's issues,
much like his promotion of family planning globally, as discussed in the
previous chapter, were rooted in an attempt to distract critics by appearing
more democratic. To finish Vargas's sentence quoted in the introduction of
this chapter, she writes, "The Fujimori government, more than any other in
[Peruvian] history, advanced women's rights in institutional terms and in
terms of placing women in visible positions, *authoritarian women with uncon-
ditional loyalty to the president*" (2008, 112, emphasis added). The complex
and low-profile work of integrating gender equity into a health system would
never give the government the kind of broad political cachet achieved by the
high profile of a women's ministry (however poorly run) or a loyal, outspoken
female congressional representative to toe the party line.

Finally, the largely urban, middle-class base of organized feminists likely
impeded them from seeing the broader gender implications of the health
reforms underway. Because reforms of the public sector affected mainly poor
women, it is possible that organized feminists did not see these reforms as a
priority. Feminists did, by contrast, join in protests against the social security
health reforms led by labor unions, perhaps an indicator of their class politics.

Conclusion

Through process tracing and comparison of six of Peru's major health reforms
of the 1990s and their relationship to transnational epistemic communities,
this chapter has advanced two arguments. First, global forces can shape the

reform process in gendered ways. The neoliberal and rights-based epistemic communities set up a gender division of labor that was reinforced by the interest groups involved in each political process. Neoliberalism dominated the "mainstream" health reforms and promoted these reforms as "gender-neutral" technocratic exercises, where gender inequalities never became a point of discussion and the reforms were considered none of feminists' business. This consensus was accepted and reinforced even by feminists who chose to ignore "mainstream" reforms. By contrast, in the "feminine" domain of family planning, rights-based discourse was most influential, and feminists were invited to participate. Rights, however, were supported in rhetoric only, based on a political calculation that such a policy would make the government appear more democratic. This gender division of labor, in turn, helps to explain why feminists did not actively attempt to "mainstream" gender equity concerns into the general health reform agenda, despite otherwise propitious circumstances. Their own networks, funding, and histories of activism led them to focus narrowly on reproductive rights and not consider the gendered impact of mainstream reforms. Other factors also impeded gender mainstreaming, including the authoritarian, characteristically neoliberal policy approach of the government, the weakness of the newly created women's ministry, and the class position of feminists.

Comparison of the politics of the reforms, in particular the divergent responses of interest groups in civil society, also underlines the gendered, classed, and racialized nature of Peru's policy legacies. The heavy political contestation by organized labor and doctors' associations over social security and the lack of contestation over public health reform demonstrates how policy legacies seek not just political advantage, but also to maintain race, class, or gender privilege. In Peru's 1990s health reforms what was reformed were the elements constructed in the neoliberal frame as the problems: working-class interests and state largesse (ironically, those interests that had previously promoted a "rights" discourse, however narrowly conceived). Gender and racial inequalities remained unaddressed, and health resource redistribution was nominal.

But what were the effects of these six reforms on gender, race, and class relations in Peru's poor communities? In the chapters that follow I provide a grounded "local welfare analysis" (Haney 2002) in which I evaluate the effects these individual policies had on equity. In this way I carry forward the objectives of previous feminist scholarship on gender and economic policy that has revealed the hidden biases of seemingly "neutral" policies.

5

Mimicking Markets: Gender Equity and Public Health System Reforms

How did the neoliberal reforms in Peru's public health system reverberate at the local level? Focusing on the intersections of gender, race, and class in poor communities, this chapter draws out the implications of market-mimicking reforms for poor, urban, and *mestizo* compared to extremely poor, rural, and indigenous women and men. These policies were not formulated with gender or women in mind, but they had important effects on gender equity, mostly negative. However, the full effects of these policies cannot be fully understood by observing gender alone; they require an intersectional analysis of the interactions of gender, race, and class. Different policies can have different effects on differently positioned people. Rural indigenous women were more negatively affected than other groups by neoliberal public health system reforms.

This chapter evaluates the effects on gender equity of the four public health reforms described in chapter 4: fees for services, means testing, the basic package of services, and administrative decentralization through the CLAS program. Fees and means testing had clear negative implications for women, especially when gender was combined with race and class. The basic health care package was not only very limited in content, it tended to exacerbate gendered patterns in the distribution of care work by relying on women's voluntary unpaid labor to meet its goals. The effects of the CLAS program were highly dependent on context. In urban areas decentralized administration opened up some spaces for leadership by *mestiza* women at the local level; in rural areas it reinforced exclusionary patterns that denied indigenous women leadership roles. However, it did lead to recognition of these women's culturally specific needs as health care users. Thus, in general, the reforms had negative effects, but they also had unintended, more positive consequences in certain contexts.

The chapter also reflects on the degree to which these reforms changed the politics of the public health system; for example, whether these policies really represented a major shift in social policy or allowed established policy legacies to endure. Several of the reforms (fees, means testing, and the basic package) drew on preexisting gendered and racialized policy legacies to further the new goal of greater "efficiency." By contrast, the CLAS may have planted the seeds for future changes in power relations in the sector. Viewed more broadly, the reforms' combined emphases on market mechanisms and efficiency indicate a possible shift in the "policy learning legacies" that inform the ways health policies in Peru are formulated—one in which market and efficiency considerations are now central, and may continue to be into the future, despite the recent "rights-based" turn discussed in chapter 4.

The effects of the neoliberal reforms are evaluated using the two components of equity discussed in chapter 1: the degrees to which reforms redistribute resources, services, and responsibilities, and recognize or value all individuals.[1] The evaluation is based on a 1998–99 study of the implementation of the reforms in four Peruvian communities: two urban communities in the Northern Cone of Lima and two rural communities in the department of Ayacucho. The urban sites included a total of six health centers, three of which were CLAS centers. The rural sites included one health center each, one CLAS and one non-CLAS. Because 72.2 percent of Peruvians lived in urban areas in 2002, and 75.9 percent in 2007, I included more urban than rural centers in my sample (INEI 2002, 2008). The urban areas were considered poor and the rural areas extremely poor; the rural sites were primarily indigenous and the urban sites mainly *mestizo*. The rural-urban mix allows comparison of racial and cultural differences in perceptions of and access to health sector reforms. The design confounds race and class to some degree, but in the same way that they are intertwined in real life.

I conducted a stratified survey of 193 residents in the four sites described above. Survey questions measured gender equity in terms of access to services,

---

1. See table 1.1 for the elements applied to health, chapter 1 for definitions, and the appendix for methodological details.

distribution of care work, and intrafamilial health dynamics such as prioritization of health services. Fifty-nine positional interviews with community leaders, health professionals, and administrators and six group interviews with residents fleshed out the relationship between health centers and communities. Finally, I logged many hours in ethnographic observation, including participating in health center events and observing center and neighborhood activities.

More than 70 percent of the population was served by the state public health system in the mid-1990s; in addition, those entitled to services in the social security sector opted to use the public sector 13.4 percent of the time, so it served the overwhelming majority of Peruvians (MINSA 1996a, 24).[2] Reforms to this sector were, therefore, of significant consequence to the population as a whole, despite, as described in chapter 4, the lack of reaction to their reform by civil society. Whereas social security sector reforms involved major cutbacks in state support, public health sector reforms brought significant increases in state funding compared to the financial crisis in the previous decade. This funding did not go unnoticed: 94.4 percent of the 193 survey respondents said the local health centers had improved over the last five years. In the early and mid-1990s the state repaired dilapidated centers and built many new facilities. In the department of Ayacucho, site of the two rural communities where I carried out the survey, the number of health establishments rose from 167 in 1992 to 320 in 1996, mostly in the public, primary care sector, where the Ministry of Health established more than 130 new health posts or centers.[3] In Lima, the site of the urban studies, the number grew from 692 in 1992 to 1,168 in 1996, again mostly in health centers and posts administered by the Ministry of Health.[4] Moreover, as discussed in chapter 4, the reforms included competitive salaries in poor urban and rural areas where personnel had previously refused to work.[5] While funding did not reach the more generous levels of the early 1980s, the mid-1990s did see important improvements over the preceding crisis.

2. My survey showed that the reason for such high filtration to the public health system was convenience; public health clinics are more numerous and often closer to people's homes.

3. Comparison of MINSA (1992, table 23, 59; 1996a, table 57, 161–67).

4. Ibid.: hospitals from 138 to 145; health centers from 282 to 560; health posts from 265 to 396.

5. Professionals under the Basic Health for All (PSBT) program make about 1.5 times more than those under the previous system of named employees. In Ayacucho PSBT doctors earned 2,800 nuevos soles a month compared to 1,980 by named doctors; other PSBT professionals 1,300 compared to 860; technicians 800 compared to 500 (data from Dirección de Salud de Ayacucho).

Along with general restoration of health services to poor communities came new health care–delivery strategies in which market mechanisms were used to generate incentives for greater efficiency, improved cost recovery, and better targeting of the poor. Because a public health system serving the poor could not be profitable, privatization was not an option. Instead, "market-mimicking" mechanisms were introduced to create market-like conditions and incentives in the public system. As noted in chapter 4, the reforms were based on market or efficiency principles—fees for services in a previously free system; means testing of those who could not pay for services; a targeted basic health care package to encourage efficient use of state resources. Clinic administration was decentralized to community boards in the CLAS program, partly to create "internal markets" so competition among state health centers would encourage efficiency. These reforms are evaluated here for their effects on gender equity.

Fees for Services

Both dimensions of gender equity, distribution and recognition, are relevant for the evaluation of the effects of fees for health care services. In terms of distribution, fees may impede some groups from accessing health care services due to inability to pay. For example, women and children are typically dependent on a male breadwinner for some economic support. Men remain the primary breadwinners, and women who work are paid significantly lower wages. Households led by single women are clustered among the poorest in Peru. One in five Peruvian households is female-headed. Of these, 89.5 percent are single-parent, female-headed households. The incidence of poverty in such households is 39.8 percent (INEI 2003–4). Thus, fees may impose a real barrier to women's access to health care because women tend to be poorer. Distribution is not just an individual consideration, however. Intrafamilial economic priorities and economic dependence also affect individual access to services. Recognition politics often play out in this arena of intrafamilial power relations. Once fees for health services are introduced, family expenses are prioritized. Are girls and boys recognized as equally deserving of health care in times of monetary scarcity? Will women internalize societal expectations to be self-sacrificing mothers and forgo their own health in favor of that of their children?

Given that women's earning power is less than men's and that women tend to be concentrated among the lowest income quintiles, feminist analysts of health reform in developing countries hypothesized that women's access to health services would drop with the introduction of fees in public health systems (Standing 1997). This hypothesis would seem applicable to Peru, yet men and women respondents in my survey responded similarly regarding their ability to pay for health care. One rural male remarked, "They charge you one sol for a visit and five to take out a molar." "Does that seem expensive to you?" I asked. "For me, ma'am, it is. Because the harvest is seasonal. The corn, for example, is only coming in May or June" (Survey 92). A rural woman reported, "Two of my sons are sick with typhoid, for two days now, but I don't have the money to take them to the health center" (Survey 82). Others could pay for the health visit, but the cost of medicines was out of reach. Another rural woman remarked, "Sometimes we don't buy the medicines at all. They charge you five soles for an injection and twenty for pills" (about U.S. one dollar and fifty cents and six dollars; Survey 45). The survey data showed that more than half the poor Peruvians surveyed could not afford basic health care: 51 percent could not pay for both medicines and the health center consultation ($N = 160$). In addition, rural residents were often asked to pay for the gas for the health center ambulance if transport to the center or hospital was required. One man described an instance when his son was gravely ill on carnival day and they took him to the health center: "The doctor said to me, 'You know what, sir, give me fifty soles [about eighteen dollars at the time] and I'll take him to Ayacucho.' Like that he said it, and where am I, a poor peasant, going to get fifty soles?" (Survey 92).

The survey also showed that a similar percentage of women and men believed medicines and health services were expensive: 51.6 percent of women and 50.7 percent of men ($N = 160$) said they did not have enough money for both consultation and medicines. Women appeared to be slightly more affected, but the difference was not statistically significant. Yet we know that fewer women than men in Peru are wage earners; they are paid less than men; and they are concentrated in lower-paid jobs or the even lower-paid informal sector. Most rural women do work—among working-age rural women in 2006, 74.6 percent were economically active, but most worked in subsistence agriculture. In Lima, by comparison, just 51.4 percent of working age women were economically active in the same year (INEI 2006, 78). Women are also concentrated in the lowest income quintiles—in 2006 women who worked in Lima earned on average 67 percent of what men earned (INEI 2006, 84).

The explanation for the discrepancy between women's self-reported ability to pay and the knowledge that women earn less most likely lies in two factors. First, women depend to a greater degree on other family members to

Table 5.1   Male and female economic responsibility for health care

				We don't pay		
	I pay	My spouse pays	Myself and my spouse pay	(insurance or exonerated)	Another relative pays	Total
Male:	52.4%	7.1%	29.8%	7.1%	3.6%	100%
	44	6	25	6	3	84
Female	47.1%	28.4%	20.6%	1.0%	2.9%	100%
	48	29	21	1	3	102
Total	49.5%	18.8%	24.7%	3.8%	3.2%	100%
	92	35	46	7	6	186

Who pays for the health consultation and medicines for your children?

$p = 0.001$. Males and females in the sample are not married/cohabitating.

help meet health expenses. Second, women tend to prioritize food, health, and other elements of family well-being at the expense of other needs. These issues lead us into the arena of intrafamilial power relations and recognition politics, since male family members often control cash assets. Women may report ability to pay for services, but further questions should include whether they can afford all the services they need or desire. For example, if the mother and a child are ill, will she put off her own illness to ensure that the child's is paid for? Will monetary help from a family member help with gynecological care?

The survey did not probe all these questions, many of which require more intense qualitative work in which significant trust is developed between researcher and respondents. Some of the data do provide insight into gender and economic dependency, however. Responses to who pays for children's health care revealed that women rely to a greater degree than men on spouses to pay for their children's health services (table 5.1).

Many Peruvian families pool their incomes, but many do not.[6] Even when income is pooled, in Peru it is common for men to withhold some of theirs for personal expenses, reducing the amount that goes to family needs such as food or health care. Women's limited income tends to go to supporting family needs.[7]

6. Studies have shown that worldwide most households do not pool their incomes (Dwyer and Bruce 1988; Haddad, Hoddinott, and Alderman 1997).

7. The self-sacrificing mother is a strong cultural theme in Latin America; see, e.g., Chaney (1974); Craske (1999). The pattern of men reserving money for personal spending was brought to my attention by several health workers (Interview Rojas Silva 1998; Interview Anon. 35 1998). For studies that find women in Latin America spend more than men on family needs, see Yoshioka (2006); Thomas (1997); Roldan (1988).

The survey set out to uncover patterns of intrafamilial priorities in two primary ways. First, it attempted to determine whether men and women and boys and girls of the same family attended different health centers of differing levels of quality, based on the hypothesis that boys or men may go to higher-quality centers. A brief family health history was recorded at the beginning of each interview, asking the respondent to recall instances of family infirmities in the past three years, and where medical attention was sought. Typically, all family members sought health care at the same establishment, with changes only when hospital care was needed or the family changed residence. Only in a few rural areas did respondents report a difference within the family. One male reported seeing a private specialist when he contracted typhoid, while he took his wife, who also had typhoid, to the public clinic to save money (Survey 173).

The second mode was through a survey question asking whom respondents would select to receive health care first if all family members were sick. Most said "all of us"; only a few would prioritize one member. When they did, however, it was usually the male breadwinner. One rural woman responded frankly, "My husband, because he works, so that we can eat" (Survey 82). A male rural resident responded, "First, I would go. Then I would send my oldest son." I followed up, "Then who would you send?"—"The next-oldest son" he said. I asked, "And your wife, when would you send her, at the end?" He corrected himself and said, "She would go after my oldest son" (Survey 93). Other sources offer quantitative data that male family members' health is often prioritized over that of females. Only 24.9 percent of girls with diarrhea are brought to a health provider, while 31.2 percent of boys are; 59 percent of boys but 33 percent of girls receive medical versus less expensive home therapies (Blondet and Montero 1995, 75).

The birth of sons is also preferred, as one doctor who had worked in a rural Andean village explained: "[The village members] continue to value the man more than the woman. For example, when a midwife assists a birth, they know that the charges will depend upon if it is male or female. If it is male it will cost 90 soles, if it is female it will be 50 soles. So if it is male they pay 90 soles and on top of that they give them a sack of potatoes and corn" (Interview Anon. 13 1998). This preference is not exclusive to rural areas; one urban mother explained, "I don't want to get my tubes tied yet, as I still hope my situation will improve and I can have my little boy" (Survey 2). To the extent that the above interview evidence and the quantitative evidence on diarrhea care demonstrate that males are more valued than females in

Peruvian society and boys' health more than girls', it is likely that when families are faced with difficulties paying for health care, recognition politics will lead to scarce funds paying for males' health needs over females'.

The fee-based system has the related potential of denying women their sex-based health needs, another point where this policy combines issues of recognition and redistribution. For example, if a husband who controls family income deems health care specific to women unnecessary, his wife may not be able to access this care. According to obstetric nurses I interviewed in these communities, many men do deny their wives or partners access to birth control based on the belief that it would allow them to be promiscuous. One rural male resident commented to me, "I don't trust anything but the condom; other forms of family planning make women ill" (Survey 29). This man may have been being protective, but it also gave him exclusive control over family planning matters. A rural woman remarked, "We don't use birth control pills or injections like they tell us to at the health clinic, our husbands don't want us to. Here there was a woman that was fixed so that she could not have children, and her husband sold his bull to take her all the way to Lima to have it reversed" (Survey 62). Such a dramatic reaction stuck in these women's minds and drove home the message that women taking charge of family planning was not something husbands condoned.

The fact that Peru's family planning program was free in the 1990s is important in that economic dependence on male partners did not jeopardize access to this service. Should family planning become fee-based, however, the connection between fees and access to reproductive health care must be kept in mind here and in relationship to other gender-based health needs as well. For example, we do not know how many women are denied checks for cervical cancer because their partners do not see this as a worthwhile expense. One woman remarked that she did not get her annual Pap smear because it was not free (Survey 63). While fees are not the only potential barrier to women receiving reproductive health care—husbands may still forbid wives to visit clinics or health providers may demand his consent—they are an important barrier.

Means Testing

In a system that charges fees to poor people, an exoneration system is an important way of providing economic access to health care. While it is clearly a distributive policy, a broader question is how means testing plays into societal recognition patterns. Means testing in which exoneration is granted based on a judgment of need, compared to a universal system in which care is received based on citizenship rights, can have a negative impact on the recognition aspect of equity by producing stigmatization rather than valuation. In evaluating gender equity and means testing, one question is how race, class, or gender differences and their intersections inform the determination of need.

Peru's public health establishments in the 1990s had no uniform policy to determine who should be exonerated from fees or receive care at reduced cost. Some establishments did not allow exoneration; others had a limit on the number of persons exonerated per month; still others had no limit. A separate study of sixty health establishments in five departments of Peru showed that on average 15 percent of patients were partly or fully exonerated from fees. When only primary health posts were considered, the number rose to 28 percent (Francke 1998, 25). Even if we accept the more generous rate of exoneration, it is much lower than the 51 percent of persons my survey found could not pay for both health services and medicines. Based on these combined numbers, it appears that more than 20 percent of the poor were left without economic access to health care, despite the exoneration safety net.

Furthermore, there were no uniform standards of means testing. In most cases decisions regarding need were made by untrained staff members using their own criteria. Some CLAS centers developed systems, and centers that had a social worker on staff had at least some system for exoneration. Social workers' education included identifying persons who could not pay, but, like the doctors and nurses charged with these decisions in centers with no social worker, they were left to their own discretion in choosing a procedure. The three centers with social workers had assessment forms ranging from a small card with a space for "prediagnostic" and "intake" to a two-page form asking questions from educational level to how often the person attended parties.

The lack of a policy or procedure left room for judgment calls on the part of untrained staff members. One Euro-descent doctor, educated at a coastal Peruvian university, had been working at a rural health center that served a primarily indigenous population for about two weeks when I asked how exonerations were determined. She responded, "I have already heard stories that the people here even have family members that live in the United

States who send them money. . . . So far I have seen fewer indigent people here than in [my previous health center]." Yet by all government poverty indicators the community was considered extremely poor, much poorer than her previous post. "So how do you decide if someone should be exonerated?" She answered, "I simply look at them" (Interview Anon. 70, 1999). The doctor charged with exoneration decisions at the other rural center (a *mestizo* man, also educated on the coast), said that "it depends on personal criteria" (Interview Anon. 37, 1999).

Not all doctors or nurses responsible for means-testing decisions had no criteria. Some devised their own systems based on where the patient lived or whether a mother had financial support from a father. However, the norm for means testing, as a nurse at an urban clinic stated to me, was "there are no norms" (Interview Rojas 1998). While formal procedures for making such determinations do not necessarily protect applicants from administrative caprice, Peru's general lack of procedures left much more room for snap judgments that often reinforced negative valuations of particular racial or gender categories.

The lack of a means-testing procedure was aggravated by pressures on local providers to generate income through fees. Regional health authorities depended on fees generated by health centers: as stated previously, nearly 20 percent of state public health costs were covered by fees. The head doctor of one rural health center explained that he needed to generate at least 100 soles (about U.S. thirty dollars) a month through fees to pay the electric bill, among basic expenses for which he was responsible (Interview Anon. 38, 1998). Pressure to generate funds was a disincentive to exonerate deserving persons, and an incentive to provide better services to fee-paying customers.

In contrast to a citizen rights–based system, means testing relies on often stigmatizing forms of inquiry that embarrass or degrade those who seek economic aid for basic human services. These methods also may rely on negative recognition judgments based on gender, class, or race. As discussed in chapter 2, Peru has a long history of viewing the poor, indigenous, and immigrant groups as carriers of disease. Means testing has invited a continuation of these negative recognition practices and has inhibited at least some of those in need from accessing health care. One female health care client commented: "I don't like the social worker. She asks me a ton of questions before exonerating me" (Survey 148). Also, consider this comment by a head doctor, regarding the cashier of his local health center: "The cashier is owner—many times she also decides if a person will be exonerated or not. Even if the social worker exonerated the person [she'll say], 'But you come every time to be exonerated. No, this time you have to pay.' There are many things that influence [economic access], so that one who is exonerated, one who is in need, thinks twice 'do I go or not?'" (Interview Anon. 13 1998).

A need to ask for exoneration can also keep away the very poor until too late. Two staff members I interviewed noted that a criterion to determine whether a person should be exonerated was whether the infirmity was an emergency (Interview Camacho 1998; Interview Cahuana 1998). Emergencies often indicate that, due to lack of economic resources or fear of asking for exoneration, the person has waited until a sickness has become serious. One doctor explained: "In the cases in which I have to give exoneration, they are people who come in a state of emergency, after the illness has gone on for a week or more. They haven't come in [sooner] first because they don't have money for the consultation, or second because they don't have money for the medicine. . . . I would say, in light of this, there is not [equitable] economic access" (Interview Camacho 1998). Yet even in emergency cases exoneration was not always granted, at least according to one urban woman, who reported: "Sometimes you need a doctor's examination, and you don't have the final 10 soles, and they won't grant you the difference . . . last year a woman died for lack of attention during her childbirth" (Survey 4).

The ideology behind means testing in Peru, similar to that in other countries, relies on highly gendered recognition politics that accept female dependence on male breadwinners as unproblematic.[8] Among staff members and social workers who carried out means testing in the eight health centers, the absence of a male breadwinner was a major criterion for exoneration (Interview Aguinaga 1998; Interview Anon. 24, 1998; Interview Marín 1998). If a male partner was determined to be in the household, exoneration was more likely to be denied. While it can be argued that such a system favored more economically vulnerable single mothers, it also overlooked potential intrafamilial power issues, as well as the possibility that the male might not be a primary income earner. One might also argue that such a criterion leads to what Carol Brown has termed trading "private patriarchy" for "public patriarchy," shifting from dependency on a male breadwinner to dependency on the state (cited in Fraser 1989, 145). Means testing was also feminine in character; most users of the public health system in Peru were adult women who came for their own health care or that of their children. Thus, it was primarily

---

8. See, e.g., Fraser (1989), drawing on the U.S. experience.

women who asked for exoneration, making them the primary "dependent" client. Means testing reinforced patriarchal forms of dependency rather than working toward women's economic autonomy or recognizing the degree to which all humans (not just women) are dependent on others.

Some questions that I observed social workers ask female clients seeking exoneration were quite invasive, reifying highly gendered double standards.[9] One day I sat in the social worker's office in an urban health post and observed interactions with the mostly women clients who asked for exoneration. One mother, with her two daughters by her side (one about ten and the other about five), sat in front of the social worker's desk explaining that she did not have the funds for a medical examination for her younger daughter. The social worker took out a form and began to fill it out, asking where she lived, whether she worked, and what items of value were in the household. She asked whether a man lived in her home and whether the daughters had the same father. She asked whether the woman had sexual relations. After observing the questioning, I asked to see the intake form, which included detailed questions regarding sexual relations, including "age of initiation of sexual relations" and "type of sexual relations." The implication was that "promiscuous" women were less deserving of exoneration. Males, by contrast, were expected to be promiscuous. In a separate event I witnessed health workers at a rural community festival hooting, "Don't forget your rain poncho!" as they passed condoms out the ambulance windows. This action displayed the workers' acceptance of male promiscuity.

Social workers' questions cause embarrassment and an invasion of privacy that only those without money, primarily women, must face. Clients who can pay for health services do not have to open their sexual lives to a stranger. This invasive questioning is based on gendered ideological assumptions that poor women are of poor moral character. It also reinforces the double standard that women should not be promiscuous. The social worker's questioning above was followed by surveillance: home visits to ensure that the client was telling the truth about her economic and sexual life. Surveillance further reinforced gendered assumptions of normality, discursive aspects of power that lead to lack of recognition of women as equal citizens.

To eliminate such discrimination, an ideal solution is a free health care system based on citizenship rights (rather than need), which would provide

9. Social worker interactions that I observed with male clients were not invasive, though I observed fewer and some fell under the "automatic" category of fee relief for clients with tuberculosis.

dignity rather than degradation to poor female health care users. While such a solution is often not possible due to fiscal constraints, a certain range of low-cost services could be declared free of charge and thus eliminate some means testing. In addition, steps are needed to train social workers and others making means testing decisions to recognize intrafamilial gendered power issues, as well as to refrain from making judgments based on sexual activity.

Basic Health Care Package

Whether a basic health care package promotes gender equity hinges on a combination of distribution and recognition criteria: whether it effectively distributes needed health care; whether it recognizes gender-based health needs; and how it affects the distribution of care responsibilities. When I asked residents what needs their local health center did *not* fulfill, they noted distributional issues such as lack of medicines, medical specialists, and medical equipment. A need for specialists was cited 17.9 percent of the time, for medicines 13.4 percent, and for equipment 10.6 percent. This was an open-ended question, with the largest frequency of response being "Nothing" (24.6 percent) or "I don't know" (21.8 percent) ($N = 179$). The responses reflected dissatisfaction with the very basic care provided by a package approach. The package guaranteed low-cost service of each package element. Care beyond these elements cost more, and may not have been locally available. While most community members cited basic infirmities such as colds as their communities' greatest health concern, their desire for greater specialization at the local clinic reflected their concerns with accessing complex health services when needed. Men and women, rural and urban, provided similar responses to these questions.

Were women's and men's specific gender-based health needs covered in the basic health care package offered by local health centers (both biologically related sex-based needs and needs resulting from gendered social factors)? In other words, were men's and women's needs equally recognized? The basic package provided for women's basic health needs related to reproductive health (see table 5.2), including detection of uterine cancer, treatment of gynecological infections, early detection of pregnancy, and safe childbirth. It provided alcoholism counseling, key for men's health in both rural and urban communities since alcoholism affects men to a greater degree than women. Some elements addressed some of Peru's most pressing health needs.

Table 5.2   Basic health care package

Children's health:
- Universal immunizations
- Adequate management of infant infectious diseases
- Prevention and recuperation from nutritional deficiencies
- Preventive and reparative dental care
- Detection and treatment of tuberculosis
- Detection and treatment of other illnesses of epidemiological importance
- Information and referrals

Adolescent and adult health:
- Counseling and voluntary and informed access to family planning methods
- Detection and treatment of sexually transmitted diseases, tuberculosis, and illnesses of epidemiological importance
- Prevention and recuperation from nutritional deficiencies
- Prevention of alcoholism and drug addiction
- Information for the development of healthy lifestyles
- Information and referrals

Women's health (in addition to that of the adult):
- Detection of breast and uterine cancer
- Early detection of pregnancy
- Treatment of gynecological infections
- Tetanus vaccination
- Information and referrals

Pregnant women's health:
- Prenatal care
- Detection and management of obstetric risk
- Safe childbirth
- Control and management of postpartum complications
- Information and referrals

SOURCE: MINSA 1994.

For example, the emphasis on pregnant women's health was appropriate, and needed, given the high maternal mortality. Emphasis on cancer detection in women was also important, given that cancer of the uterus and of the breasts were the main causes of death for twenty- to fifty-nine-year-olds in 1996–2000 (PAHO 2002) and Peru has the third-highest rate of cervical cancer in Latin America (WHO/ICO 2007, 6).

Yet even in these areas comprehensive coverage was lacking. For example, as Alicia Yamin points out, the basic package did not cover obstetric complications such as hemorrhage, the leading factor in maternal mortality. Moreover, fees for normal birth, despite its inclusion in the basic package, averaged U.S. 100 dollars in public hospitals, beyond the reach of a population whose average monthly salary was 120 dollars (Yamin 2003, 121, 105).

Moreover, a number of gender-specific basic health concerns were not addressed by the package. One was prevention and counseling with regard to violence against women. In the year 2000, a national survey found that 41 percent of women in a relationship had been physically abused by their spouse or partner, 34 percent the object of psychological control, and 48 percent verbally abused or threatened (UNIFEM 2005, 2). Second, while detection of sexually transmitted diseases was included, I observed little attention to AIDS in the local clinics, whereas several other components of the package were vigorously applied. AIDS in Peru began as a disease that affected mostly males, but the male-female ratio declined from 11:1 in 1990 to 3:0 in 2006 (PAHO 2007).[10] Men's cancer, such as prostate cancer, a leading health problem in Peru, was also not addressed in the basic package. Finally, while prevention of alcoholism and drug addiction was listed as part of the basic package, it did not occur in practice. At one rural clinic I observed doctors and other center personnel drinking to excess at community festivities, indicating a need for health professionals' as well as community education on the issue.

Family planning and sexually transmitted disease elements of the basic package were important, but in practice they remained far from an attempt to cultivate reproductive health, as agreed on at the 1994 Cairo Conference. The ICPD accords instruct governments to promote overall healthy and satisfying sexual relations free of coercion. Reproductive health counseling is listed under "Adult Health Care" as opposed to "Women's Health" in the basic package, but in the 1990s women were the almost exclusive target of family planning initiatives. This rural man's response about men's experience with family planning at the local center was typical: "They haven't talked to me about it, they only gather the women" (Survey 87). Moreover, the family planning program's thrust in practice was population control rather than broader reproductive health, as discussed in chapter 4. The control objective is clear in the sterilization campaigns led by local health clinics, discussed in chapter 6. It is also clear in the neglect of infertility. The basic package did not offer aid for infertility, despite its inclusion in the ICPD accords, and despite the fact that infertility can be a major social and economic hardship, especially in rural indigenous communities. This fact was brought to my attention by a rural couple who desperately wanted children and had not

---

10. Since the late 1990s AIDS care has taken on a much higher profile in Peru, funded in part by the Global Fund and probably influenced by the UN Millennium Development Goals, one of which specifically focuses on AIDS.

been able to conceive. At the health center and even the city hospital they found health professionals unwilling to offer help or advice.

The basic package also depended on women's unpaid labor for several elements; playing on the preexisting gender division of labor and cultural suppositions that women's time is "free," it placed a greater burden of social responsibility on women than on men or the state. In the children's basic package, universal immunization depended in large part on women's voluntary labor during vaccination campaigns. A major campaign was underway at the time of this research. To meet their quotas, health center professionals mobilized women from mothers' clubs and community kitchens to help reach the population. Infant infectious diseases were managed by training mothers and women volunteers to watch for these illnesses and dispense oral-rehydration therapies when health centers were closed. Finally, prevention and recuperation from nutritional deficiencies were heavily dependent on mothers charged with family nutrition.

These policies had some important negative consequences for women. Many women participated in these voluntary activities with instrumental interests of their own, usually left unfulfilled. One woman whom I met during one of my urban community studies volunteered her house as an emergency rehydration station for children with diarrhea in her *pueblo joven*. She had hoped her volunteer work would be a stepping-stone to a paid position at the clinic, a path to personal development and family financial security. After three years, however, she realized that no such opportunities were forthcoming. While this woman had the time to invest in the hopes of it leading to a paid position, rural women had less time and energy to spare from home and field on voluntary social service labor. This finding confirms the conclusions of researchers in other Latin American countries that neoliberal policies increasingly look to poor women "as the 'answer' to a weak welfare state as well as a source of cheap labor" (Lind 2002, 229).

CLAS Administrative Decentralization

Administrative decentralization also has the potential to affect the distributive and recognition aspects of gender equity. As described in chapter 4, CLAS decentralized administration of local health clinics to community members rather than to municipal or state authorities, as several other countries (such as Chile or Argentina) did. This decentralization had several unintended

effects on gender equity. In the rural CLAS, which served largely indigenous communities, administrative boards were dominated by men, reflecting patriarchal recognition politics and reinforcing men's decision-making
power. Only one of the six community board members of the rural CLAS was
a woman, a pattern ministry staff confirmed was true for most rural CLAS.[11]
The status of this sole female board member helps explain how she became
the exception to the rule (Interview Barboza 1999). Miriam Barboza, a single
mestiza schoolteacher in her late twenties, was elected to the CLAS board
because of her prior leadership in her community's *ronderos*. The *ronderos*
were local militias organized with government support to defend rural communities from Shining Path guerrillas. Barboza was one of few women active
in *ronderos* in her village, and among very few with a leadership role. As a
schoolteacher she was more educated than most women in her district. Moreover, her *mestiza* status made her different from the indigenous women; she
was culturally more similar to local and national elites. Other women in this
community did not have her education or the status, respect, and leadership
experience she had gained through her class, race, education, and participation in the male-dominated militia.

Figure 5.1 shows a district meeting in Vinchos, one of the rural sites. This
was not a CLAS meeting (the town was not a CLAS site), but a district meeting for the town and outlying settlements. It was called and led by the mayor,
with his assistants. The photo illustrates the typical gendered patterns of
politics in rural communities in Ayacucho. Note that it is almost entirely men
who are seated on the chairs carefully lined in the street that surrounds the
town plaza and faces the mayor's office. Men also lead this meeting. Women
are largely seated on the far curb. They not only lack seats, but sit a good
distance away, as if they are uninvited guests. Wittingly or not, the CLAS
programs in rural areas reinforced negative forms of recognition in indigenous communities by accepting male domination of the CLAS boards, much
like the male political domination illustrated in this photo.

The urban CLAS boards, by contrast, were dominated by women. Urban
mestiza women responded to the 1980s economic crisis by organizing a dense
network of survival-oriented organizations such as community kitchens and
mothers' clubs. They had the leadership experience and social capital to take
advantage of the participatory administration offered by the CLAS. They were
also better educated than poor rural women: 65 percent of the urban women

11. Personal communication with Ricardo Díaz Romero, February 19, 2001.

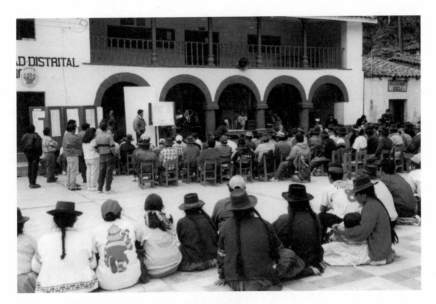

Fig. 5.1   District meeting, Vinchos Ayacucho

surveyed had at least a partial high school education, compared to 12.8 percent of rural women.[12] They were therefore better prepared to take on the
administrative responsibilities CLAS membership entailed, and had already
gained community acceptance of their leadership in "feminine" areas such as
nutrition and health.

The CLAS largely failed to provide such empowerment opportunities for
rural, indigenous women. By empowerment, I mean the real decision-making
and agenda-setting powers bestowed on these women as board members.
They could hire and fire local personnel, decide how client fees would be
spent, and approve an annual local health plan, and they gained positive
community recognition and status for the leadership role they played as CLAS
members. Part of the reason behind the failure to empower rural indigenous
women is that program staff did not consider the gender dynamics in rural
communities, thus effectively excluding women from public leadership positions. In addition, it did not address the fact that a large percentage of rural
women are monolingual Quechua or Aymara speakers, while health personnel were mostly Spanish-speaking. Nor did these women have sufficient formal education to carry out the human resource and financial administration

12. $N = 107$, $p = 0.000$. These percentages are consistent with education levels reported
by national surveys.

required. If we use literacy rates as a proxy for Spanish language skills, in 1995 in rural areas of Peru 43 percent of women were monolingual Quechua speakers compared to 17 percent of men (Blondet and Montero 1995, 61). This figure only improved in 2006 to 34.4 percent illiteracy rate among rural women and 11.9 percent among rural men (INEI 2007b). Rural women's lack of Spanish capability and low levels of formal education have their roots in local patriarchal gender relations, which favor boys' education over that of girls.

A second unintended consequence of the CLAS program was its effect on relations between the urban, *mestizo* health personnel and the largely indigenous populations they served in the rural areas. The shared administration model provided staff members some incentives to be more culturally sensitive. CLAS members hired health center staff from a pool of candidates presented by the regional health authority and were therefore able to make language and cultural understanding a job requirement, if this was their priority. A nurse at one rural CLAS described his hiring experience: "It shocked me when part of the hiring committee was a community member. He would ask you things not necessarily related to health. . . . He asked me, for example, 'Do you know how to speak Quechua?' and 'What would you do if a resident was a monolingual Quechua speaker?' . . . He also asked me questions about their general culture" (Interview Bermudo 1999).

By hiring staff who spoke Quechua and understood Quechua health concepts, these CLAS members addressed severe inequities in health care access based on recognition. Quechua culture has its own health concepts, often not understood by the medical professionals serving these communities, which leads many community members to give up asking the health center for help. "They don't understand those sicknesses," they would tell me (Survey 30). For that reason, some preferred local traditional healers, "Here we cure ourselves with a medicine man. In the health center they don't know this sickness – if they give you an injection you'll die. Here we get sick with *susto* but we cure ourselves with our herbs" (Survey 72).[13] CLAS board members' demand that local health professionals speak their language and understand their culture was a major step in improving equity along the dimension of recognition. At the non-CLAS rural center, by contrast, residents complained of being treated "like animals," and respondents expressed a desire for doctors and nurses

13. *Susto* is identified by lack of energy, restless sleep, high fever, and droopy eyes (PRATEC 2002, 195).

from the community rather than from the coast (Survey 136). By forcing some cultural recognition and understanding, the CLAS improved provider-client relations in a context in which state health professionals have histori-cally disparaged indigenous populations.

Sensitivity to cultural practices also has a gender correlate in rural Peru. Women are more likely to maintain their native language and dress than men (de la Cadena 1996). When I asked interviewees to explain why they felt comfortable or uncomfortable in the non-CLAS health center, rural women often responded that they felt "uncomfortable, because I am scared, I do not know how to speak, nor do I understand Spanish" (Survey 71). This inability to communicate and resultant fear kept some community members—mostly women—away from the health post altogether and inhibited many from ask-ing questions or receiving important information. When we asked one woman if she could talk in confidence with the health professionals, she said, "No, they don't understand you in Quechua. For that reason, you can't express all that you feel. I have difficulties with Spanish, a few words, no more" (Survey 45). Furthermore, many staff efforts at health education were wasted as a result of the language barrier. One woman described a lecture on family plan-ning this way: "They spoke in vain. I didn't even understand them because they spoke in Spanish" (Survey 112).

The CLAS efforts to bridge the cultural divide in rural areas between staff and clients is an important step in terms of cultural recognition, and of even greater consequence to rural Peruvian women due to women's greater main-tenance of indigenous cultural practices than men. Respect for culture does not always promote gender equity and in fact may work against it, as aca-demic debates over gender and culture have highlighted.[14] Gender, culture, and the CLAS in Peru show the importance of considering how culture and gender interact and create barriers for particular people. In evaluating poli-cies, an intersectional analysis is critical—we must keep in mind how policies may affect different people differently depending on race, class, *and* gender.

The final aspect of the CLAS program that affected gender equity relates to distribution of care work. While zeal for efficiency can limit availability of health care in important ways, it may also positively affect women by reduc-ing some of their care work burden. Women in Peru and elsewhere are usu-ally the primary adult responsible for their children's health (see table 5.3).

14. See, e.g., Nussbaum and Glover (1995); Okin et al. (1999); Shachar (2000); Phillips (2002).

Table 5.3   Women's compared to men's care of sick children

				Another		
		My spouse	Myself and my	family member	The child goes in by	
	I do	does	spouse do	does	him/herself	Total
Male	16.9%	42.2%	34.9%	3.6%	2.4%	100%
	14	35	29	3	2	83
Female	72.5%	8.8%	16.7%	2.0%	0%	100%
	74	9	17	2	0	102
Total	47.6%	23.8%	24.9%	2.7%	1.1%	100%
	88	44	46	5	2	185

When a child is sick, who takes him or her to the health establishment?

$p = 0.000$. Males and females in the sample are not married/cohabitating.

Therefore, waiting times and clinic hours are key to alleviating women's care work burden.

Unfortunately, women's unpaid work is often unrecognized and undervalued. One doctor commented: "Women are the ones that have to look after nutrition, clothing, health, education. . . . If you look at the work of the women here, it is tremendous. But it is not valued because it does not have an economic benefit. It seems we opt to think that they don't work. . . . When a woman comes in they say, 'The Mrs. has all the time in the world, she doesn't work.' When a man comes in they try to attend to him more quickly because they think that he is missing work" (Interview Anon. 13 1998). This attitude may explain why 46.2 percent of the women I surveyed but only 25.7 percent of the men felt that waiting times were long or very long ($N = 161$, $p = 0.002$). A gender-positive side effect of shared administration was overall shorter waiting times than non-CLAS centers, according to survey respondents. The average waiting time at a CLAS center was reported to be 34 minutes, compared to 46 at the non-CLAS centers, with 46.4 percent of non-CLAS, compared to 27.1 percent of CLAS clients feeling that their wait was long or very long ($N = 161$, $p = 0.055$).

Clinic hours can also alleviate care work burdens, or provide the potential for redistribution to men. Paid work in Peru is usually performed from eight to five, Mondays through Saturdays.[15] Because most health clinics were also open only during these hours, working women and men had to take time off work to access care for themselves or their children. A male urban resident

15.   Based on observation of formal and informal sector work habits during my eighteen-month residence in Peru.

told me "the post is closed on Sundays, but Sundays are important for men" (Survey 176). A single father commented that, although he had social security health coverage, he took his kids to the local CLAS health post because it is open on Sunday (Survey 191). Indeed, I found that I had to go to urban neighborhoods on Sundays expressly to find men to survey—there were never men at home during the week or on Saturdays. Expanded and Sunday hours would offer the opportunity for *men* who work outside the home to take a greater role in family health care responsibilities. Only one center in my study, a CLAS center, offered expanded hours of operation. In rural areas the centers were open on Sundays, which tended to be their busiest days because families felt they could not leave their farms and animals during the week. Moreover, families could combine the long trip to the health center with shopping at the weekly market. But the center was open only half a day Sunday, and often clients were turned away at closing time after walking up to five hours to reach it.

A related problem was staff absenteeism, especially chronic in rural isolated areas. This was a particular problem when patients traveled long distances to find the health center closed, even during regular working hours. Staff absenteeism was the chief complaint among residents near the rural non-CLAS center. One woman remarked, "Whenever there is an emergency, no one is there. When there are serious illnesses, because of them, we die" (Survey 155). The vigilance of community board members in the CLAS model was an effective means of deterring absenteeism. CLAS members stopped in to make sure staff members were at work and ensured that staff arrived at work punctually. In one CLAS a punch clock was introduced by the board to counteract tardiness. Reduced waiting times, expanded hours of service in some CLAS, and deterring staff absenteeism and tardiness helped relieve some of women's care work burdens and the distributive inequities these entail.

Market-Mimicking Reforms and Gender Equity

Market-mimicking reforms sometimes had a negative impact on women; sometimes they reified unequal gender relations; sometimes they opened up spaces for positive change. Fees and means testing clearly worked against gender equity along both redistributive and recognition dimensions. Compared to a system where all receive services on the basis of citizenship rather than need, fees presented a barrier to health care for the poor and for women and girls, who are concentrated among the poor. Moreover, recognition politics within families potentially led to prioritization of male over female health care. Exoneration was insufficient; means testing increased negative recognition between social groups along intersecting class, gender, and racial lines. The basic health package recognized some of men's and women's specific health needs, but it ignored other important needs, reified gendered patterns in care work, and distributed only the most basic forms of health care. Administrative decentralization through the CLAS had a number of unintended positive consequences for gender equity: recognition aspects such as spaces for new patterns of community leadership and responding to culturally specific health needs, and distributional aspects such as greater levels of efficiency that translated into lesser care work burdens. The degree to which the program succeeded, however, depended crucially on context.

The shorter CLAS wait times alleviated some of women's care work burden, but not because of policy makers' recognition of this burden; it was an unintended side effect. Neoliberal social policy reforms, like the economic reforms that preceded them, continue to ignore the importance and costs of women's social reproductive role. The basic package was more representative of the way neoliberal reforms play on gender divisions of labor, in that it depended on women's unpaid labor.

These reforms and the policy makers who designed them also paid little attention to another key area of feminist inquiry: intrafamilial power relations and dependency. While neoliberal reforms may have led to the "self-sufficiency" of health centers, they failed to recognize that human life is inherently interdependent. Their definition of self-sufficiency does not account for the degree to which these centers depend on women and communities for their success. Nor do they recognize that it is not entirely possible (or necessarily desirable) for individuals to be self-sufficient. Women, due to structural and familial interdependence, are often less able to pay for particular gender-based health services in particular. How policies may be reinterpreted through dependence and intrafamilial power relations needs to be explored.

This grounded local analysis also reaffirms the importance of an intersectional analysis that pays attention to the interlocking relations among gender, race, class, and other markers of difference. Women face different barriers to health care. Women in Peru, Marisol de la Cadena writes, "are more indigenous," meaning that they tend to maintain their indigenous culture more than men do, making the relationship between cultural and gender recognition tight (de la Cadena, 1996). Policy makers need to be attentive to the ways race and gender may work together. Indigenous women in Peru face particular needs that are a product of their culture. Recognition of needs of differently positioned women is crucial for gender equity in health care.

Finally, the health policies examined in this chapter had ramifications for both redistribution and recognition. In health sector reforms in the 1990s, it is clear that women lost out in terms of distribution. They were less likely to be able to access services in a fee-based system, and the basic package generated more unpaid health-related care work, the burden of which fell on women. In terms of recognition, the effects were more complex. Fees and means testing had clearly negative implications, while decentralization opened some spaces for recognizing urban women in community leadership and recognizing culturally specific health needs in rural areas. The bulk of the evidence, however, points toward a negative impact of neoliberal health reforms on women and gender equity. Of the four reforms, only the CLAS had some (unintended) positive effects. The CLAS was a product of the peculiar alignment between democracy advocates and neoliberal thinking in the post–Washington Consensus period. Even this reform, however, was not entirely positive for gender equity.

Did These Policies Affect Politics?

Several of the policies discussed in this chapter reinforced preexisting gendered and racialized policy legacies in the health sector. The CLAS, however, may have introduced some seeds for future change. Fees and means-testing policies brought a new layer of negative recognition politics to a public system originally conceived of for second-class citizens—the poor, the indigenous, and the majority of women. In particular, the lack of a clear system of means testing allowed old forms of discrimination against poor women and indigenous populations to continue. But this discrimination now took place under the new watchword that "all must pay their own way." The basic package also was in keeping with the public health system's historical emphasis on promoting public health for the primary purpose of improving economic development, rather than promoting healthful lives in and of themselves. This emphasis on economic development is evidenced in the motivations behind the reform (global and national) described in the previous chapter, and in the very basic services offered. Fees, means testing, and the basic health approach modified the daily procedures of the health system, but by and large left the general politics of Peru's public health sector intact.

In contrast to fees, means testing, and the basic package, the CLAS program did disrupt long-standing power relations in the health sector, in which doctors and the government dictated the content and quality of public health services. The CLAS reform combined a focus on efficiency with softened neoliberal concern with "participation." It thus allowed average community residents a voice that they had never had before in the public health system in Peru.[16] This shift in power toward average citizens and away from doctors and government administrators may explain the resistance (discussed in chapter 4) the CLAS reform faced in the late 1990s and early 2000s from ministry officials who refused to let the program expand. This resistance, in and of itself, proves that the CLAS was a dramatic challenge to existing hierarchies in Peru's health system and held significant promise for disrupting the policy legacy of the poor, acquiescent, silent public health system client.

The CLAS disrupted doctor-patient and government-community power divides in a positive way by working toward equalizing power between the two, but it did so in a highly gendered and racialized manner. In rural areas such contestation drew on existing patriarchal power relations, increasing rural men's political authority while doing little to increase the voice of indigenous women. In urban areas women were the most vocal, but dominance of women in these areas ran the risk of local health care politics being ghettoized as a feminine, less important political arena. CLAS effects on general politics of the health sector were positive but not pathbreaking. Nevertheless, the CLAS may have planted some seeds of future change.

The market orientation of all these reforms may signify a broader and lasting shift in the politics of the health sector in Peru. The idea that social services—even services for the poor, which are unprofitable—ought to incorporate market or market-mimicking mechanisms was a concept introduced by the neoliberal juncture of the 1990s. This market-oriented approach appears to be enduring and may represent a shift in policy learning legacies for the sector. Even as Peru's health policies have become more populist, preferences for efficiency over human well-being have continued, as the story of free school insurance in the chapter 7 demonstrates.

---

16. There were participatory programs in the health sector in Peru prior to CLAS; none afforded such decision-making power to community members.

6

Controlling Poor Women's Bodies: Intersections of Race, Gender, and Family Planning Policy

María Vilcahuamán was twenty-five years old when she opted for "voluntary surgical contraception" via a tubal ligation.[1] Along with other mothers in her rural highland community, she had been participating in a state aid program run by her local public health center that distributed children's food supplements to the mothers of malnourished children. One day in 1996 the nurse-midwife of the health center singled out women in the program who had three or more children and encouraged them to consider tubal ligation, showing them an illustrated brochure of the procedure. After three subsequent visits by the nurse to her home, Mrs. Vilcahuamán finally agreed to the procedure, and she was escorted by the clinic ambulance to the closest hospital for surgery. As we sat in her house talking, this is how Mrs. Vilcahuamán described her experience to me:

> It was a two-day campaign, and they say that Friday there were something like ninety people in the hospital, and in the beds they put them up and down, face up and face down, because there weren't enough beds. And we had even come on Saturday, and they still put us two to a bed. They did five men that day, five males [and the rest were] women, Miss, they were women. And a woman from Pichiurara was trying to

1. Pseudonym. This information and the quote which follows are from an interview with author (A1).

escape. . . . [Afterwards], all the ladies in the beds in the room that I was in were crying and they gave them shots, shots—each one of us got shot. And a nurse midwife from Huanta said "even though you are like rabbits, you won't have children," laughing at us as she said this.

Mrs. Vilcahuamán was one of many women targeted for sterilization by the reformed family planning program, which staged "sterilization campaigns" in poor communities. Her account is horrific, yet because she speaks Spanish and did understand the explanation of the procedure that she ultimately consented to, her experience was better than others. Many other rural Peruvian women who underwent state-provided tubal ligations were never transferred to hospitals for the procedure and instead were operated upon in poorly supplied health posts. Many who spoke only Quechua did not understand the procedure as explained in Spanish, nor did they give informed consent for it. Still others died due to the lack of sanitary conditions in which these surgeries took place.

In chapter 4 I recounted how the reformed family planning program, in its official documents, significantly reflected the rights-based discourse of reproductive health that was developed at the 1994 ICPD conference in Cairo. Feminists in civil society had even won the creation of a tripartite committee (the Mesa Tripartita), in which they participated, to monitor the program's adherence to the Cairo accords. Moreover, I explained that the president's speeches and the program's advertising campaign in urban areas specifically targeted feminists and the feminist-minded population by asserting that the reformed family planning program would help achieve the objectives of the ICPD and Beijing Women's Conferences. However, I also demonstrated that a contradictory undercurrent was evident: the reformed family planning program was linked to a broader government policy of poverty reduction, in which the president and the highest echelons of his administration covertly favored population control over reproductive rights. This underlying objective of population control is all too apparent in Mrs. Vilcahuamán's story. The large number of women who were herded into an overcrowded hospital, with insufficient beds to accommodate the patients waiting for the procedure and the callous attitudes of the health professionals, testifies to pressures to control these women's bodies rather than fulfill their reproductive rights.

In this chapter I explain how the abuses like those experienced by María Vilcahuamán occurred in spite of strong feminist advocacy at the time for reproductive rights and feminists' oversight role through the Mesa Tripartita.

I follow this explanation with an analysis of the reactions of feminists and the Catholic Church to the family planning program once the program's abuses had been revealed. Due to their urban and middle-class base, as well as their own cooperation with the government in "monitoring" the family planning program, feminists were slow to defend the primarily rural, indigenous women who had been denied their reproductive freedom. Feminists' responses were even more complicated by the fact that the Catholic Church and conservative politicians sought to use the abuses as a platform to advance their anti–family planning agenda. The shorter-term politics surrounding the sterilizations provides some important strategic lessons for feminists in the realm of body politics. Viewed over the long term, these politics also provide some clues as to why a rights-based policy was so hard to implement in Peru, even when the letter of the policy was quite positive. Over the long term, the sterilizations reveal that old policy legacies continue to have strength—specifically the historical exclusion of the poor (and especially poor indigenous women) from an active voice in politics and learning legacies that use women's bodies for economic objectives.

Denial of Rights

The reform of the family planning program in the 1990s was potentially revolutionary in both distributive and recognition terms. In terms of distribution, it promised wide dispersal of a range of family planning methods to poor and rural women who before this time had had very limited access to contraception. Moreover, with the legalization of voluntary surgical sterilization, a new form of birth control was available. In terms of recognition, the rights-based principles upon which the program was based did not distinguish between people of different races, regions, or classes. Rather, in the letter of its policy, the family planning program confirmed the free decision of the number and spacing of children as a right of all couples. In practice, the distribution of contraceptive supplies and even sterilizations was abundant, even in the most remote regions and among the poorest echelons. They targeted primarily women, however, and few men, leaving the burden and risk of surgical sterilization largely to women (tubal ligation carries more risk than vasectomy). Numbers available from early in the campaigns show a total of 65,065 tubal ligations being performed from January 1995 through August 1996, compared to 4,800 vasectomies (CLADEM/CRLP/DEMUS 1998,

17–18). The quality of these services was uneven; the poorest, rural and indigenous populations received the worst quality of care. And, in practice, the same recognition of the right to make decisions about reproduction was not granted equally to all: the poorest, rural and indigenous women were at times deceived or cajoled into the procedure.

In 1996 and 1997 Giulia Tamayo, a lawyer with the feminist human rights group Comité de América Latina y el Caribe para la Defensa de los Derechos de la Mujer (Latin American and Caribbean Committee for the Defense of Women's Rights, CLADEM), was the first to expose patient grievances with the government family planning program. Her report (CLADEM 1999) documents 243 cases of sterilization under questionable circumstances in nineteen departments, and it led Peru's human rights ombuds office, the Defensoría del Pueblo, to launch a full investigation of the program. Between 1996 and 1998 217,446 people in Peru were surgically sterilized by the state family planning program (Defensoría del Pueblo 1999, 289). The impressive number was achieved in part through the system of staff productivity quotas described in chapter 4, while the quality of care, as we can tell from Mrs. Vilcahuamán's story, was less than adequate.

According to the Defensoría del Pueblo, the family planning program displayed systematic deficiencies in gaining voluntary and informed consent for surgical sterilization.[2] Of 157 cases investigated in 1999, forty-one had no consent procedure at all. Of the ninety cases that took place when a consent procedure was part of the program's policy, the procedure was not used by staff in seventy-one.[3] Finally, of the nineteen cases where the consent form was used, it was filled out properly only eleven times (Defensoría del Pueblo 1999, 43–45). Consent forms and updated manuals on sterilization procedures were not prepared and distributed prior to the launching of the program, and when they were produced, they were not distributed to all health centers and posts in a timely manner, or sometimes at all (Defensoría del Pueblo 1999; Interview Anon. 26, 1999). Moreover, the Defensoría found twenty-seven different consent forms, many of which were confusing (Interview Mantilla 1999).

The Defensoría investigated twenty-four cases of death or serious injury as a result of surgical sterilization and found the majority due to low-quality

---

2. The General Health Law of Peru (Ley 26842), passed in July 1997, specifies a patient's right to consent prior to any medical or surgical procedure except in the case of an emergency.

3. The twenty-six remaining cases involved complaints about reproductive health procedures that did not require a consent procedure.

care, such as a lack of sanitary conditions and thus infection; poor medical practices, including damage to other bodily organs during the procedure; or a lack of follow-up care (Defensoría del Pueblo 1999). From 1996 to 1998 the Defensoría del Pueblo documented sixteen deaths as a result of female sterilizations; or a rate of 7.35 deaths per every 100,000 operations (Defensoría del Pueblo 2000).[4]

There were a number of factors that led to the abuses of women's reproductive health and rights by the reformed family planning program. They occurred due to a combination of underlying neo-Malthusian policy objectives; direct pressures on staff from the office of the president; additional pressures on staff from health sector labor reforms; and enduring sexist and racist attitudes of some health professionals toward the indigenous women they served. Moreover, all of these were embedded in a highly gendered and racialized policy context in which sexist and racist policy learning legacies of using indigenous women's bodies as instruments of economic policy endured.

As discussed in chapter 4, beneath its feminist-inspired rights-oriented rhetoric, the primary goals of the family planning program under Fujimori were economic growth and poverty reduction, not reproductive health and rights. The government logic was that a reduction in population would lead to an increase in GDP per capita. Thus, elite, primarily white, male policy makers sought control of women's bodies as a means to meet their goals of economic growth.

These policy goals contributed to the record of mounting abuses. The president pressured family planning program staff to meet sterilization quotas, and the precarious working conditions of state health employees led to low-quality care and human rights abuses. As evidenced in the government policy documents discussed in chapter 4, the state used the number of women sterilized as an indicator of successful poverty alleviation. According to former staff of the program, the president's personal family planning advisor, Dr. Eduardo Yong Motta, would contact the program weekly to set increased quotas for surgical sterilizations. Furthermore, the president or Dr. Yong Motta would attend the program's weekly meetings to monitor achievement of the quotas (Interview Anon. 6 1998). The president himself also took a direct interest, as the then director of family planning related: "When the office sends him the results, not only of voluntary surgical contraception,

4. For comparison, the risk ratio of tubal ligation in the United States is 3.9 per 100,000 procedures. Vasectomies in the United States carry a much lower risk of 1 per 100,000 (Smith, Taylor, and Smith 1985).

but of all things related to reproductive health . . . the president takes the time to review it" (Interview Pachas 1998). The president even met directly with directors of the health system at the subregional level in an effort to promote the surgical sterilizations at the local level (Interview Anon. 6 1998). One doctor working in a state health post at the time described the consequences of these pressures: "The family planning program is a very good program, but at times it has been interfered with by political decisions. They require quotas and deadlines that they oblige us to meet. As a result, there have been some cases—I can't be specific as to whether they constitute a lot or a little—that have arrived at extremes . . . [the health professionals] overstepped the norms in order to fulfill a quota, and touched people who should not have been touched" (Interview Anon. 13 1998).

Another factor contributing to heavy pressures to recruit women was the precarious position of state health employees, who were largely hired on contracts that were renewed based on productivity levels. As explained in chapter 4, the shift from guaranteed jobs, or "named" positions, to short-term contracted positions renewed based on productivity was part of the broader reforms of the health sector. If quotas for sterilizations were not met, then within this labor structure professionals risked losing their jobs.[5] Given the overabundance of health professionals in Peru and the small number of health sector jobs at this time, possibilities for finding another position were very slim. In addition to these pressures, some employees were given financial incentives to meet or beat the quotas in local sterilization campaigns.[6] One professional midwife who formerly worked in the Ayacucho region stated to me that she personally received ten Peruvian soles (about U.S. three dollars and fifty cents at the time) for each mother she recruited. Even after the national program ordered a halt to sterilization campaigns, the regional authority for one of the health centers in which I conducted fieldwork offered the health center one hundred Peruvian soles for each woman recruited for sterilization (about U.S. thirty-five dollars).

But the horrible treatment experienced by the women targeted by the campaigns was not simply due to the population control objectives, the executive-level pressures, or the productivity quotas imposed on health workers. These

---

5. See also "Médico admite campaña del gobierno," *El Comercio,* February 23, 1998, A14 and "Denuncian en EE.UU. plan de esterilización," *El Sol,* Febrero 25, 1998, 3A for doctors' testimonies of these contract obligations.

6. These campaigns and financial incentives were documented in the three volumes of reports put together by the Defensoría (1998, 1999, 2000).

combined with the racist and sexist attitudes of some state health workers toward rural indigenous women, attitudes that significantly impacted local health care worker–patient relations. It was the nurse in Mrs. Vilcahuamán's story who ridiculed the women who underwent tubal ligation. She literally added insult to these women's injuries and, by doing so, revealed her own racism and classism and reinforced gendered and racialized stereotypes of poor indigenous Peruvian women as animal-like and sexually unrestrained. This nurse's views were common among the staff that I interviewed in the rural health posts included in my study. A deep class and racial divide existed between the primarily *mestizo* staff, born in the cities and educated on the coast, and the indigenous peoples whom they served in the Andean rural areas.

Because rural indigenous women were also among the poorest and least formally educated in Peruvian society, they were the most easily deceived by staff members who were seeking to fulfill quotas or receive financial rewards and cared little about these women due to their own disparaging views. This comment from one rural woman recruited for a sterilization illustrates how such deception worked in practice: "No, they didn't explain it to me, I didn't understand anyway. I told them I couldn't, I had to work in my field. . . . I didn't know that they were going to operate on me" (Interview A2 1999). Other women told of the health care workers convincing them with explanations like "It will be two stitches, no more" and "Two hours and you will be back at work" (Interviews A1 and A3 1999). While these are just a few examples drawn from my interviews, Peru's Defensoría del Pueblo documented such deceptions at length in its official reports.

The following analysis of the advertising imagery targeted at poor women further illustrates how the family planning policy, rather than practicing reproductive health and rights, continued old policy learning legacies of controlling poor women's bodies as a means of achieving broader national economic and social objectives. Moreover, it shows the deeply gendered and racialized aspects of this policy. While the general urban populace was exposed to feminist-inspired radio and newspaper ads proclaiming women's and couple's right to choose how many children they wanted, an entirely different form of advertising targeted the low-income and poor clientele of state-run public health clinics. In the form of posters, billboards, and calendars hung on state health clinic walls, advertising in poor urban neighborhoods, in a neo-Malthusian vein, emphasized that more children would cause greater poverty. In rural areas, where the population was largely indigenous, the program's imagery was even eugenicist.

Posters and large calendars that hung in the waiting areas of state health clinics typically depicted two contrasting pictures side by side. In Lima's poor neighborhoods the posters featured a happy, clean family with a boy and a girl, in a house with a neatly kept green yard, juxtaposed with a picture of a straw shack jammed with a family with many sad children in a dusty, dirty neighborhood (see figure 6.1, contrasting pictures). The posters read: "Only you can decide how many children to have." At times these posters only showed the picture of squalid conditions, with the slogan "For Life and Health. FAMILY PLANNING. Only you can decide."

The contrasting images of poor and middle-class urban life send the message that fertility control can lead to an elevation in class status. Lima is

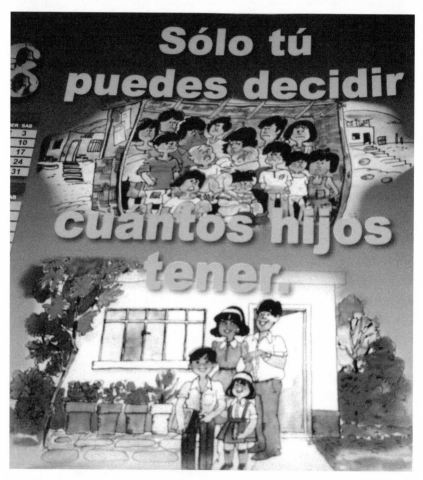

Fig. 6.1   Family planning poster in an urban health post

situated in a desert, and in some poor neighborhoods water for cooking and bathing is brought in by truck, delivered and stored in large metal drums. Only the wealthy could afford the irrigated green lawns, flowers, and trees depicted in the small family picture. The children in this family are dressed in school uniforms and hold books in their arms, indicating they have been able to pay the fees for uniforms and materials.

In a rural province in the department of Ayacucho, the billboard pictured in figure 6.2 was clearly racialized. On the right side of the billboard, in the center of the "O" in the word "NO," a typical rural, highland indigenous family is depicted, with mother and daughter wearing traditional skirts and long, braided hair. The parents' faces express panic and exhaustion, apparently due to the five children surrounding them. The billboard contrasts this family of seven with a family of four who appear to be of European descent: the parents are tall and fair, and the mother's short-cropped, curly hair is blonde. The mother's Western-style dress is clearly impractical for the physically demanding agricultural work of rural Ayacucho. Finally, the better-off, white family has two boys and no girls. Girls in rural areas of Peru are less valued and are often considered a burden. This billboard implies that family planning could lead to having only sons.

The billboard telescopes a racialized message. By controlling one's fertility, one will "Live Happily," as the billboard states—and apparently simultaneously

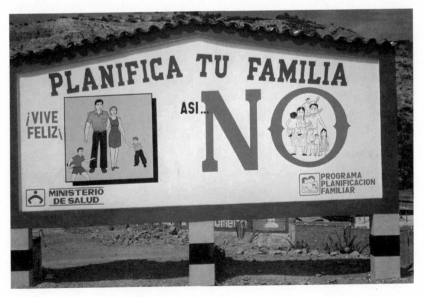

Fig. 6.2   Family planning billboard in rural Ayacucho

become white and lose indigenous cultural traditions. The proposed transformation is also gendered. In rural Peru women protect and preserve indigenous cultural traditions, and only the mother and daughter in the pictured indigenous family maintain traditional dress. The proposed transition to "whiteness" then imposes a much greater burden on women, who have also been more resistant to giving up their cultural traditions.

The above combination of factors, embedded in a highly gendered and racialized context that demeaned poor and indigenous women, provided a very poor context for the provision of true reproductive health services in which voluntary and informed consent was central. While these factors explain how and why the abuses occurred, they also point to the centrality of the intersections of gender, race, and class. It was not just women, but poor women and indigenous women, who were denied rights by the family planning program.

Uncomfortable Allies Respond

Once these abuses were revealed, groups in civil society attempted to hold the government accountable but members of the president's party and his ministers denied any wrongdoing. Two women congressional members, Beatriz Merino of the Frente Independiente Movilizador party and Anel Townsend of Unión Por el Perú, who had in the past supported women's political rights, demanded that the Women's Commission of the Congress take action and investigate the quotas for sterilizations and other abuses. The commission did begin an inquiry, including visits by commission members directly to health centers.[7] However, the head of the commission, Luz Salgado, a staunch member of the president's party, defended the program and vehemently denied the existence of quotas.[8] The Minister of Health did the same when called upon to testify.[9]

Thus, groups in civil society resorted primarily to outside means to demand change in the government family planning policy. An unusual alliance began

7. "Comisión de la Mujer visitó centros de Salud," El Comercio, January 26, 1998, A4.
8. "Congresistas piden investigar compañas de esterilización," El Comercio, January 13, 1998, A4.
9. Presentations by Minister of Health Marino Costa Bauer before the Commissions of Health, Population and the Family and Women, Human Development and Sports, January 16, 1998, and March 10, 1998, respectively. See also "Entrevista a Marino Costa Bauer," El Comercio, April 3, 1998.

to coalesce in opposition to the program: the Catholic hierarchy and Peruvian feminists.[10] Juan Julio Wicht, a Peruvian priest and intellectual active in debates on population, stated in an interview in 1998: "The institutions and the parties are very debilitated. All that is left is the press and the means of communication" (Interview Wicht 1998). Indeed, in 1998–99 few mechanisms of accountability existed in Peru because the Fujimori regime had grown increasingly authoritarian. For feminists, the task of responding to the government abuses was made more complicated by their implicit alliance with Fujimori since Beijing, and their explicit engagement with the state and international population agencies through the Mesa Tripartita.

The hierarchy of the Catholic Church, which had opposed the family planning program since the start, took advantage of the newspaper reports of program inconsistencies and abuses to launch its own campaign against government-provided family planning services. The Church hierarchy ferreted out stories of abuses in the family planning program and provided these to the media. Cardinal Augusto Vargas Alzamora appeared on television news shows and made regular statements to the major newspapers denouncing the family planning program.[11] Vargas and his successor, Cardinal Luis Cipriani, also used Sunday Masses to sway the public against the program and to place pressure on the government. In addition, religiously conservative congressional members, such as Rafael Rey, a member of the conservative Catholic Opus Dei, demanded an investigation of the program on religious grounds.[12] Church agitation against the program led to the inclusion of "natural" family planning methods in the family planning program's array of contraceptive choices.

A number of factors compromised feminists' responses to the abuses by the family planning program. Feminists faced the dilemma of speaking out against the family planning program, for whose expanded services they had advocated for decades prior. Criticizing the program ran the risk of harming the cause of reproductive rights in the public eye and placed feminists in

10. Other groups later joined these two central actors as well, including the Colegio Médico and USAID, who because of its historic support of family planning in Peru also fell under scrutiny. USAID eventually called upon Peruvians involved with the implementation of the policy to testify before the U.S. Congress. My discussion will be limited to the actions of the Church and feminists.

11. Vargas was interviewed, e.g., on the show "Panorama" of Panamerican Television (Channel 5) on Easter, April 12, 1998. See also "La ley divina está por encima de las leyes humanas," *El Comercio*, May 8, 1998, A9. On Cipriani see "La sociedad debe proteger la vida," *Cambio*, April 5, 1999, 11.

12. "Demandan que se paralicen campañas de esterilización," *El Comercio*, January 26, 1998, A4.

the unsavory position of apparent agreement with the Catholic hierarchy. Second, they faced the political problem of criticizing a very popular government. Third, feminists themselves were divided. Although some backed the regime, most did not; and among Fujimori's feminist opponents, some felt that problems in the family planning program were secondary to the larger fight against an authoritarian regime.[13] Feminists' positions were further complicated by the involvement of Peru's major feminist organizations—Manuela Ramos, Flora Tristán, and the Red Nacional de Promoción de la Mujer—in the Mesa Tripartita. These feminist organizations were caught in a web of political and financial relationships with the Peruvian state and the international population agencies. Their dependence on both good relations with state actors and financial support from international population agencies to carry out their work compromised their ability to speak out directly and quickly against abuses in the state family planning program.

The Mesa Tripartita was intended to represent the interests of the state, international institutions, and civil society in determining specific steps to carry forward the Cairo accords. The brainchild of the Latin American Women's Health Network, it was successfully implemented in Peru as a result of the combined efforts of Flora Tristán and Manuela Ramos (Interview Carrasco 1998). Its first steps, in 1997 and 1998, were to map out existing activities of the government, civil society, and international agencies in the field of reproductive health. The three sectors then prioritized which aspects of the Cairo accords would be implemented immediately (Interview Cambria 1998). Finally, the Mesa developed indicators and mechanisms to monitor the implementation of the accords.

Some feminists felt that "the space decidedly allowed feminists to enter and present initiatives, or at least to promote debate and make proposals" (Interview Carrasco 1998). Moreover, it was a means of holding the state accountable to the Cairo accords (Interview Cambria 1998). The Mesa was seen by these sectors as a means to influence an authoritarian regime otherwise closed to input from civil society. Other feminists outside the Mesa disagreed with its premise altogether, arguing that reproductive rights should not be negotiated.

When abuses in the family planning program came to light, feminists on the Mesa had the difficult task of demanding government accountability while still preserving the institution as an important access point for information,

---

13. This position was particularly strong among feminists in Flora Tristán.

communication, and negotiation. Feminists' reactions and positions were varied. Some feminists on the Mesa felt that their role was to defend the state family planning program. According to one, "[in the Mesa Tripartita] the majority of people did not have a clear idea of their role as 'civil society,' on the contrary, they had the idea that 'we are all part of the Family Planning Program' and therefore, the enemies of the Program are our enemies" (quoted in Barrig 1999). Manuela Ramos needed to maintain good relations with local government health offices for the success of its multimillion-dollar reproductive health project, Reprosalud, while simultaneously defending women's rights. Moreover, Reprosalud was financed by USAID, which also sat on the Mesa. USAID, for its part, was concerned about the Peruvian family planning program, especially when its abuses were brought to light. However, as a bilateral agency, it was committed to working with the government to improve the program (Interview Anon. 41). Due to Manuela's cross-cutting relationships with the state and USAID, speaking out against the family planning program was risky.[14] Similarly, the Red Nacional de Promoción de la Mujer received a good portion of its financing from UNFPA, which directed the Mesa Tripartita (Interview Fernandez-Castilla 1998). UNFPA's response to abuses in the family planning program, similar to USAID, was to work more closely with government administrators to improve the program, rather than critique it.[15] According to some observers, the dependency of the Red Nacional on UNFPA financing moderated the feminist organization's approach (Interview Palomino 2005). Thus, for some feminists the connection with the state and international agencies that the Mesa provided, while initially designed to empower feminists, instead undermined their autonomy and ability to speak critically.

The three feminist NGOs on the Mesa attempted to hold to a middle position between protecting advances in family planning and pushing the Mesa to respond to the problems in the program. Some followed the UNFPA lead and sought to use the Mesa as a space to work with the government in improving its family planning practices. The feminist organizations debated whether

14. Reprosalud was a multiyear reproductive health project financed by USAID. The program was given the largest sum ever granted to an NGO in Peru. There was disagreement among members of Manuela whom I interviewed in June of 2005 on whether Reprosalud hampered Manuela's response to government abuses to sterilizations; some felt this was not an issue, others felt that there indeed were fears that speaking out against the government would harm Manuela's relationship with local health offices.

15. The UNFPA-Peru representative explained, "I believe the [family planning] strategy of the government is clear: to give options to those that do not have options . . . they are providing an important tool for empowerment" (Interview Fernandez-Castilla 1998).

each case of questionable sterilization ought to be brought to the Mesa for negotiation, or whether new cases should be taken directly to the Defensoría del Pueblo for investigation (Interview Dador 2005). Over time, and with pressure from other feminists, feminists on the Mesa became more outspoken. Representatives of Manuela Ramos, for example, eventually asked for the resignation of the minister of health. Overall, however, these feminist organizations responded to the abuses in family planning only slowly. The web of relations that they had with the state and international population agencies compromised their ability to hold the state accountable to the Cairo accords.

Feminist groups not involved with the Mesa spoke out most strongly against the abuses in the family planning program. Some lobbied Congress to utilize its constitutional powers to oversee the ministries. Some supported the Defensoría del Pueblo in an effort to strengthen this institution as a mechanism of horizontal accountability (Interview Tamayo 1998). The Defensoría documented the cases of death, uninformed consent, and other irregularities in the program. It made accurate information available and spoke out as an independent voice within the state, demanding an end to the sterilization campaigns, a waiting period prior to the surgeries, and the revision of some family planning documents. However, the Defensoría's powers of enforcement were limited to publicizing and denouncing the government's errors.

Ultimately, CLADEM and a consortium of smaller Peruvian NGOs utilized an international source of accountability, the United Nations. After receiving a critical report on the policy prepared by CLADEM's Lima office, the Center for Reproductive Law and Policy in New York, and the Lima office of the Estudio para la Defensa de los Derechos de la Mujer (Center for the Defense of Women's Rights, DEMUS), the UN Committee on Elimination of Discrimination Against Women, which oversees signatories' adherence to the CEDAW, called upon Peru to justify its family planning policy.[16] The government sent representatives of the Women's Ministry to respond to the questioning. Although the UN action was effective in forcing the government to explain its actions publicly for the first time, this approach depended on Peru's voluntary agreement to the international accords, with no guarantees for future compliance. As Peru did with a similar human rights accord with the Organization of American States in 1999, it could simply pull out of the accords altogether.

The feminists who did speak out against the government did so in an increasingly authoritarian political context. By the late 1990s the Fujimori

16. See CLADEM/CRLP/DEMUS (1998), as well as UN proceedings.

government censored much of the media and denied its opponents basic civil and human rights. In 1998 Giulia Tamayo, the activist who first broke the story of abuses in the program and who was a central figure in bringing the abuses to the attention of the CEDAW commission, was physically threatened, her home was broken into, and videos of testimonials that she had been gathering as evidence of wrongdoing in the family planning program were stolen.

Curiously absent from the debates over family planning in the 1990s were the voices of the women most affected. Poor, rural, and indigenous women did not collectively organize to voice their opinions on family planning policy. Instead, their voices were primarily heard in the individual testimonials of abuses collected by Tamayo and the Defensoría del Pueblo.[17] The collective response of indigenous and peasant women came much later, in 2001, from the Mujeres de Anta—twelve peasant and Quechua-speaking women of Anta, in the department of Cuzco. Organized by the feminist umbrella organization Movimiento Amplio de Mujeres, these rural women traveled from Cuzco to Lima to demand indemnification for the sterilization abuses that they had suffered at the hands of the family planning program (Mogollón 2003). The Toledo government, in response to the actions of the Mujeres de Anta, granted that women who were negatively affected by the sterilization campaigns and practices were eligible for free state health insurance under the Seguro Integral de Salud, discussed in chapter 7.

The general lack of organized response by poor, indigenous and peasant women is reflective of a number of factors. Peru is notable among countries with large indigenous populations for its lack of an indigenous movement and organization. The strongest rural organizations to emerge in the 1990s were the *rondas campesinas,* or peasant militias, which were formed in self-defense against the threat of the Shining Path. The *rondas,* with their mostly male membership, did not address family planning policy, perhaps because they perceived it as a personal and female issue. Furthermore, many of the *rondas* supported the Fujimori government. Finally, it is worth noting that many rural and poor women "prefer" sterilization as a contraceptive choice; in fact, one of the major arguments of proponents of Fujimori's family planning program was that its emphasis on sterilization was a logical response to a large and long-standing unmet demand. Although there are no statistics to prove what the real demand for sterilization was, some poor women, in

17. One such case, of María Mamérita Mestanza Chávez, a peasant woman from Cajamarca who died from complications as a result of forced sterilization, was taken by CLADEM and the CRLP to the Inter-American Commission on Human Rights.

the face of few alternatives and in a context of material deprivation, did see sterilization as a reliable method to end cycles of unwanted pregnancies.

Re-reform and Reaction

As a result of the efforts of feminist whistle-blowers and the proactive position of the Defensoría del Pueblo as well as international agencies, Peru's family planning program was substantially overhauled in 1999 (Interview Anon. 41). Moreover, demand for a range of family planning options continued to be strong in post-Fujimori Peru.[18] However, the Fujimori population-control agenda did damage the cause of reproductive rights. Following President Fujimori's flight into exile due to a corruption scandal and a brief transition under Valentín Paniagua, in 2001 Peruvians elected Alejandro Toledo president of Peru by a very small margin (53.1 percent of the vote) in a runoff election.[19] Due to his weak political support, Toledo sought allies among conservative politicians.

Toledo's first two health ministers belonged to conservative Catholic groups. His first minister of health, Luis Solari de la Fuente, belonged to the Sodalicio de Vida Cristiana, and his second, Fernando Carbone Campoverde, to Opus Dei. Both Solari and Carbone actively sought to reduce the scope of reproductive rights in Peru, in part by taking advantage of the family planning scandals of the 1990s. In his writings prior to becoming minister of health, Solari asserted that a "social alliance" bound "Northern nations" with feminists interested in controlling birth rates. In 2001 Solari introduced legislation, which never passed, that would have allowed health care providers "conscientious objection" to carrying out any medical act that was against their personal moral or ethical views. He also introduced successful legislation making "the Day of the Unborn" an official national commemorative day (Chávez 2004, 33, 34, 36).

When Fernando Carbone became minister, he reopened the sterilization debate, claiming that under Fujimori there had been three hundred thousand cases of forced sterilization. His attempt to hold Fujimori accountable

18. While the percentage of women of fertile age in union using a modern form of contraception has grown from 41.3 percent in 1996 to 47.6 percent in 2004/5 (INEI 1996, 2007), unsatisfied need for contraception remains high. In 2000 25.5 percent of sexually active women were inadequately protected against unwanted pregnancy (INEI 2000).

19. Election data from Base de Datos Políticos de las Américas, http://www.georgetown.edu/pdba/Elecdata/Peru.

was based on questionable facts and an obvious underlying political agenda. Clearly Carbone sought to use the family planning scandal under Fujimori to severely weaken state family planning in Peru. Moreover, he did so by again invoking rights rhetoric: he labeled Fujimori's family planning actions "genocide" and set up a "truth commission" to investigate them (Chávez 2004, 44). Under Solari and Carbone, many health ministry personnel, including those who worked in reproductive health, were replaced by religious conservatives. Minister Carbone banned the use of the word "gender" in any health ministry documents, reflecting the Catholic hierarchy's opposition to the term.

In its 2002 and 2005 investigative reports on family planning in Peru, the office of the Defensoría del Pueblo found that since 2001 there had been an increase in health establishments denying both access to surgical sterilization and full information on the range of contraceptive methods available. It also found that since 2001 stocks of contraceptives in state health establishments had decreased and patients were being charged for contraception, in violation of Peruvian law (Defensoría del Pueblo 2002). Moreover, the Defensoría found that the ministry had refused to make the emergency contraception pill (legalized in 2001 before Toledo took office) available in public health establishments (Defensoría del Pueblo 2002, 143). Carbone also argued that intrauterine devices were abortive and attempted to remove them from public health centers. A congressional commission in 2002 called for making voluntary surgical sterilization again illegal. In 2003 the Health Ministry implemented a "Peru-Life Strategy" that emphasized the "rights" of the unborn (Chávez 2004, 42, 47, 37). The effects of these policies became apparent in national statistics on contraceptive use. Peruvians' use of all artificial forms of contraception dropped by 26 percent between 2002 and 2004,[20] likely due to instances of illegal fees, some doctors' refusals to provide contraception, and perhaps most importantly, Solari and Carbone's refusals to restock contraceptive supplies.

In 2003 feminists and public health activists successfully lobbied Toledo to remove Carbone from the ministry. Again, rights language was invoked, this time to support sexual and reproductive rights.[21] This second wave of

20. Percentages calculated from raw figures provided in Defensoría del Pueblo (2005, 46–67: 1,411,646 in 2002 and 1,047,521 in 2004).

21. In addition to feminist NGOs like Flora Tristán, Manuela Ramos, and CLADEM, the struggle against conservatives in the Ministry of Health generated new organizations in civil society, such as the Mesa de Vigilancia en Derechos Sexuales y Reproductivos (the Sexual and Reproductive Rights Vigilance Committee) of the ForoSalud (Health Forum), which was active in pushing Carbone out of office.

battles over family planning again underlines how global human rights and feminist discourses were employed to shape national political agendas. The succeeding health minister, Dr. Pilar Mazetti, who was appointed in 2003, actively repaired the damage done by her predecessors to state family planning programs. That damage was extensive: religious conservatives gained direct power within the Ministry of Health and significantly weakened the state family planning program. Their influence on governmental attitudes outlasted conservative ministers. Even in 2007, after Minister Mazetti left the post, reports emerged in the Peruvian media of religiously conservative policy makers maintaining a grip on Ministry of Health reproductive health policies.[22] The refusal of the ministry in 2007 to approve a clear protocol for legal, therapeutic abortion, despite the development of such a protocol by the major mother-child hospital in Lima, is further evidence of the enduring legacy of religious conservatism.[23]

Short-Term Lessons, Long-Term Legacies

The family planning debacle in Peru raises theoretical questions regarding both short-term feminist politics and long-term policy legacies. For feminist politics, it raises questions regarding the relationship between feminists and the state and the viability of mixed state–civil society–international institutions like the Mesa Tripartita. It also highlights the weak political connection that feminists have made with poor, indigenous women, which in turn allowed a legacy of rural, indigenous women's silence in the political arena to perpetuate itself. In terms of legacies, the debacle highlights the irony that the "rights"-based language that has been so successfully promoted by feminists has yet to change policy practice, in which poor women's bodies are still considered appropriate terrain for national economic objectives.

In terms of state-feminist relations, the family planning debacle demonstrates the need for multiple feminist locations. Although the Peruvian feminists who participated in the Mesa were constrained by their relationship

22. Specifically, Enrique Chávez, "La agenda escondida: Especialistas denuncian graves deficiencias en políticas de salud sexual y reproductiva," *Caretas,* May 18, 2007.

23. In January 2007 a protocol developed by the major women's hospital in Lima, the Instituto Nacional Materno-Perinatal, clarified the conditions under which a therapeutic abortion would be granted (DIRECTIVA N°-DG-INMP-2007, January 2007). This might have represented progress, except that in April 2007 Vice Minister of Health José Calderón issued a resolution declaring the protocol void (RVM 336-2007-SA, April 2007).

with the state and international population agencies, the same relationships allowed them access to information on state policy and practices. In the increasingly authoritarian context of Peru in the late 1990s, the ties that feminists forged with the state were in fact some of the only bridges that existed between the state and Peruvian civil society. The Mesa was therefore a key point for information and negotiation that other groups, such as labor unions, lacked altogether.[24] Yet participation in the Mesa also muted the extent to which these feminists could be critical. On the other hand, feminists outside the Mesa, who were free of compromises with state and international agencies, were key in bringing international attention to the national problem of sterilization campaigns. In what Margaret Keck and Kathryn Sikkink call the "boomerang pattern," these feminists responded to an authoritarian national context by using international mechanisms to pressure the state (1998). Both pragmatic feminist groups willing to interact with the state and autonomous, radical feminist groups able to strongly criticize state actions are essential to success of feminist policy positions.[25]

In Peru's family planning program, a hidden population-control agenda was masked by the disingenuous use of feminist discourse. Recognition of this agenda was not obtained through administrative monitoring but through actual observations of the program in action in remote rural villages. Such efforts require state cooperation coupled with an autonomous base for investigation and contestation as well as willingness to move beyond the urban centers to observe the effects of policies in remote areas. The fact that it took over a year for abuses in the family planning program to be discovered indicates a lack connection between Peruvian feminist NGOs and the rural, indigenous women they hoped to serve. Peruvian feminists are concentrated in Lima, and poor and indigenous women are poorly represented in the feminist movement, whereas government co-optation of feminist discourse was facilitated by feminists' own relative privilege.

Poor rural women have traditionally been excluded from Peruvian politics, and in this case follow the same contours of the poor in general in the context of Peru's health reforms: poor, indigenous women remained excluded from the public health policy making that would greatly impact their everyday

---

24. By contrast, leaders of labor unions, health-related NGOs, university professors, and business representatives whom I interviewed during this time (1998–99) expressed that they felt completely shut out by the government and lacked the mechanisms for negotiation that the feminists had forged in the Mesa Tripartita.

25. See also Lycklama á Nijeholt et al. (1998) and Stetson and Mazur (1995).

health care experiences and instead were seen as objects of reform. In the neoliberal health reform policies described in chapter 5, the poor were targeted in order to increase the nation's "human capital." In the case of family planning, the policy takes on a stronger gendered and racialized expression in that poor indigenous women's reproduction was to be controlled in the name of economic development. Poor indigenous women, like the poor more broadly, lacked the organizing capacity to respond in a united front to the government's policies. But unlike the rest of the poor, these women had purported allies: urban-based feminists. The ties between these groups, however, remained tenuous. While feminists ultimately did support indigenous women, they did so slowly and as a result served as ineffective spokespeople for their rural sisters. Legacies of political silence were reinforced in a continuing dynamic in which class and racial privilege served some (feminists) with more voice than others (indigenous women).

The events surrounding the family planning program in the 1990s also raise a number of questions with regard to policy learning legacies. Family planning was the only major health reform that appeared to follow a rights-based, rather than a neoliberal, emphasis. Its reforms appeared to respond to strong rights-based pressures from feminists on both the national and international fronts. Yet, in this one policy reform area that seemed to hold the greatest potential for improving gender equity, we instead find discrimination and the violation of rights.

In the end, the shift to "rights" in this arena was only discursive. The fact that a significant sterilization campaign occurred in a context such as the 1990s, when the Peruvian feminist movement was active and strong and international discourse militated against population-control policies, is testament to the endurance of the belief among state technocrats, politicians, and even health care workers themselves that poor women's bodies can serve as instruments in the service of national economic development strategies. The durability of these legacies—the policy learning legacy of controlling poor women's bodies combined with a legacy of silencing the political voices of rural indigenous women—raises important questions regarding the political strategies necessary for the successful implementation of rights-based policies even in cases where their acceptance by elites in government may be more sincere. Policy learning legacies in complex areas like health care may be more difficult to reverse when they are absorbed not just by policy makers but by the health care workers themselves. They may be especially hard to reverse when they signify race, class, or gender privilege as well.

7

Insuring Gender Equity? Public and Private Insurance Schemes

Two of Peru's health reforms had important consequences for gender equity and possibly health sector politics over the long term: the introduction of private insurers into the social security health insurance system and the populist establishment of Seguro Escolar Gratuito (Free School Health Insurance, SEG), which eventually became broader, general-targeted health insurance for the poor, Seguro Integral de Salud (Integral Health Insurance, SIS). Viewed side by side, private insurance for the wealthy and state-targeted insurance for the poor offer a contrast in market-oriented and state-oriented approaches. As detailed in chapter 4, they also stemmed from very different political objectives and policy processes. The reform of social security health insurance was a decidedly neoliberal process concerned with making room for the market in the health sector, whereas the establishment of state-targeted health insurance (as SEG and eventually SIS) was a neopopulist process concerned with generating political support through providing a tangible state benefit. The implications of these reforms for gender equity, however, cannot be read directly from their divergent state/market origins.

This chapter evaluates these reforms according to their abilities to redistribute and recognize. It also analyzes their political evolution, especially the evolution of the targeted free school insurance into general insurance for the poor. It concentrates on distributive issues such as economic and geographic access, as there are limited data available to evaluate implications for the distribution of care work.[1] In terms of recognition, this chapter considers the degree to which these reforms recognize the distinct health needs of men and women, promote a sense of "common humanity" by reducing stratification, and give citizens a voice in their health care system.

To some extent, the implications of these reforms for gender equity map onto state/market differences, but in other ways they surprisingly converge, despite their very different origins. Each is deficient in attending to women's health needs through the life cycle; each tends to prejudice women's basic health care needs in quests for greater "efficiency"; and each at different moments has succumbed to socially or religiously conservative demands that tend to limit women's access to reproductive health care—in spite of the fact that these limitations, over the long term, are quite *in*efficient. Thus, they share nonrecognition of women's health needs, despite one being a statist and the other a market-oriented reform. They diverge on economic and geographic distribution and the recognition and promotion of a common humanity. The market-oriented social security reform has introduced new economic barriers and increased stratification by class, race, and gender; the SIS, especially in its more recent evolution, appears to be moving toward universal care where all citizens have a right to health care, including greater insurance coverage for women and indigenous people.

Reconfigured Social Security

The fundamental 1990s health sector reform was the introduction of private sector health provider entities (EPS) to compete with the state social security health system. EPS were allowed to function alongside the state health social security provider, which in 1999 was renamed from IPSS (Instituto Peruano de Seguridad Social) to EsSalud. Workers selected an EPS on a company basis, voting collectively to select a private insurer to serve the health needs of all employees or to remain with EsSalud. Collective choice was intended to minimize adverse selection by private insurers of only the wealthiest and

---

1. Available data do not allow measuring the effects of insurance reforms on care work. One way this might be done is to compare days a patient stays in the hospital for the same procedure from time period to time period or carrier to carrier. Shorter hospital stays often imply more home-based care, the bulk of which falls on female family members. An additional indicator could also be developed in national surveys, in which the respondent is asked how many days in a given time period were dedicated to care for a sick or recovering family member.

healthiest clients. The fact that the private insurer would cover only basic services (*capa simple*) and the state insurer, EsSalud, would cover complex care (*capa compleja*) was intended to help pool and control the costs of the most expensive health care by maintaining complex care in one state system.

In addition to introducing private EPS, EsSalud began a process of internal reform. Law 27506 of 1999 placed new personnel working for the agency on a private sector contract regimen similar to that of the Ministry of Health Basic Health for All program, discussed in chapter 4. The law extended coverage to a variety of previously uncovered populations, in particular, informal sector workers, who could now buy insurance through EsSalud. (The economic crisis of the 1980s and 1990s had swelled the informal workforce as formal sector jobs disappeared. In 2003 56.8 percent of Peru's economically active population worked in the informal sector; ECLAC 2005.)[2] EsSalud also instituted complementary worker compensation insurance, added representatives from retired persons and small and microenterprises to the agency's tripartite board of directors, eliminated state contributions to social security financing, and strengthened the authority of the agencies' general manager.[3] It also separated financing and provision, following reform recommendations of the time (Carbajal and Francke 2003, 518, 516).

In keeping with previous work on gender and welfare regimes and gender and economic policy, evaluation of the distributional effects of the EPS reform requires examining whether the costs of insurance have been shifted from state to market or from market to individuals or families, and if so, how those shifts may affect women and men differently. Male and female workers enrolled in either EsSalud or the private EPS option have 9 percent of their salary deducted from their paycheck. For those who opt for EPS, the deduction is split, with 2.25 percent going to the EPS and the remainder to EsSalud. That male and female workers pay the same percentage is better

2. For statistical purposes, the International Labor Organization (ILO) defines the informal sector as own-account workers (but excluding administrative workers, professionals, and technicians), unpaid family workers, and employers and employees working in establishments with less than five or ten persons engaged. Paid domestic workers are excluded. ILO Web site, http://www.ilo.org/public/english/employment/skills/informal/who.htm (accessed June 8, 2006). For estimates of Peru's informal sector I have used ECLAC statistics (Statistical Annex of ECLAC 2004) combining own-account and unpaid family workers (excluding professional and technical) with those in nonprofessional and nontechnical establishments employing under five persons.

3. For details see *Diario de los Debates*, Primera Legislatura Ordinaria de 1998 26a Sesión Miercoles, January 27, 1999. The law also ostensibly makes the institution economically and administratively autonomous, a characteristic that legally also applied to IPSS but was rarely enforced. For a discussion of the shortcomings of this law see *Análisis Laboral* (1999).

for gender equity than in neighboring Chile, whose private providers have charged women 3.2 times more than men for the same health insurance, especially in their reproductive years (Pollack 2002, 20). The percentage basis also allows for women (who generally earn less than men) to pay in proportion to their earnings rather than a flat fee. Thus, the salary deduction system protects women to some extent from market forces, which in other countries have shifted responsibility for health and human reproduction disproportionately to women.

In addition to the salary deduction, private insurers (but not EsSalud) charge copayments for services. These do raise gender equity concerns. A private insurer may charge copays and deductibles for services, as long as these do not exceed 2 percent of the insured person's monthly income for ambulatory services, or 10 percent income for hospitalizations (Ley 26790, Article 17). The regulation also states that copays must not exceed 10 percent of the cost of treatment (Reglamento, Article 42). By tying copays to a percentage of income, this system is more equitable than a straight copays system, but it still generates some gender inequities. Copayments affect women more than men because women use health care facilities more than men due to biological factors such as greater reproductive health care needs, longevity, and morbidity (Gómez Gómez 2002). Social factors also play a role; women have lower independent incomes and higher rates of dependency on males and disproportionately pay for children's health care needs (see chapter 5; Yoshioka 2006; Thomas 1997; Roldan 1988). All these factors make copays a heavier burden on women and put them at a disadvantage compared to men in the private insurance scheme.

Statistics specific to Peru fit this broader pattern of women's economic disadvantage in fee-based health systems. Women's sickness rate is higher: in 2008 35 percent of women versus 27 percent of men reported having been sick recently (ENAHO 2008). Women use health care services more; in 2004 58 percent of all health consultations with private insurers were provided to women, compared to 42 percent to men (SEPS 2005, 40). Yet women also earn less—in 2006 women who worked in Lima earned on average 67 percent of what men earned, and only 51.4 percent of women of working age were employed (INEI 2006, 84, 78). Women's higher unemployment rates (10.6 percent versus 7.8 percent for men in 2006; INEI 2006, 80) are in part due to discrimination, child care responsibilities, and tradition. These factors, plus women's responsibility to pay for the bulk of children's care, likely underlie the fact that in 2008 women were significantly more likely than men to not seek health care due to lack of funds.[4] Peru's limits on copayments, tied to salary, are an important step toward greater gender equity, but they do not address the fact that women pay for health care more often than men despite lower financial independence.

Another regulation provides some relief to women's greater usage rates and their related copays. This regulation stipulates that the EPS insurer may not charge copayments for emergency care, preventive care (which includes routine gynecology), or maternity care. Women enrolled in an EPS do tend to use health services most in their reproductive years (SEPS 2005, 40). The prohibition of copays for routine gynecological and maternity care makes the system more gender-equitable than if all care were subject to them, as in Colombia, for example, where sliding-scale copays apply to all services (Ewig and Hernández 2009). Copays for other health needs are still discriminatory toward women because they are lower income earners and use health care more over their lifetime due to greater morbidity and longevity than males (female longevity in 2008 in Peru was 74.3 years compared to males' 69.2; PAHO 2007).[5] Peruvian women's use of health services continues to be higher than men's into old age (SEPS 2005, 40). In upper age brackets no copay exclusions exist, since these apply mainly to reproductive care.

Coverage of dependents under the private insurance system generates new distributional gender inequities. In EsSalud dependents are automatically covered by the same basic salary deduction. In private plans, however, there is an extra charge for each dependent covered, often wives, female partners, or children.[6] Table 7.1 shows that in 2006 59.5 percent of females covered by an EPS were covered as dependents, compared to 46.3 percent of males. Women's higher dependency rate puts them in a more precarious position for lack of health coverage should their marriage or partnership dissolve. Moreover, the higher cost of covering dependents under the EPS system puts women at greater risk of being dropped from insurance in times of economic stress. Even in EsSalud dependency can be an issue, despite no increase in cost, for the same reasons of strained or dissolved relationships. Dependency

---

4. Based on author's calculations using third trimester 2008 Encuesta Nacional de Hogares Sobre Condiciones de Vida y Pobreza survey data; 16.3 percent of men and 18.5 percent of women reported not seeking care due to lack of money, a statistically significant difference, $p = 0.008$, $N = 22,330$.

5. For a review of gender and morbidity research globally, see Sen, George, and Östlin (2002a).

6. The specific extra amount charged is determined by the individual EPS and presented along with other plan specifics to workers prior to the company vote.

Table 7.1   Sex and insurance dependency, EPS and EsSalud, 2006 (adults and children)

	EPS direct affiliate	EPS dependent	Total EPS	EsSalud direct affiliate	EsSalud dependent	Total EsSalud
Male	53.5%	46.3%	100%	62.2%	37.8%	100%
	23	20	43	4,504	2,734	7,238
Female	40.5%	59.5%	100%	32.6%	67.4%	100%
	15	22	37	2,407	4,965	7,372
	$p = 0.339$			$p = 0.000$		
	$N = 80$			$N = 14{,}610$		

SOURCE: Author's calculations from ENAHO 2006. Latest available data; questions regarding dependency were eliminated in the 2007 and 2008 surveys.

rates in EsSalud among females are even higher than in the EPS: 67.4 percent of female affiliates. One health advocate indicated that in strained partnerships women or children would often be denied care through EsSalud because the male partner would not share the insurance card required for services (Interview Olea 2007). A 2007 move to an electronic database of affiliates may have helped alleviate this problem.

The distributive effects of the EPS reform include the geographic distribution of services. The private social security insurance system is extremely limited in its geographic reach. The EPS serve almost exclusively urban areas; 61 percent of EPS-affiliated health establishments are in Lima and Callao, as are 67 percent of their health personnel (SEPS 2005, 28–29). Almost all EPS health establishments are in the major coastal cities. The urban bias is explained in part by the fact that the largest companies in Peru are in urban areas and the population is also over 70 percent urban, while the rural economy, except in mining towns, is predominantly based on small-scale and subsistence agriculture. Yet not having facilities in rural areas denies the rural population the choice of higher-quality private health care.

Shifting to the degree to which the health social security system reform addresses recognition concerns, a first step is to determine whether the basic health needs of both men and women are provided for, and thus recognized. According to Law 26790, each EPS must provide a "minimal plan," a state-mandated basket of basic health of services whose content is outlined in the regulations.[7] Legally, all medical needs are covered by either the state or

7. Reglamento de la ley de Modernización de la Seguridad Social en Salud, Decreto Supremo No. 009-97-SA, published in *El Peruano*, September 9, 1997. The minimum plan in

private social security providers, with EsSalud paying for or directly providing any service not covered in the minimal plan. The minimal plan provided by private insurers covers many women's gender-based health needs, such as treatment of diabetes mellitus (which has a higher incidence in women than men), a yearly gynecological exam, basic family planning consultation, and insertion of an IUD.[8] It covers normal childbirth, including multiple births and caesarean section. In addition, the state social security agency covers the cost of a ninety-day maternity leave and a subsidy for lactation for those covered by the social security system (enrolled in an EPS or EsSalud). The plan does not, however, cover a complicated birth. Men's and boys' specific basic health needs are also generally covered by the basic plan, including inguinal hernia for boys, prostate care, and a wide range of emergency care addressing men's greater likelihood of death or injury as a result of accidents.[9] Anything not included in the minimal plan, officially, is to be provided by EsSalud, with the exception of abortion, which is in general illegal except to save the life of the woman; but even in these cases this right is rarely granted (Interview Chávez 2007). An estimated 22 percent of Peru's maternal mortalities are due to complications from abortion (Yamin 2003, 105), and women with complications from illegal abortions are often treated discriminatorily in the health system (54).

Officially the state social security health system, EsSalud, is supposed to cover all care outside the minimal plan required of private insurers, but there is good reason to believe it does not always do so. According to Peruvian law, EsSalud may deny any health care it deems to be "high cost" and with "low chance for recovery" (Decreto Supremo 001-98-SA). There is no protocol for determining what care is "high cost" or when a patient is deemed to have "low chance for recovery" (Interview Garavito 2007). How much this loophole is used, and whether all services are covered in practice, would require separate data collection via patient health records to compare services required

---

appendix 2 is to be updated every two years. As of this writing, the contents of the plan have not been updated since 1997. The law has only been modified by changing subsidy rates for injury, maternity, and breastfeeding.

8. In Peru, similar to other countries, the diabetes mellitus death rate for women has traditionally been higher than that of men. For example, in 2003 the rate was 14.3 in 100,000 compared to 13.1 for men. In 2008, however, the rate for men was slightly higher, 13.8 compared to 13.7 for women (PAHO 2007).

9. Men's death rate due to accidents in 2004 (other than transport accidents) was 32.9 in 100,000 compared to 13.2 for women; for transport accidents the rates were 18.2 and 6.2 (PAHO 2007).

and services actually provided. The poor financial situation of the state social security agency, however, may very well mean that not all services are regularly offered. EsSalud has been plagued by budget deficits and underfinancing: in 2005 the government owed EsSalud over a billion soles (about U.S. 300 million dollars) in contributions, which resulted in long lines and lack of medical supplies (Díaz 2006). As a result, EsSalud began to prioritize some types of health care services over others, based on cost-effectiveness criteria (EsSalud Memoria 2004, 11).

Another dimension of recognition is the promotion of a "common humanity" among health care users. By failing to serve the informal sector, the EPS contribute to gendered stratification. Most income-earning women in Peru work in the informal sector, due to discrimination in the formal sector and the fact that informal sector jobs tend to be more flexible, allowing women simultaneously to care for children and earn income. In 2003 35.8 percent of economically active urban Peruvian men and 49.7 percent of women were employed in the informal sector (ECLAC 2007, 348, 352). The percentage of independent workers (of which informal sector workers are a subset[10]) who buy insurance through the EPS has fluctuated, from 2.6 percent of all insured by an EPS in 1999 to 3.4 percent in 2005 to just 1.6 percent in 2008; most of them are more likely highly skilled independent professionals.[11]

The low enrollment is indicative of the fact that private health insurance is too costly for the majority of independent workers. The annual health insurance rate for a twenty-seven-year-old in 2008 from one of the major health insurers, RIMAC, for its basic plan was 518 dollars. For the same company's more expensive "Full Salud" package the cost was U.S. 678 dollars. Independent workers pay a set fee, with cost dependent on risk. Similar to Chile, which allows risk to be calculated based on sex and age and has resulted in higher premiums for women and the elderly, Peru allows private insurers to discriminate based on sex and age, but only when insurance is purchased independently. For example, the cost of the Full Salud package mentioned above doubles to U.S. 1,290 dollars if maternity coverage is included. For a fifty-five-year-old, the same package (minus maternity) is U.S. 1,476 dollars. Dependent child coverage from this company costs an additional 342 dollars

10. Independent workers work for themselves rather than others. ECLAC defines informal sector workers as a subset of independent workers: workers with low education and skill levels, unpaid workers, owners of microenterprises, and domestic workers (ECLAC 2008, chaps. 2, 10).

11. Calculated from SEPS affiliation statistics at http://www.seps.gob.pe/estadisticas/afiliaciones.asp (accessed June 6, 2006, December 21, 2008).

to 456 dollars, depending on the age of the child.[12] These costs are prohibitive, given that Peru's average monthly income in 2004–5 was about U.S. 200 dollars for women and for U.S. 300 dollars for men (INEI 2005). Some newer companies have entered the market with slightly cheaper rates, but the rates remain beyond the means of average Peruvian informal sector workers.[13] In addition to higher costs for the middle-aged and elderly, many private plans are not available for persons over sixty.[14]

The EsSalud social security system is less costly and more economically accessible for some independent workers. Yet these workers make up a minuscule portion of EsSalud affiliates—only 1 percent in 2006 (EsSalud 2007, 13). Independent workers may opt to purchase EsSalud coverage and pay according to their age and the number of family members they wish to cover, at significantly lower rates than EPS coverage. Annual rates for an individual EsSalud plan range from 816 soles for those aged twenty-five to thirty-four years of age to 1,680 soles for those over sixty-five (U.S. 263 dollars and 542 dollars), about half the cost of private independent coverage. Like private insurers, EsSalud charges more for elderly persons in an inverse relationship to income; maternity care, however, carries no extra charge. The system does charge copayments for independent workers, amounting to ten soles (U.S. three dollars and twenty-two cents in December 2008) for each ambulatory visit and the cost of the first night of hospital care.[15] As in the private system for formal sector workers, EsSalud copayments for independent workers do not apply to maternity, emergency, or preventive care. While much smaller, the copays for independent workers raise the same concerns of gender-based inequalities as in the EPS system.

In terms of promoting a common humanity, the social security health reforms have done little to address the vulnerability of domestic workers.

12. Calculated on RIMAC rates calculator, http://www.rimac.com.pe/, December 21, 2008, for a twenty-seven-year-old: 1,601 soles for the basic plan, 2103 soles for Full Salud, 4,000 soles for Full Salud with maternity coverage; for a fifty-five-year-old, 4,578 soles for Full Salud (December 2008 exchange, 3.10 soles to a dollar). Dependent coverage based on table at http://www.rimac.com.pe/ilwwcm/connect/PR_PortalRimac/P%C3%A1gina+Principal/Rimac+Seguros/Seguros+Personales/Salud/Full+Salud/Full+Salud+-+Benef (accessed December 21, 2008).

13. Mapfre charges 1,496 soles or 482 dollars annually for a client under forty years of age. See http://www.mapfreperu.com/portal/productos/salud/trebol_salud/index.asp (accessed December 21, 2008).

14. Based on a review of plan costs and rules on insurers' Web sites, June 2006, December 2008.

15. http://www.essalud.gob.pe/seguros/potestativo/pvital.htm (accessed December 21, 2008).

Domestic work is almost entirely female in Peru, and in 2003 11.5 percent of all economically active urban women worked in this sector (ECLAC 2007). According to a Peruvian NGO that advocates on behalf of domestic workers, 90 percent of these workers are indigenous, making this an issue of intersectionality, where gender and race come together and define a particular class of workers.[16] The former state social security law mandated that domestic workers be covered by their employers, though at lower contribution levels than for other workers. The 1997 reforms put domestic workers in the same category as other formal sector workers, eligible for social security health coverage through the state system, in which employers are obliged to pay a 9 percent salary contribution, based on a minimum wage of 500 soles per month. The employee pays an additional 4 percent, for a 13 percent total contribution.[17] Mandatory coverage of these women helps equalize male and female rates of health insurance coverage. Contributions by home employers, however, have rarely been enforced, and the higher rate under the revised law may make them even less likely to do so.[18] According to the Training Center for Domestic Workers, only 4 percent of domestic workers are enrolled in social security, despite the obligation that employers enroll their employees (Gurgurevich 2005). Moreover, many domestic workers are paid less than the minimum wage of 500 soles a month (about U.S. 160 dollars), and often as little as 200 (about U.S. 64 dollars). A 9 percent contribution on the minimum wage would be 45 soles, which applied to a 200-sol salary results in a contribution that many employers refuse to pay.[19] This almost entirely female and indigenous workforce is highly vulnerable and often unable to demand its rights due to lack of power vis-à-vis employers. Many domestic workers use the public health system rather than pursuing their right to higher-quality state social security services.

Finally, there is little evidence of real voice for patients in the reformed social security system, especially in recognizing the range of voices that need to be heard. The 1990s reform added representatives from microenterprises

16. Cited by Centro de Capacitación para Trabajadoras de Hogar, http://www.globalwomenstrike.net/English2006/JournalPeru.htm.

17. Ministerio de Trabajo, http://www.mintra.gob.pe/trabajadoras_hogar_faqs.php (accessed June 1, 2006).

18. There is substantial employer evasion in social security contributions for the general workforce. In July 2006 the government tax institute, SUNAT, found that on average employers did not declare 30 percent of their workers. Peru.com, http://www.peru.com/finanzas/idocs2/2006/7/25/DetalleDocumento_323104.asp (accessed July 26, 2006).

19. Personal communication with Sofia Mauricio, director of Casa de Panchita, an advocacy and employment agency for domestic workers in Lima, June 8, 2007.

and retired people to the EsSalud board of directors. These were important steps in recognizing informal sector workers and the aged. There is little evidence, however, that the board has significant influence over EsSalud policies. For example, the union leader who sat on the board in 1998 found that it did serve as a platform from which she could advocate for workers' rights, but it gave little space for debate on actual reforms (Interview Baca 1998). This lack of influence is perhaps seen most clearly in that the groups given representation in the 1990s are still the most negatively affected by EsSalud policies. The EPS have no formal participatory mechanism at all.

The Evolution of Targeted Health Insurance for the Poor

Given that most empirical studies on gender and health sector reform have found markets to have a negative impact on gender equity, one would expect Peru's targeted health insurance reforms, due to their statist orientation, to perform much better than its market-oriented social security reform.[20] Unlike the classically neoliberal political process that led to the latter, the process that resulted in the Seguro Escolar Gratuito (Free School Health Insurance, SEG) was born largely of presidential, populist motives. It expanded in the later years of the Fujimori administration into the Seguro Materno Infantil (Mother-Infant Insurance, SMI) and under Alejandro Toledo (2001–6) into more general Seguro Integral de Salud (Integral Health Insurance, SIS), further expanded by president Alán García (2006–12). This expansion points to a possible new "policy learning legacy" as well as changing international and regional trends in health reform toward broader, more generous coverage. Below, I examine the implications for gender equity of each iteration of this insurance.

Free School Health Insurance

SEG was a positive development for health care coverage for school-age children, but more for boys than girls and more for the poor than the extremely poor. All Peruvians have a right to health services in the public health system, but they must pay the associated fees unless they request and receive

---

20. Including Pollack (2002); Gómez Gómez (2002); Forget et al. (2005); Ewig and Hernández (2009).

exoneration. The SEG allowed a target group of children to receive health care through the public system free of charge. With a budget of 30 million dollars in 1998, this insurance targeted about six million children aged three to seventeen and attending public schools (World Bank 1999, 44). The program provided a positive alternative to means testing, but maintained the efficiency of targeting: by serving only children who attended public schools, it targeted poor and working-class families and excluded wealthier families with children in private schools. The positive aspects of the program are reflected in the statement of one rural mother who, after taking her children to the health center for care, commented, "I never paid the consultation fee, everything was free. My son went with his school health insurance and I never paid even for medicines. Even for my daughter they pulled her tooth with the school insurance" (Survey 42). This insurance not only alleviated some of the inequities generated by fees, but was meant as an incentive to keep children in school.

Yet, in practice, recognition politics within families served to skew the degree to which this reform was actually able to distribute health care to all children in need. The reform did not treat girls and boys differently; it was targeted simply at schoolchildren. But by not recognizing the social relations within families faced by boys and girls, or the health practices of the very poor, policy makers overlooked how the reform might interact with class and gendered recognition practices in poor rural Peruvian communities. While some of the residents of urban shantytowns and rural areas were quite pleased with the program, as evidenced in the quote above, in rural areas I began to pick out a pattern of responses when I asked what residents thought about SEG. Many families could not take full advantage of SEG because their daughters were not enrolled in school. "My daughters don't study," remarked one woman (Survey 62). Another, when I asked, "Does your daughter have school insurance?" responded, "The rest of my children study and have it, but my daughter does not study" (Survey 29).

In rural areas of Peru, education of boys is prioritized over that of girls. Boys are viewed as future family breadwinners, for whom education is important. Girls are expected to carry out domestic chores and broader social reproductive activities such as tending animals or small-scale household production. Many families perceive that traditional female tasks do not require much formal education, so girls are thought to be of greater benefit to families if they engage full time in family social reproduction at a young age.

Many rural girls are sent to school for only a few years, which made many ineligible for SEG insurance.[21]

An encounter during the rural portion of the survey illustrates this household gender dynamic. As my Quechua-speaking assistant, Madeleine, and I trekked rural Ayacucho carrying out the survey, we stopped at a home where we saw an older woman cooking breakfast in a cooking shelter. The thin woman stirred her kettle of soup alongside her granddaughter, age eleven. Our presence attracted the attention of the woman's adult son, who made clear that he was the patriarch of the family. He claimed to need to get to work in the fields—no time to answer questions about health—yet out of curiosity he hung around answering a number of the survey questions before his mother had a chance to respond. When I asked about recent family health issues and where care was sought for these, the man's young daughter complained that she had a toothache. I asked why she had not sought dental care at the local clinic down the mountain. The father intervened—"If she goes to the clinic, then who would be left to tend to the animals?" This encounter illustrates two related gender issues in many families of the rural highlands. One is dependency; how this father controls his daughter's access to health care. The other is what it says about girls and schooling. His daughter should have been in school that day, a Tuesday. For this father, however, it was more important that his daughter tend to the animals than attend school *or* take care of her own health needs.

The disparity in girls' and boys' education is evident in national statistics. According to national survey data for the period when SEG was operating, 8.2 percent of men and 14.2 percent of women did not have access to education (ENAHO 1997, cited by CARE/USAID). This difference was more dramatic in rural areas, where the average number of years a girl studied in school was 3.7, compared to 8.3 years in urban areas. In 2006 34.4 percent of rural women and 11.9 percent of rural men were illiterate (INEI 2007b). In 2000 national household data the skew in SEG affiliations becomes apparent once girls are able to help around the house. For children aged nine and under, there was not a significant difference between boys and girls in school attendance or SEG enrollment. At age ten and over, however, girls' school attendance dropped significantly; 19.9 percent of rural girls between

---

21. On gendered attitudes toward education in the Department of Ayacucho see Thiedon (1999).

ten and seventeen did not attend school in 2000, compared to 16 percent of boys in the same age range.[22] Of the girls who did not attend school, 9.9 percent reported that they didn't attend because of housework responsibilities (no boys reported this reason) and another 13.4 percent reported "family problems" (boys gave this reason only 0.8 percent of the time).[23] At the same age, a statistically significant gap appears in boys' and girls' affiliations with SEG; 76 percent of rural girls compared to 80 percent of boys age ten to seventeen reported affiliation with the SEG in 2000.[24] One might argue that the program provided an incentive for these families to send their girls to school. However, if it had such an objective, it would have had to reach out to these families and encourage the enrollment of girls in school, something it did not do.

In addition to this unintended gender discrimination, a socioeconomic bias resulted from this form of targeting. SEG increased access to health care among the best-off recipients, but not among the poorest of the poor, who were excluded because they do not send their children (boys or girls) to school at all (Jaramillo and Parodi 2004, 53, 16).

Mother-Infant Insurance

In 1998 Peruvian policy makers approved a new targeted health insurance to complement free school health insurance. In contrast to SEG, which was set up on an entirely populist basis and with little preplanning or even legal basis, Seguro Materno Infantil (Mother-Infant Insurance, SMI) was carefully planned. Similar to the other reforms of the period, it was designed by a small set of consultants contracted by the Program to Strengthen Health Services—an economist and a public health doctor who worked in relative isolation from the rest of the ministry (Espinoza 2002). The neoliberal epistemic community also played an important role in the development of this insurance. It was inspired by a similar insurance in Bolivia, and modified for Peru by a combination of actors from the IDB, World Bank, and Peru. The World Bank and IDB viewed the Bolivian reform positively for its success in reducing maternal mortality, and members of Peru's health ministry

22. Author's calculations from ENAHO (2000), cross-tabulation of sex and school attendance for children ages ten to seventen, $N = 1,472$, $p = 0.049$.

23. Author's calculations from ENAHO (2000), $N = 262$.

24. Author's calculations from ENAHO (2000), cross-tabulation of sex and SEG coverage ages ten to seventeen, $N = 1,472$, $p = 0.04$.

visited Bolivia in the process of developing maternal-infant insurance.[25] In addition, Peruvian health expert David Tejada was formerly head of Bolivian maternal health insurance and returned to Peru to help start the insurance model at home (Espinoza 2002; Interview Tejada 2002). Pilot maternal health insurance was initiated in 1998 with IDB financing (Espinoza 2002; Yamin 2003). The insurance began in 5 provinces in two departments and gradually expanded to 160 provinces in eighteen departments (ParSalud 2007, 2). It was followed by permanent national SMI in 1999. The expansion was to be financed in its first three years by a parallel IDB–World Bank loan of U.S. 87 million dollars from each bank, later reduced to 27 and 28 million dollars, respectively.[26]

Through SMI the Ministry of Health subsidized maternal-child health by reimbursing local health providers for these costs, providing an incentive for greater coverage and for reaching those most at risk of maternal mortality (Espinoza 2002; Yamin 2003). Those eligible for the insurance were children under four and all pregnant or postnatal women within forty-two days of giving birth who were not covered by private or state social security health insurance and, initially, lived in specified geographic areas. Normal deliveries were covered, with a symbolic fee of ten soles (about U.S. three dollars) for obstetric complications (Espinoza 2002). The SMI aimed to cover 80 percent of all affiliates with institutional births and to reduce maternal mortality from 265 to 128 per 100,000 live births in the first three years (Yamin 2003, 149).

The IFIs sought to use the insurance to move Peru's health reform process in what they saw as a more positive direction. The IFIs saw the mother-infant insurance idea, along with the CLAS, as among the most promising ideas to come out of the health reform process, and thought they would have the greatest impact.[27] The IFIs also saw this insurance as a way to subtly nudge the government away from its emphasis on the populist school health insurance, which they saw as serving a population (schoolchildren) with few critical health needs compared to other demographic groups. However, contrary to the IFI objectives, which had urged careful targeting of beneficiaries, the SMI, like free school health insurance, became a largely populist program

25. Bolivian insurance had increased that country's rate of institutional births by one-third in eighteen months (World Bank 1999, xiii).

26. The change in amount was at least in part because the Ministry of Finance did not want to use loan money for continuing costs, preferring treasury money (Interview Garavito 2007). Yamin (2003, 148) writes that multiple problems with implementation led to the reduced financing.

27. Interview Anon. 16; interview Anon. 17; interview Anon. 18.

promoted by President Fujimori on the eve of the 2000 election with little careful targeting (Weyland 2007, chap. 5).

Domestic political factors also drove the establishment of this new targeted insurance. Among these were Peru's alarmingly high maternal mortality indicators. According to one account, this insurance was designed at the behest of the health minister, urged by the president to do something about these rates (Espinoza 2002).[28] Maternal mortality was Peru's worst health indicator overall, a point of international embarrassment for the Fujimori government and a rallying call for feminist groups (Yamin 2003, 145). Some ministry technocrats who agreed that maternal mortality should be a priority asked the IFIs to include maternal-infant insurance in loan conditions, as a way to ensure the success of the insurance concept (Weyland 2006, chap. 5). Another reason the insurance was finally approved by the president was that the government hoped to use it to deflect national and international attention from the debacle of Peru's family planning reforms.[29] Health insurance for mothers and children would place a more positive face on the efforts of the Ministry of Health to serve women, less than a year before presidential elections.

The program should have improved gender equity by making health care more available to poor women and children and by combating Peru's egregiously high maternal mortality rates. In practice, however, the program was not very successful in distributing care to those most in need, and the quality of the care distributed was low. Moreover, although the program recognized the vital health need of expert care during pregnancy and childbirth, this is only one health need of women throughout their life cycles.

In terms of distribution of basic health services, the program failed to reach large numbers of women due to its limited financing. Even if the initial bank financing had been fulfilled, the program would not have had the funds to reach even a fraction of the women most in need (Yamin 2003, 150; Espinoza 2002, 37). Given its limited finances, the program sought to target the poorest women, but it lacked the technical ability to identify these women (Yamin 2003, 151; Espinoza 2002). Implementation was poor: slow

28. The government also established a multisectoral committee on safe and healthy maternity in 1998 (Mesa Multisectoral por una Maternidad Saludable y Segura) and in 2000 formalized a contingency plan for reducing maternal mortality, supported by USAID's main health project in Peru, Proyecto 2000 (Yamin 2003, 157–58).

29. Yamin confirmed with multiple informants that the SMI was approved primarily to deflect attention from problems in the family planning program at the time (2003, 153–54).

reimbursement of local facilities by the ministry led to shortages of medicines and basic supplies and frustration by providers (Yamin 2003, 151). Finally, the insurance faced resistance within the ministry by those who viewed it as imposed by the IFIs. Perhaps due to its administrative and financial weaknesses, it reached only 21.6 percent of its target population (Jaramillo and Parodi 2004, 40).

The program increased insurance coverage among pregnant women and infants on a highly uneven basis. The program was piloted in a few (not necessarily poor) areas, which contributed to uneven geographic and socioeconomic coverage (Yamin 2003; Jaramillo and Parodi 2004). For example, in the relatively well-off region of Tacna, where the program was first piloted, 75.6 percent of mothers and children were covered by maternal-infant insurance in 2000, compared to 23.3 percent in Ayacucho and 13.2 percent in Huancavelica—the two poorest regions of the country.[30] Moreover, one in three of those covered by the maternal-infant program were not poor at all (Jaramillo and Parodi 2004, 40). Like school health insurance, mother-infant insurance increased overall access to health care among those who were close to the poverty line but not among the extremely poor.

The program was also criticized on public health grounds. SMI sought to reduce maternal mortality primarily through prenatal controls, identification of "high-risk" pregnancies, and institutional rather than home births. But the majority of maternal deaths do not occur among those classified as "high risk" in the prenatal stage, making prenatal controls no guarantee of safe childbirth (Yamin 2003). Safe childbirth and reduction of maternal mortality depends essentially on the availability of necessary equipment and expert health personnel in the case of an obstetric emergency. Postpartum hemorrhage, which cannot be detected beforehand, is the leading cause (45.2 percent) of maternal deaths in Peru (Yamin 2003, 160). Yet very few health centers or hospitals—especially in rural areas—had the services necessary for dealing with an obstetric emergency such as postpartum hemorrhage, and thus the ability to save endangered mothers' lives in childbirth.[31]

In terms of recognition, while SMI, with some prodding from the international sphere, recognized a very specific gender-based health need women

30. Numbers from Jaramillo and Parodi (2004, 37), based on their analysis of ENDES (2000) data.
31. Yamin (2003, chap. 4), shows that the UN guidelines for availability of basic and comprehensive essential obstetric care services were not met under the SMI program. For UN definitions and guidelines see Yamin and Maine (1999).

face—expert assistance during childbirth—it also only recognized the needs of gestating mothers. Other aspects of women's health care throughout the life cycle were not incorporated into this program. (Distribution of care work, societal stratification, and "voice" were not significantly changed by this reform.) The program did not last long due to a number of factors, the largest being a change in government.

Integral Health Insurance

Following Fujimori's flight into exile in 2000 on charges of corruption, the transitional government of Valentín Paniagua (2000–2001) combined SEG and SMI into one program in 2001. The combination was consolidated in 2002 when Toledo's government renamed the combined program Seguro Integral de Salud (Integral Health Insurance, SIS). SIS covered five major population groups, three of them covered under the previous targeted programs. Plan A covered general health care for children zero to four years of age, Plan B covered general health care for children ages five to seventeen, and Plan C offered coverage of pregnant women, childbirth, and forty-two days of postpartum care. Plans D and E added groups not covered by the previous insurance plans. Plan D offered care to adults in need of emergency services. Plan E was aimed at adults in extreme poverty, and also specified several special beneficiary groups: victims of forced sterilizations from the 1990s; women who worked in community organizations such as mothers' clubs and communal day cares; local health promoters and midwives; members of the shoeshine guild; victims of political violence; and residents of remote areas of the Amazon and the Andes. In March 2007, under the presidency of Alan García (but planned under Toledo), a "semisubsidized" option was added, where low-income persons could apply for integral health insurance and receive it at low cost.[32]

The SIS extended its target group as presidents also sought to increase their populist base of support. Under Toledo, several groups covered by the new insurance were clearly populist additions, such as the "shoe-shiners" (Toledo himself had been a shoe-shiner as a boy, a point he emphasized in

---

32. Persons with incomes less than seven hundred soles a month pay ten soles a month, and for incomes between seven hundred and one thousand soles per month pay twenty soles. Family coverage for anyone with an income less than sixteen hundred soles a month costs thirty soles a month. SIS Web site, http://www.sis.gob.pe/mercadeo/index_2.htm (accessed June 25, 2007). The exchange rate in 2008 was 3.10 to the U.S. dollar.

his election campaign) and women's community organizations, which have historically been used in a clientelistic manner by Peruvian presidents (Barrig 1989, 1992). García removed some groups as beneficiaries (such as shoeshiners and the aforementioned women's organizations) but added his own interest groups: in 2007 mototaxi, tricycle taxi, and public transport operators, and in 2008 a select group of poor neighborhood leaders.[33]

The expansion of integral insurance under Toledo and García was also due to broader national political pressures. Although the term "universal" has been used in Peru since at least the early 1990s, it often has simply meant health care coverage for all, of varying qualities, not a single-payer or single-provider system for all. By the mid-2000s there was growing sentiment among political parties, activists in civil society, and health policy experts that universal health insurance was the right policy direction, and expansion of integral health insurance seemed to be the appropriate road toward this goal. In the lead-up to the 2006 elections, an Acuerdo Político en Salud (Political Accord in Health) was formulated under the leadership of UNFPA, CARE, and the National Democratic Institute in Peru, and agreed to by consensus by fifteen political parties. In this accord, "universal" health care, meaning universal insurance coverage, was a major political priority. Health activist organizations such as the ForoSalud and the Peruvian Medical Association (Colegio Médico) also called for universal insurance, and continued to lobby for it after García was elected. Perhaps in response to these pressures, García's 2006 address to the nation promised the state would work toward universal health coverage, and went beyond the accord by declaring the goal of a "single

---

33. The Plan E recipient list was significantly revised in Decreto Supremo 004-2007, passed in March 2007. In the implementing regulations (Directiva No. 2007/SIS-J), May 2007, shoe-shiners, "organizaciones socials de base" (primarily women's grassroots organizations such as community kitchens and mothers' clubs), and day care providers through the state Wawa-Wasi program were no longer included. Groups of victims previously delineated as victims of human rights abuses, forced sterilization, and political violence were no longer separately specified. The regulations state a single group "beneficiaries of health reparations." Local voluntary health promoters (*agentes comunitarios de salud*) and other groups such as Andean and Amazonian rural populations maintained their benefits. In December 2008 García declared that two thousand neighborhood leaders (the majority men) who attended a political event in their honor would receive SIS coverage for themselves and their families (*El Comercio,* December 7, 2008).

34. Speech, July 28, 2006, reprinted in *El Comercio,* October 13, 2006, http://www .elcomercio.com.pe/EdicionOnline/Html/2006-07-28/onlPolitica0549038.html (accessed June 28, 2007).

system" (*sistema único*).[34] Peru's strong economic performance through the mid-2000s also afforded a positive economic context to expand the insurance.

There were regional influences for the shift toward more universal options as well. Broader health insurance mechanisms for the poor had been introduced in other countries, such as Plan Auge in Chile and Seguro Popular in Mexico. The accord was similar to these in its emphasis on universal insurance but not a single system, and in its call for a basic plan of guaranteed services. The Chilean and Mexican programs have been of interest to Peru's policy makers as models on which to refashion and expand integral health insurance. Officials from the Chilean and Mexican health systems have come to Peru to consult on the issue, displaying the continuing strength of regional transnational networking on health reform (Interview Cuentas 2007; Interview Garavito 2007).

But how well did the insurance perform with regard to gender equity? An important distributional aspect of gender equity is how beneficiaries are identified. Integral insurance changed its mode of beneficiary identification several times between its inception in 2001 and 2007. When the two previous insurance programs were combined in 2001, health insurance was no longer tied to school attendance and effectively became universal for all school-age children whether or not they attended school. (The switch was political as well, as school-based insurance was a hallmark of the Fujimori era.) In March 2002 the mother-infant aspect of the insurance shifted from geographic targets to universal insurance for all gestating mothers and children under four. In the third trimester of 2003 the program implemented a means-testing mechanism applied to all beneficiaries individually. In the second semester of 2004 means testing was abandoned in rural areas but maintained in urban areas (ParSalud 2007, 2).

These changes in beneficiary identification have important consequences. First, as discussed previously, school insurance identification based on school attendance worked against rural girls. After the delinking of school attendance and health insurance, by 2008 there was no longer a significant gap in coverage between rural boys and girls. Among rural children ages ten to seventeen, 77.2 percent of boys and 76.5 percent of girls reported coverage under the SIS program, a negligible difference and an improvement over the SEG.[35] This coverage has also translated into greater user rates of health care services. A rural child affiliate of SIS is 2.9 times more likely than a

---

35. Author's calculations from ENAHO (2008), cross-tabulation of sex and SIS coverage among children ages ten to seventeen, $N = 1,456$, $p = 0.737$.

nonaffiliate rural child to use health services (ParSalud 2007, 14). Second, the regionally targeted form of mother-child insurance missed many of the mothers most in need. The expansion of mother-child insurance to all poor gestating mothers was important for equity in that it now reached more mothers in need. Insurance affiliations demonstrate that by 2008 the SIS program had led to significantly greater numbers of women covered by health insurance, effectively reversing earlier trends of undercoverage (table 7.2).

The new insurance had a single means-testing instrument, the Socioeconomic Evaluation Form (Ficha de Evaluación Socioeconómica, FESE), a vast improvement over the haphazard methods described in chapter 5. Again, the neoliberal epistemic community played a role. The instrument was developed with the financial support of USAID, through its health reform projects in Peru, Proyecto 2000 and Partners for Health Reform Plus. Peru's instrument was based in large part on the Colombian one.[36] USAID financed a number of studies that tested its ability to accurately identify and differentiate between poor and extremely poor households (Madueño, Linares, and Zurita 2004). Rather than poverty-line or income-measurement methods, it used a statistical index of economic well-being in which beneficiaries were assigned points for variables such as location, composition, and size of their dwelling; plumbing, electrical, and telephone connections; ownership of appliances such as refrigerators and televisions; sex, age, and education level of household head; and number of household members who work versus number of dependents (Interview Cuentas 2007).

Although the instrument is a significant improvement over those I observed in the late 1990s, it still has a number of shortcomings. In terms of design, it fails to capture two important aspects of poverty. First, and critical for gender equity, it does not capture intrafamilial poverty or power relations (discussed in chapter 5) that may deny especially women and girls the resources to pay for health services in families that are categorized as nonpoor. Second, the instrument does not capture the temporarily poor. An estimated 25 percent of Peru's population have been classified as poor at least once in a four-year period, making this a significant oversight (Chacaltana 2002, cited in Madueño, Linares, and Zurita 2004, 25). A third questionable design aspect is that it asks whether the person making the request for the insurance uses contraception, and if so, what type (SIS 2004). The addition is curious in that none of the studies that led to the design of the instrument

---

36. The Colombian instrument, the Sistema de Selección de Beneficiarios (SISBEN), is used for health and general poverty alleviation programs.

Table 7.2 Sex and insurance affiliations over time

	1991 Prereform and midcrisis			1994 Postcrisis and midreform			2008 Postreform		
	Male	Female	Total	Male	Female	Total	Male	Female	Total
Private insurance	4.9%	7.6%	5.8%	1.3%	1.3%	1.3%	1.4%	1.2%	1.3%
	64	47	111	121	128	249	153	132	285
EPS	n/a	n/a	n/a	n/a	n/a	n/a	0.2%	0.2%	0.2%
							22	22	44
IPSS or EsSalud	54.3%	49.6%	52.8%	19.4%	19.6%	19.5%	18.7%	18.3%	18.4%
	711	307	1,018	1,771	1,883	3,654	2,047	2,033	4,080
Military/police insurance	4.3%	0.3%	3.0%	1.6%	1.9%	1.7%	1.8%	1.4%	1.6%
	56	2	58	142	178	320	198	161	359
SIS	n/a	n/a	n/a	n/a	n/a	n/a	33.2%	38.8%	35.8%
							3,632	4,319	7,951
None/de facto public system	36.6%	42.5%	38.5%	77.0%	76.3%	76.6%	45.7%	41.1%	43.2%
	479	263	742	7,014	7,309	14,323	5,004	4,576	9,580
	$p = 0.000$ $N = 1,929$			$p = 0.223$ $N = 19,285$			$p = 0.000$ $N = 22,072$		

SOURCES: Author's calculations from ENAHO 1991, 1994, 2008.

identified family planning use as integral to determining poverty level; in fact, the question is not included in the eligibility criteria (Interview Cuentas 2007). One can speculate that the addition has more to do with government demographic objectives than with determining poverty level. It is thus a questionable and invasive addition.

In its implementation, the means-testing instrument also has a number of shortcomings. First, those charged with implementation were often health professionals untrained in means testing (Defensoría del Pueblo 2007, 116). According to one study of six sample districts in three departments, of those charged with filling out the instrument, 43 percent had received only one training session and 10 percent had no training at all (Sabhaperu 2007, 25). This study and an investigation by the Defensoría del Pueblo found that the instrument was often inaccurately filled out. In 2004 91.5 percent of the applications in the Defensoría's sample of 200 applications from a variety of health establishments were missing at least one variable related to dwelling, and 91.5 percent did not register the educational level of the head of household. Based on a sample of five hundred applications from 2006, the Defensoría found marked improvement, but still 27 percent did not contain all relevant variables with regard to dwelling (Defensoría 2007, 154). Such inaccuracies mean that determinations of poverty level are suspect in spite of what may be a well-intentioned design.[37]

A comparison of the period in which the insurance was universally granted to the one in which all beneficiaries were subject to means testing is also instructive as to the efficacy of the instrument in practice. Data compiled by ParSalud (the office financed by the IDB and World Bank to support implementation of the insurance) from insurance affiliation records show that introducing the means-testing instrument in 2004 led to a dramatic drop in affiliations across all economic levels—a drop only mitigated when the instrument was dispensed with in rural areas later that year. For example, affiliates to Plan C, for gestating mothers, dropped by more than half when the instrument was introduced. The largest drop in affiliations of children under five also occurred in this time period (ParSalud 2007, 4, 9). The fact that the drops occurred as much among the poor as among the nonpoor raises serious questions about the utility of the means-testing instrument, and whether some of the "snap judgments" described in chapter 5 still reign.

37. Providing insurance automatically to victims of past political violence, as stipulated by the law, appears to be a major shortcoming of the program. According to the Defensoría, local health professionals have frequently not granted these victims automatic coverage (2007, 75–77).

In addition to distributional concerns, there is some emerging evidence that the means-testing instrument is causing rifts in recognition between different members of society. These are alluded to in the report by the Defensoría del Pueblo, which finds that health professionals have preferred to treat patients who pay out of pocket rather than those covered by integral insurance. These practices are in part a result of the central office tendency not to fully reimburse costs or to reimburse very slowly (Defensoría del Pueblo 2007; ParSalud 2007). One citizen's 2008 testimonial mirrors some of the tensions I observed in the late 1990s between patients and health center cashiers: "The attention of the administrative personnel is a bit cold. . . . Because we go with a piece of paper that the government has given us doesn't mean that we deserve mistreatment . . . because you don't have any money you have to wait until the end to be seen" (quoted in ForoSalud 2008, 11). Treating integral health insurance beneficiaries poorly, regardless of cause, feeds into a larger cycle of creating social divisions, with some citizens viewed as more deserving than others.

Another contributor to these recognition divisions is the central concern of policy makers and aid agencies with "filtrations"—persons receiving free insurance who are not poor (see Defensoría del Pueblo 2007; ParSalud 2007; Sabhaperu 2007). Given the scarcity of resources and the desire to reach those most in need, this concern is valid. However, an overemphasis on "free riders" can have negative consequences, demonizing those who receive free benefits as "undeserving" (as seems to be a practice among some health professionals) or creating negative feelings between those who do and do not receive them, as evidenced in other social programs.[38]

Finally, fees and their gender-inequitable features have not disappeared with integral insurance. A 2008 study by the civil society organization ForoSalud reported that 37 percent of those surveyed in metropolitan Lima were charged a fee for joining SIS (contrary to the law), and another 29 percent reported that all their consultation and treatment costs were not covered as they should have been (ForoSalud 2008, 9, 14).[39] One mother described taking her daughter to have a tooth pulled: "And they told me no, the insurance doesn't cover that. I paid for the consultation, but the insurance did not

38. In the parallel Juntos program, where cash transfers are given to mothers as an incentive to keep children in school and take them to clinics regularly, researchers found antipathy between those who did and did not receive the benefit (Jones, Vargas, and Villar 2007).

39. Fees were an ongoing problem in SIS. For 2002 figures, see ENAHO (2002), cited in Minsa-OPS (2003, 53).

cover the extraction. . . . I opted to give her a pain reliever, because I don't have the money to pay for the treatment" (quoted in ForoSalud 2008, 15).

As discussed in chapter 5 and in the section on social security system copays, fees impose a greater burden on women because they tend to need health care services more, dedicate financial resources to children's health care, and have smaller independent incomes. Contributing to the tendency to charge fees is the fact that local health centers and health posts still face significant pressures to generate fees for services (Amnesty International 2006). Slow reimbursements from the central SIS office also create the incentives discussed above to seek fee-paying clients, and even to deceive patients into paying fees they rightfully should not have to pay (Defensoría del Pueblo 2007, 77–78; Interview Olea 2007; Interview Garavito 2007).

SIS has been fairly successful in providing insurance to the poorest, especially the rural populations, which are those most in need. In 2006 50.5 of all affiliates were rural residents, while another 27.7 percent were in poor urban communities (Defensoría del Pueblo 2007, 66); by 2008 the number of rural affiliates (also majority indigenous) had risen to 66.2 percent (author's calculation from ENAHO 2008). As an insurance mechanism rather than actual health facilities and equipment, integral health insurance is easy to disseminate to rural and marginal areas. This also means that while affiliates may have the right, based on insurance, to care, the program has not necessarily changed the quality or distribution of existing health services. This shortcoming was addressed to some degree in 2006 when President Toledo decreed that the insurance would cover transport from local health establishments to regional or national establishments.[40] This change was significant for rural populations, who otherwise had to bear the transport cost individually, as described in chapter 5. While its rate of rural coverage is good for equity, better-off regions have higher affiliation rates, indicating continuing inequities in access to health care between rich and poor and from region to region (Vera la Torre 2003, 42–43). Moreover, the program has had more success serving the merely poor than its target group of the extremely poor (Defensoría del Pueblo 2007, 118–39).

The program also faces major financial difficulties in achieving coverage of its target population. Full coverage of current target beneficiaries will require significant increases in government allocations to the health sector. Early in

40. Decreto Supremo No. 006-2006SA, March 21, 2006, cited in Defensoría del Pueblo (2007).

the program, budget increases were substantial (28.7 percent in its first year over school health and maternal-infant allocations; Vera la Torre 2003, 28), but the insurance required continual economic growth, political support, and careful fiscal management at the ministry level (OPS-Perú 2002). Perhaps the most significant finding in a 2007 report by the Defensoría del Pueblo was that the insurance has been vastly underfunded with respect to the needs of its beneficiary population. Funding actually dropped between 2006 and 2007 (from 271 million to 267 nuevos soles) despite plans to broaden coverage, including to those in the semisubsidized plan.

Although the SIS reform did not significantly change the distribution of care work between the state and society, until May 2007 it did provide free health care to women volunteers in poor communities.[41] It thus provided some recognition of and compensation for the vital social reproductive role these women play. However political the motivation, health insurance for the thousands of poor women who dedicate significant time and personal resources to maintaining the social and human fabric of poor communities is a small price for the important benefits Peru reaps from their unpaid labor. The 2007 discontinuation of this benefit to the community volunteers may be a cost savings or a shift away from populism. It also may have been a way to stop a process of negative neighborhood politicization: leaders of base organizations had the authority to select members from their organization to receive the benefit, leading to infighting. In its place, however, policy makers should consider other ways of compensating these women for their vital social reproductive work.

SIS also has had significant gaps in recognizing gender-based health needs throughout the life cycle. Plan C, which targets gestating women, does recognize the vital need for expert assistance during pregnancy and childbirth. Moreover, there is some evidence of improvement over the previous mother-child insurance. For example, use of the drug oxytocin to reduce postpartum hemorrhage has increased from 44 to 93 percent of births among affiliates to the integral insurance, while training of personnel for better quality childbirths has also increased (ParSalud 2007, 24). The plan also includes coverage of birth complications such as hemorrhaging, the leading cause of maternal mortality.[42]

With the exception of gestating mothers, however, until March 2007 SIS ignored most other gender-based health needs, and, most critically, did not

41. See above, note 33.
42. This coverage also allows for treating incomplete abortions that result in hemorrhaging.

offer general reproductive health care. The care package in place until 2007 for extremely poor adults was limited to emergency care, topical care, surgery, and hospital stays. Basic reproductive health care for both men and women and detection of cervical cancer for women were left uncovered. Moreover, given that the insurance works as a reimbursement of costs, reimbursement only for care of gestating women arguably served as a disincentive to serve other health needs, including women's reproductive care.

This glaring gap in coverage—in spite of the fact that it would be more cost-efficient and relatively low-cost to provide such care—may be explained by the fact that the minister of health at the time the SIS was formulated was Fernando Carbone Campoverde, who belonged to the ultraconservative Catholic sect Opus Dei. The ParSalud program was charged by the World Bank to devise the original package of services for integral health insurance in 2001–2. The team originally included reproductive health care, but this element was removed by the ministry before the package was finalized (Interview Garavito 2007). The exact motivation behind finally including reproductive health care is unclear, though it may have been due to change in the director and in the policy direction of the insurance toward more integral rather than targeted health needs (Interview Cuentas 2007). The change may also have been due to critiques of the lack of inclusion of reproductive health care from international agencies such as UNFPA and feminist organizations.[43] Still, some restrictions remained. Emergency contraception, for example, as of 2007 was provided only in cases such as rape, not on demand, in spite of its legality in Peru (Interview Cuentas 2007).

While the noninclusion of reproductive health care and even the current restrictions on emergency contraception are extremely inefficient over the long term, there are other examples in which "efficiency" concerns have led to health care exclusions that are gender-inequitable.[44] In the revised 2007 list of allowed treatments (which differentiates between subsidized and semisubsidized regimens), there are limitations on birthing coverage in the semisubsidized regimen. A beneficiary cannot be pregnant at the time of signing up for the insurance and cannot use the prenatal and birthing benefits for the first ten months of the insurance contract. Given that the

43. UNFPA did not directly lobby for the change, but in public forums had systematically critiqued the lack of inclusion of reproductive health care in the previous package (Interview Zamora 2007).
44. A check for cervical cancer is much less costly than treatment of advanced intra-uterine cancer; emergency contraception is much less costly than childbirth (especially an unwanted birth).

coverage contract is renewed annually, the way this exclusion is currently written means that there is only a two-month window during the year in which pregnant women in the semisubsidized regime can receive prenatal and birthing care—effectively excluding most beneficiaries from the birthing benefit. Moreover, this exclusion appears not to be an oversight, but a cost-saving calculation (Interview Garavito 2007).[45]

The focus on women only as gestating mothers is striking in the way treatment of AIDS was incorporated into the program. Previously, testing for AIDS had been voluntary. In June 2004 Law 28243 made HIV/AIDS testing obligatory for pregnant women, denying them the choice for testing that others were given.[46] Although the test is mandatory, it is not free, with hospitals and health posts charging from fifteen to twenty-five soles (U.S. five to eight dollars; Interview Olea 2007). A pregnant woman found to have HIV/AIDS was treated for the disease only during pregnancy, to avoid mother-child transmission (CESIP and Manuela Ramos 2005, 22–23). Nonpregnant adults (men and women) were specifically excluded from AIDS treatment under the insurance plan. The effect was to value women's health only to the extent that it affected that of her fetus; once the child was born or prior to pregnancy the woman's health condition was unimportant. The 2007 revised package of services removed AIDS treatment altogether, providing just prevention services. The limited treatment provided until 2007 and now the lack of treatment altogether work against a sense of common humanity among Peruvians because only those with social security health care coverage are guaranteed AIDS treatment. Finally, integral health insurance has no mechanism for providing affiliates a voice in their health care system.

Gendered Convergences and Divergent Legacies

Although the social security insurance and public insurance reforms seem to move in different directions (toward greater private sector care versus greater state-provided care), and despite their radically different political roots, the two insurances present similar problems with regard to gender equity. In terms of distribution, both reforms present concerns. In the reconfigured social security health system, although several of Peru's norms and

45. The revised package is outlined in Decreto Supremo 004-2007-SA, March 2007. Other questionable aspects are vague exclusions such as "aggressions" (*agresiones*) and complications of medical or surgical care—effectively excluding care for mistakes by health personnel.
46. This law modified the preexisting AIDS law, Law 26626.

regulations protect women from the egregious economic discrimination they face in other largely privatized systems, such as Chile's and Colombia's, barriers to gender equity remain. The copays in the EPS system and for informal sector workers affiliated with EsSalud discriminate against women. In addition, EPS has no services for the rural sector. In the evolution of targeted insurance, there have been distinct distribution issues in each phase. In the SEG the focus on school-attending children interacted with gender biases in rural communities to skew the insurance benefit toward boys. Maternal child insurance simply did not reach the poorest regions. The SIS program is broader in reach, but lack of funding and old modes of discrimination on the ground have led to illegal fees being charged with regularity, affecting women more than men. Neither reform really addressed the distribution of care work, though the free insurance to women volunteers in poor communities was a short-lived nod to the valuable community care these women provide.

In terms of recognition, neither reform has attended well to women's health through the life cycle. Important laws are in place requiring private insurers to cover basic reproductive care for women, but care for older women through private insurers is costly due to higher copays in the EsSalud system and higher deductibles or exclusions by the private insurers. In the maternal-infant and SIS targeted insurances, the focus has been solely on pregnant women, ignoring health needs during other parts of their life cycle. Second, the drive for "cost savings" often cuts corners precisely on the gender-based health needs women require. This is most evident in the ten-month pregnancy waiting period in the semisubsidized insurance regime, and in the previous limits on AIDS treatment to only gestating mothers.[47] Private insurance packages offered to independent workers also charge additional fees for maternity coverage. Such strategies may save the state or private companies money, but ultimately these costs fall on the women and families in need, a shift in burden rather than a savings.

Finally, both private and state-provided insurance have important exclusions that arise not from cost incentives, but from politically or religiously conservative politics. Many of these exclusions, ironically, are *inefficient*. The exclusion of reproductive health services from the SIS program until 2007 is one example, as is the limited distribution of emergency contraception.

---

47. To see if this is a pattern in the social security system as well, a study of instances when the vague EsSalud policy not to treat "high-cost" illnesses is applied, and whether women's health needs are compromised in the process, would be warranted.

The limits in care for abortion complications in both insurances are more examples, as is the fact that therapeutic abortion is rarely granted in the social security system.

Thus, these reforms converge in some surprising ways, despite their distinct genesis and approaches. Yet they also diverge in ways that may be quite consequential for long-term gender, class, and racial stratification. The entry of private health care providers, rather than creating greater commonalities among Peruvians, has led to greater stratification with class, gender, and race components. The private EPS system is of higher quality than state social security health services; 90 percent of EPS affiliates surveyed in a study by the superintendent of health considered EPS health services better than those of EsSalud (SEPS 2005, 24). Yet this system serves the upper class, primarily formal sector workers in the largest, wealthiest companies—and only these employees have a choice of health provider (Carbajal and Francke 2003, 523). This class composition has a racial correlate; according to 2008 household survey data, no indigenous persons are served by the EPS system (table 7.3). The EPS system also privileges males slightly more than females, and places females to a greater degree in more precarious dependent insured status. But this reform has remained quite limited in its reach. As the data on changes in insurance affiliations over time by sex and race presented in tables 7.2 and 7.3 show, the EPS serve less than 1 percent of the Peruvian population.

The SIS, while its means-testing instrument creates some stigmatization, has the potential to reduce stratification in the long term. The statistical trends on sex and insurance coverage in tables 7.2 and 7.3 show that the SIS demonstrates a tendency toward less stratification and greater universalization. One can observe a shift from "before reform," in which the state social security system, which served a majority of *mestizo* males, had more than 50 percent of the health insurance market, to a flattening of gender distinctions between health systems due to the economic crisis. In 1994 *mestizos* still dominated the social security system, but the dramatic informalization of the Peruvian economy as a result of the economic crisis meant that females and males were now equally represented in both the social security and public health systems. Moreover, the public system came to serve more than 75 percent of the population. In the postreform period, especially with the SIS reform, we see numbers of women and—to the extent that statistics can capture the fluid notion of race in Peru—indigenous peoples with health insurance jump dramatically, reversing earlier underinsurance trends.

Table 7.3 Race and insurance affiliations over time*

	1991 Prereform and midcrisis			1994 Postcrisis and midreform			2008 Postreform		
	Mestizo	Indigenous	Total	Mestizo	Indigenous	Total	Mestizo	Indigenous	Total
Private insurance	6.0% 107	2.8% 4	5.8% 111	1.4% 209	1.1% 33	1.3% 242	1.6% 267	0.2% 10	1.3% 277
EPS	n/a	n/a	n/a	n/a	n/a	n/a	0.3% 42	0% 0	0.2% 42
IPSS or EsSalud	53.6% 957	42.1% 61	52.8% 1,018	20.9% 3,113	13.8% 428	19.7% 3,541	21.3% 3,465	9.6% 436	18.7% 3,901
Military/police insurance	3.1% 56	1.4% 2	3.0% 58	1.8% 276	1.3% 39	1.7% 315	2.0% 322	0.6% 29	1.7% 351
SIS	n/a	n/a	n/a	n/a	n/a	n/a	30.5% 4,964	47.6% 2,157	34.1% 7,121
None/de facto public system	37.2% 664	53.8% 78	38.5% 742	75.0% 11,198	83.2% 2,576	76.4% 13,774	45.6% 7,417	42.0% 1,901	44.6% 9,318
	p = 0.001 N = 1,929			p = 0.000 N = 18,020			p = 0.000 N = 20,799		

*Race is measured by mother tongue. Quechua, Aymara, and other indigenous languages are coded as indigenous, Spanish mother tongue is coded as mestizo.
SOURCES: Author's calculations from ENAHO 1991, 1994, 2008.

This statistical trend is limited to one aspect of health care, however: insurance coverage and related stratification. The insurance is for free coverage in the same public health system which has traditionally served these groups, and which is of significantly lower quality than the EPS or EsSalud options. Insurance has not changed the quality or distributional reach of the public health system. Moreover, women's health coverage is largely restricted to birthing care under Plan C of the program. Finally, insurance is only one factor related to access to health care; as outlined in chapter 5, other factors, such as geography, language, staff attitudes, and availability of services (including gender-specific services), are also important.

The fact that the one reform that appears to be having a positive effect on stratification stemmed from a populist political impulse may also serve as a lesson. While the relationship between populism and gender is far from predictable (Kampwirth, forthcoming), in this case the extension of greater social rights through populist means bodes well for this one aspect of gender equity. The interest in reaching out to broad groups of the poor can have the side effect of alleviating class stratification and potentially gender and race stratification. While populism is usually condemned due to its associated authoritarianism and lack of democratic channels, political rights in the absence of social rights, as Ruth Lister notes, are meaningless (Lister 1997). The SIS reform at least appears to be extending social rights.

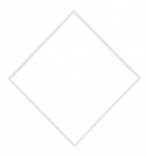

Conclusion

In the mid-1990s the "Washington Consensus" was on the cusp of change. The major international financial institutions had begun to respond to critiques of their top-down policy making style and their orthodox approach to economic stabilization in developing nations. Their response included loosening loan conditions to allow for government spending on social policies such as health care and education, as long as this spending fit new efficiency standards and priorities. With this shift in the nature of neoliberalism also came a wave of social policy reforms that sought to apply market principles to state social policies. These reforms reconfigured social policy systems in important ways and also introduced new political dynamics. Despite the high profile of transnational feminism in this period, however, gender equity was not a priority of the reform agenda.

As Latin American reformers set about reforming health systems, they saw inefficiencies and inequalities between rich and poor. Policy makers even recognized historic policy interest group legacies—labor unions and doctors' associations—that they would have to contend with to reform the health system. These inefficiencies and class-based inequalities were real and critical. What reformers did not see were the ways in which health systems were historically *not just* a product of class contestation and co-optation and a perpetuation of class-based inequalities in access to health care. Gender and race inequities were also fundamental to those political and social dynamics.

In this book I have exposed the role of gender and race in both the long-term policy formation processes and the shorter-term politics of Peru's health sector reforms at the turn of the twenty-first century. I have also demonstrated how the neoliberal reforms of the 1990s and 2000s in Peru had significant ramifications for gender and racial as well as economic equity. These inequalities are intertwined, and thus one cannot simply combat one without recognizing their intersectionality.

The Peruvian experience of health reform provides several broad theoretical lessons. The longer-term story of health reform in Peru helps develop an improved theory of policy legacies that understands policy legacies not as neutral political factors, but as factors that carry with them clear implications for gender, race, and class inequality. The shorter-term politics of reform furthers our understanding of these legacies by demonstrating when and how some legacies can be overcome while others remain in place. Analysis of the failure of gender mainstreaming in these politics of reform, moreover, helps identify the key elements necessary for successful gender mainstreaming. Examination of the impact of these reforms on the everyday lives of Peruvians provides broader lessons in the ways in which market-oriented reforms impact gender equity. Finally, the Peruvian case demonstrates the value of an intersectional approach, while showing that assumptions about gender, race, and class developed in one context will not necessarily be the same in another.

Gendered and Racialized Legacies

The longer-term view afforded by a policy legacies approach to understanding social policy reform allows one to see the lasting and therefore more powerful influences of policy feedbacks over time. More than simply reinforcing or strengthening the power of particular political actors or serving to reinforce the policy "status quo," as previous theorists have conceived of them, policy legacies also entrench the class, gender, and race inequalities on which they arise. In the process of Peru's health sector reform, some legacies were defeated, others were left in place, while others, possibly new legacies, were spawned. Each of these legacies carried particular gender, race, or class implications.

The masculine and *mestizo* class-based power of labor unions and doctors was severely curtailed in the reform process. These interest groups were legacies of the early history of co-optation in the health sector as well as the growth of the health system itself. They were the state's greatest adversaries in the reform process, especially in the reforms to the social security health system that affected these groups' particular privileges. A combination of factors led to the overcoming of these once-powerful legacies, including a consensus among those engaged in the neoliberal epistemic community that these groups were the major threat to reforms and needed to be overcome. In addition, the growing authoritarianism of the Fujimori government and the relative insulation of the reform process facilitated reformers' ability to defeat these interest groups. Although doctors and unions are still organized as interest groups in Peru, their powers over health sector politics have diminished markedly from their prereform status.

Yet reformers were quite comfortable maintaining other legacies. The class- and race-based legacy of political silence among Peru's poor and indigenous populations fit quite comfortably with the technocratic, closed approach to policy making of the reform era. As in the past, contemporary reformers viewed these groups as "human capital" rather than rights-bearing citizens. These groups lacked the political power that unions, doctors, or other key actors of the sector have traditionally had, and thus their needs and demands did not figure centrally in the reform agenda except as human capital measures. The continuing lack of a broader commitment to racial equity in the health system is evidenced in a growing dissatisfaction with public health care facilities, dissatisfaction in part rooted in lack of cultural understanding between health care users and the professionals that serve them.[1]

The policy learning legacy of controlling women's bodies for economic or demographic targets also continued through the reform period, as tragically illustrated by the family planning program's sterilization campaigns. While the letter of this policy was significantly rights-based, key government documents revealed that the underlying neo-Malthusian agenda of the government remained unchanged. Instead, the Fujimori government hijacked reproductive rights discourse disingenuously to appear more democratic. The ineffectiveness of the rights-based epistemic community, of which feminists were a part, was part of the reason behind this ironic turn of events.

---

1. In a survey conducted by Peru's Defensoría del Pueblo, the number dissatisfied with the "acceptability" of state health services grew from 20 percent of their sample in 2004 to 65 percent in 2006. Some of this dissatisfaction was strictly related to cultural factors, such as language barriers or lack of respect by medical providers for indigenous health practices (Defensoría 2007, 220–22).

But it was also stymied due to the authoritarian and neoliberal character of policy making in this regime. At the same time, the new neoliberal emphasis on cost-efficiency and tying health policies to overall economic goals fit quite comfortably with this old historical learning legacy.

The reform process itself may have also spawned "new" policy interest and learning legacies. In other words, the new policies created in the reform period may in the future feed back into the policy process. The one reform that already seems to have created what Paul Pierson calls a "lock-in" effect, in which a popular expectation that the program will continue cements a particular policy approach, is the targeted insurance for the poor, the SIS. This insurance, which began as populist-inspired school health insurance under President Fujimori, has persisted through three iterations and three presidents, and has come to represent the future of the Peru's health sector. Perhaps the greatest evidence of the power of this "new" legacy is that despite the identification of SIS with his predecessor, President García has vowed to expand it.

Identifying changes and continuities in policy legacies helps us to better understand the politics of the reform period and its potential impact into the future. But the gendered and racialized patterns of policy legacies stemming from the reform period do more: they provide clues to assessing the future potential for gender, class, and racial equity. In Peru the defeat of the masculine and *mestizo* interests of unions and doctors' associations, combined with the political popularity of the SIS targeted insurance, which has already proven to ameliorate some gender and racial stratification, has opened up the possibility for the future consolidation of the social security and the public health systems. In December of 2008 the government of Alan García presented to the Congress a bill for "Universal Health Insurance," which was passed by Congress in March 2009. The law builds on and extends the SIS program to still wider groups and provides a legal basis for an eventual basic health insurance for all.[2]

---

2. Reported in major Peruvian media outlets, e.g., RPP Noticias, "Gobierno aprueba Ley Marco del Seguro Universal de Salud," December 17, 2008, http://www.rpp.com.pe/2009-03-18-minsa-costo-de-atencion-por-aseguramiento-universal-sera-de-280-soles-al-ano-noticia_170867. html; La Republica, "Aprueban Ley de Aseguramiento Universal de Salud," December 17, 2008, http://www.larepublica.pe/sociedad/17/12/2008/aprueban-ley-de-aseguramiento-universal-de-salud; *RPP Noticias,* "Minsa: Costo de atención por aseguramiento universal será de 280 soles al año," March 18, 2009, http://www.rpp.com.pe/2008/10/30/una_japonesa_fue_secuestrada_ocho_a%C3%B10s_por_su_madre_esquizofrenica/2009-03-18-minsa-costo-de-atencion-por-aseguramiento-universal-sera-de-280-soles-al-ano-noticia_170867.html.

But there are other "new" policy legacies that may block progress toward equity. The likelihood of bringing the privately insured into a consolidated system is very low, due to the new interest group legacies created in the reform period. While the EPS are politically weak given their very small market of wealthy consumers, private sector interests are exceedingly hard to remove once lodged in state social policy systems, as the experiences of the United States and Chile demonstrate (Hacker 2002; Ewig and Kay 2008). Private providers will want to protect their profitability, and their insured will oppose losing their privilege of better-quality health care. The block that such interests would pose to full system consolidation is an important one for full equity, given that financial solidarity of the wealthy is necessary for the viability of a single, universal system. In addition, the interests and institutions created by the old social security system, although politically much weaker now than before, still may pose an important obstacle to a single health system.

Even though a single system would address important aspects of gender equity, such as the promotion of common citizenship rights, it is no guarantee of other aspects of gender equity. A universal system, for example, will likely continue the relatively new policy legacy of making decisions on a cost-efficiency basis. Given that cost-efficiency concerns often choose to be more "efficient" at the expense of women's health needs, this potential legacy does not bode well for gender equity, even in a "universal" system. In the short term, part of the key to addressing this risk is vigilant gender mainstreaming. In the long term it requires a defeat of the old policy learning legacies of the mother-child dyad approach to health care and of the view among both economic and social conservatives that women's bodies are appropriate terrains of control rather than vested with human dignity. If means testing becomes a legacy, it also may aggravate gender-, class-, and race-based inequalities. As such, any combined system must not only be universal in its coverage, but access to it must be based on citizen rights rather than income.[3] Moreover, it must be gender-aware in the content of its services.

Policy legacies not only uphold particular group interests, public expectations, or old policy tools, but also have real effects on equity and stratification by upholding gender, class, or racial interests. For feminist researchers

3. Fiscal constraints pose an obstacle to providing health care based on citizenship. However, better tax collection and equitable distribution of resources between health systems (or consolidation into one system) are two steps that can be taken to address fiscal limitations.

of social policy, legacies are critically important for recognizing how gender, race, and class play into political processes, and at the same time how negative legacies might be overcome in order to work toward a more equitable future.

The Gendered Politics of Reform

This analysis of the politics of Peru's health sector reform sought to understand why some policy legacies were overcome, but not others, and why feminists did not pursue "gender mainstreaming" in the area of health sector reform, despite their high profile and influence at the time, globally and nationally. The theory of epistemic communities, in which there must be not only a strong network of like-principled professionals, but also a context of crisis where these professionals are seen as the ones with the "answers" to a particular policy problem, helps to explain why some legacies were overcome in the reform period while others were not. The Peruvian government turned to the neoliberal epistemic community—composed of individuals working in IFIs, other international organizations, and Peruvian experts—for its market-based solutions to Peru's health problems at a time when the need to reform was perceived as one of crisis proportions. Significantly, this collusion led to the defeat of key policy interest legacies. The influence of this community waned as critics of neoliberalism questioned its principles and as the Peruvian state no longer perceived a crisis in health care, but in its decade of influence it had remarkable impact. By contrast, in areas where legacies were maintained, such as Malthusian-oriented population policies, despite a well-developed rights-based transnational epistemic community with clear interests in overturning this legacy, this community failed to have a real impact. Its links to the Peruvian bureaucracy were weaker, in part due to weaker financial ties. Perhaps more important, because there was not a perceived crisis in reproductive health care in the same way that there did exist such a crisis in basic public health care provision, the rights-based community was not viewed as needed expertise to resolve a pressing problem, but rather as a convenient set of attractive discourses that could be co-opted for political purposes, but not implemented in good faith.

One of the major roadblocks to gender mainstreaming was the competing influence of these two epistemic communities. The neoliberal community successfully framed some reforms as "gender-neutral" and thus without need for gender expertise. By contrast, family planning was viewed as an appropriately feminist domain, where feminists were invited to actively participate in its reform and oversee its implementation through the Mesa Tripartita. As a result, a gendered division of labor developed in the political process between "masculine" mainstream reforms and "feminine" family planning policy. Surprisingly, feminists themselves, due to their own networks and financial ties, accepted this division—that is, until global organizations like PAHO and the Ford Foundation encouraged interest in "mainstream" health reforms and a few feminists followed this call. Mainstreaming was made even more difficult by other factors. The insulated mode by which most of these reforms were formulated (a function of growing authoritarianism under Fujimori but also characteristic of neoliberalism) made influence difficult to achieve. And, ironically, feminist interests were also not facilitated by supposedly women-friendly state institutions, such as the Women's Ministry established under Fujimori.

The closed nature of policy making in the 1990s makes the input gained by feminists in the more rights-based family planning reform and their permanent dialogue with the government on family planning policy through the Mesa Tripartita all the more impressive. This was a rare instance of political access in an otherwise closed political process, and of successful gender mainstreaming. Yet the story of the family planning debacle in Peru also demonstrated that while this inside track of the Mesa Tripartita was important for gaining information from an otherwise insulated political system, equally important for confronting abuses in the family planning program was an autonomous base of feminist activism unconnected to the government.

Three key elements emerge from this analysis as necessary components for successful gender mainstreaming by feminist activists: global financial and discursive support for mainstreaming efforts; strong feminist connections in lateral spheres of political influence where policies are formulated and implemented; and an autonomous base in civil society for vigilance in the process of implementation. These elements will surely find resonance in the experience of other countries and other policy areas as well.

The Impact of Health Sector Reforms on Gender Equity

By documenting the effects of neoliberal health reforms on equity, conceived of intersectionally, I have sought to extend feminist studies of neoliberalism beyond structural adjustment to an understanding of the implications of "second-wave" social policy reforms for gender equity. Guided by a modified form of Nancy Fraser's twofold conceptualization of justice as redistribution and recognition, I conclude that neoliberal health policies, on the whole, have had a negative impact on women, the poor, and indigenous groups. Fully understanding the effects of market-based health reform and why it has had such negative impacts, however, requires the disaggregation of the broader package of reforms into the individual policies. These distinct policies had negative impacts on gender equity for different reasons and in different ways. Moreover, not all reforms were negative for gender equity; a few, unintentionally, had positive impacts.

Market-oriented health sector reforms have led to five main types of gender inequities, which span distributive and recognition aspects of justice: (1) inequities of economic access; (2) inequities in the distribution of care work; (3) inequities in serving gender-specific health needs; (4) inequities of voice in the health care system; (5) and inequities in full citizenship, whereby some health care users are denied the same common humanity as others (stratification). Not all of the reforms discussed in this book led to each of these inequities; most contributed to one or two. Taken as a whole, however, these are the five main ways that market-oriented health sector reforms impacted gender equity in Peru. Due to the similarity of health sector reforms across Latin America and even globally, these five main forms of gender inequity are likely to be encountered in other countries as well.

Economic access is not simply a class-related phenomenon, though the poor suffer more that the rich. It is also a highly gendered issue. Women, in Peru as in most countries, participate in paid work at lower percentages than men. When they are in the paid workforce they tend to be paid less than men and are more likely to work part-time and take more time off work to take care of children, the disabled, or the elderly. In Latin America working women tend to be concentrated in the informal sector, which pays less and affords no benefits. Women use health services more because of their reproductive health needs and their greater levels of morbidity than men, and because they live longer than men and thus need health services more in old age. Equity in economic access to health care, therefore, requires compensation for women's labor market discrimination, their lesser participation in the labor market due to their social reproductive roles, and their greater health care usage rates, which are largely biologically determined. Moreover, a gender analysis of economic access must also consider internal family gender dynamics and how male control of family cash assets or intrafamily gender power relations between men and women might affect the economic access of women or girls to health care services.

The drive for profitability or cost recovery through fees for services and through private, for-profit health care imposes a particular burden on women. In Peru, gender inequity in economic access manifested itself quite clearly in the case of the fees imposed in the public health system as well as the copays in the state social security health system. In both systems fees imposed a greater burden on women due to their higher usage rates combined with their greater dependency on family members to help pay health care costs. Women whose husbands refused to share the cost of fees were at greatest risk of not accessing care. Such risks were moderated somewhat in Peru's social security system, where providers were required by law to not charge copays for reproductive health care and care related to pregnancy. The social security and public health system, however, did not recognize women's greater health needs than men in old age due to greater longevity, and the fact that fees as a result pose a greater inequity for older women who also have lower incomes. In addition to inequities generated by fees, reforms that opened the insurance market to private, for-profit insurers also posed particular risks to gender equity. High-quality health services in Peru became even more tightly linked to an individual's insertion in the labor market, and in turn served to devalue the unpaid social reproductive work that women carry out. Moreover, many of the women who are affiliated with private insurers in Peru tend to be in the more precarious position of dependents on spousal policies.

The market does not recognize differences in male and female structural positions in the economy, nor does it recognize that intrafamilial gender relations may play a role in ability to pay. Moreover, insurers tend to view women's higher usage rates as risks of higher cost to the insurer rather than fundamental human needs. As a result, fees for services, copays, and market-based insurance programs tend to discriminate against women; this is a lesson that carries well beyond Peru to the majority of countries where gendered labor market inequalities and health utilization patterns also exist.

More equitable reforms would redistribute care work more evenly between women and men and shift family care work burdens to the state or the market. Ignoring the wealth of scholarship condemning the burden placed on women by economic shock therapies during the first-wave economic reforms, Peru's health reform policy makers showed little concern for the burden of care work that fell disproportionately on women as a result of market-mimicking health reforms. In fact, the use of women's unpaid labor continued to be a central strategy of cost savings, and the shift in care-work burden from states to families intensified. This shift was most evident in the Basic Health for All Program, which relied heavily on women's unpaid voluntary labor to meet health care goals such as vaccinations of children, child nutrition, and other basic elements of the basic package of services that it offered. In addition to a tremendous burden, such practices reify existing unequal gender relations, in which women's time is viewed as "free." Social policies throughout the world that tout "participation" must also be critically evaluated for the degree to which such participation may actually be reinforcing gendered care work patterns.

A third major gender inequity generated by Peru's reforms was a lack of recognition of both women's and men's essential gender-specific health needs. Women and men have different health needs based on biology, such as women's reproductive health needs. Other health needs are socially produced, and often such needs are influenced by gender, such as the social ill of violence, which manifests itself differently for men and women (more domestic violence aimed at women, and public, street violence among men). Moreover, women and men have specific health needs throughout their life cycle. Several of Peru's reforms entailed providing a specific package of services (in the Basic Health for All Program, the EPS minimal plan, and the SIS), but very often those packages did not cover crucial women's health services due to cost concerns. In the case of the Basic Health Package and in the original SIS, for example, complicated birth was not covered. The limitations on birthing coverage in the semisubsidized plan of the SIS also displayed this pattern, where women were essentially excluded from any birthing care at all. The proliferation of health reforms throughout the Latin American region that offer a "package" of services determined based on cost-effectiveness factors poses the same risk as those evident in Peru, that one or more critical gender-specific health needs will not be covered in these packages due to costs.

In curious contradiction to the otherwise fairly uniform drive for low-cost, high-impact health services in these packages, at times religiously conservative political powers or previous policy legacies were able to derail the drive for efficiency and prevent the inclusion of other women's health needs—such as screening for cervical cancer or provision of contraception—into the package, despite their low cost and large health benefits. The 2002 SIS package, for example, offered no reproductive health benefits outside of prenatal and natal care. The package was not only lacking in their coverage of full reproductive health care, but it also displayed a tendency to view women's health care *only* as reproductive health care, and ignored women's health needs in other moments of their life cycles. In other words, the policy legacy of the mother-child dyad became symbolic of women's health, to the point of erasing women's identities and rights to health care outside of motherhood. Perhaps the most disturbing example of this was the treatment of women for AIDS in the 2002 SIS package only when they were gestating mothers. The fact that such tendencies toward religious conservatism or viewing women's health as fundamentally mother's health are not exclusive to Peru, but worldwide, also shows the importance of vigilance toward these risks in other contexts, though the solutions for overcoming them may vary.

Full equity requires a voice in one's health system, including input into the policies as they are formulated and the right to shape and question services in their delivery stage. Peru's reforms were broadly inequitable on this point—little voice was allowed to health care users overall—but in those instances in which voice was allowed it was often gender-inequitable in practice. The only reform to explicitly incorporate health care users in decision-making roles was the CLAS. Yet the success of the CLAS in involving the participation of both men and women was highly contextual. In the rural areas CLAS committees were dominated by men, and the program accepted largely patriarchal practices that viewed decision making as men's domain. By contrast, in urban areas, where women were more organized in grassroots organizations, more women participated. This division also had a strong racial character, as language and cultural barriers worked against indigenous women's participation in the CLAS in rural areas. The CLAS program shows more broadly that even when providing channels for "voice," previous gender-, race-, and class-based patterns of political representation may interfere with seemingly gender-neutral policies, leading to unintended inequities.

The final major way in which these reforms generated inequity was in shaping a broader sense of citizenship or common humanity among Peruvians. Historically, Peru's health system has been highly stratified into separate and unequal systems, with the beneficiaries of the better-quality systems being largely working and middle class, male, urban, and either *mestizo* or white. Women, the poor, and rural indigenous peoples were clustered in the poor-quality public health system. The reform period had three main effects on stratification: economic, gendered, and racialized. The separate, higher-quality private EPS health system, available only to those who worked in the largest companies, served to further stratify Peruvians. This stratification was not just a question of economic status, but also gendered due to women's lesser participation in the formal workforce, lower salaries, and concentration in the informal sector. It was racialized for similar reasons, and also because the EPS private system serves only the primarily urban, largely *mestizo* and white-populated geographic areas of Peru. In the public system the means testing applied in the 1990s as well as the more sophisticated means-testing instrument developed in the 2000s also served to further divide Peruvians into "deserving" and "nondeserving" citizens. Means testing, as has been shown in other cases around the world, undermines a sense of common humanity, marking recipients as "defective" or "pathological" in contrast to the "independent" and "upstanding" individuals who do not seek state support.[4] The only reform that has begun to alleviate stratification (but with important caveats) was the one reform born of populist motives, the SIS, which has significantly altered the previous patterns of economic, gender, and racial stratification in insurance coverage.

Given the high level of regional and even transnational diffusion of "model" health reforms—such as Peru's borrowing of the Bolivian maternal-infant health insurance model or its modification of the Chilean private health insurer model—the findings in this book with regard to the impact of health reforms on gender equity have tremendous relevance for other countries. Maternal-child insurance programs in Bolivia and Ecuador (which like Peru based its program on the Bolivian model) ignore women's health needs throughout the life cycle, overlooking in particular the needs of older women, and thus present similar issues as the Peruvian case with regard to servicing all of women's health needs. Chile's private health insurance system has proven to be even less economically accessible to women than the Peruvian one, due to a lack of state regulation over private health providers, which allows them to charge women more for their higher "risk" of needing reproductive health services (Pollack 2002). It has also led to greater gender stratification than in Peru (Ewig 2008). Similar to Peru, Colombia cut costs by denying women critical health services such as mammograms and full diagnosis of cervical cancer (Ewig and Hernández 2009). The basic health care package implemented in Mexico was similar to Peru's in its dependence on women's unpaid care work for its success (Martínez et al. 2002). Finally, fees for health services have been shown to be negative for women's access to health care elsewhere in Latin America (Gómez Gómez 2002; Ewig and Hernández 2009).

---

4. For a rich discussion of this phenomenon in the Hungarian context, see Haney (2002).

While the specific rules and effects may vary, the broad patterns of second-wave health reforms are quite similar across the Latin American region and to some extent across the globe. The five major forms of gender inequities produced by market-oriented reforms are likely to hold true for most health sector reform experiences. In addition, I hope the framework that I present in chapter 1 for evaluating gender equity in health sector reforms along redistributive and recognition dimensions will prove useful for evaluations of reforms across Latin America and beyond.

An Intersectional Approach

While each of these five major forms of inequity generated by the neoliberal reforms fundamentally impacted *gender* equity, when analyzing gender equity we must remain aware of the diversity of women's and men's experiences and the ways that gender interacts with other factors such as class and race. By employing an intersectional analysis, I have been careful to specify *which* women and *which* men have the best access or the fullest citizenship with respect to health care. Although theories of intersectionality abound, empirical intersectional analyses are still rare. My findings demonstrate the importance of distinguishing among women and men of different race, class, and geographic backgrounds. For example, the CLAS reform affected rural, indigenous women's voice in the health care process quite differently from that of urban, largely *mestiza* women. The EPS reforms offered an opportunity of better-quality care for primarily elite, urban, and *mestizo* or white men, and to a lesser extent for women of similar economic and racial backgrounds. These distinctions provide a more fine-grained understanding of the effects of reforms on equity.

An intersectional approach can also provide insights into politics. For example, because the family planning program explicitly targeted poor urban and rural indigenous women, the problems with the program remained invisible to the mainly urban and *mestizo* feminists for some time. The interactions between gender, race, and class help, then, to explain feminists' slow reaction to the abuses of the program.

Applying an intersectional approach to Peru, far from its theoretical origins in the United States, also points to the need for some care when traveling with this particular theory. Assumptions about the impacts of combinations of race, class, and gender in the United States would not work in Peru, where race is understood quite differently and where its interactions with gender and class are also distinct. An intersectional analysis requires careful contextual knowledge of local understandings of race, class, and gender. Categorical approaches to intersectional analysis that utilize broad statistical data are useful in this endeavor, but may be meaningless or misunderstood in the absence of careful, intracategorical qualitative work that seeks to understand the meanings behind these categories.

Final Words

Perhaps most significant, this research has shown the importance of universal, yet difference-sensitive social policies as the key to gender equity, understood intersectionally. An ideal rights-based health system would be of universal quality and granted to all based on citizenship rather than income or occupation. It would also entail substantial financial solidarity across classes, genders, and races and provide voice to all. Finally, it would recognize specific gender-based health needs of men and women and strive to disrupt, rather than reinforce, inequitable patterns of care work, where women have faced the greatest burdens with the least amount of recognition.

As I write this conclusion, we are faced with a political moment when the rights-based epistemic community seems to be gaining ground, but when it is also still unclear what their full vision of "universal" health care might entail. Moreover, it is still unknown what role the policy legacies of the neoliberal era might play in struggles for greater equity into the future. In this new context, many countries in the Americas find themselves at a crossroads—they can remain with market-oriented models of health care or some version of these, or they can take a leap toward truly equitable, universal models of health care as a human right, and fight the political battles necessary to make this vision a reality. But what this book should have made clear by now is that the choice of market-oriented or rights-oriented health care is not just a question of addressing the gulf between rich and poor. Nor does a rights-based approach automatically resolve all inequities. Gender and its relationship to race and class need to be put squarely on future health policy reform agendas in order to truly promote equity and full health care rights.

methodological appendix

Critical to this study is a methodology that combines top-down analysis of policy formation with bottom-up, qualitative and quantitative analysis of policy implementation. In chapter 2 I provide a historical perspective on gender, race, and class in health policy formation in Peru, based on secondary historical materials. My findings regarding the politics of neoliberal reform, presented in chapter 3, are based upon process tracing the health reform process in Peru (George and McKeown 1985; George and Bennett 2005; Hall 2003). Using positional and reputational methods, I interviewed thirty-six national-level policy figures, some on more than one occasion. Most of these individuals were mid- and upper-level bureaucrats active in health reform formulation and implementation, but also included were three former ministers and one congressional representative. I also interviewed fourteen representatives of bilateral and multilateral institutions such as the World Bank, the Inter-American Development Bank, the United Nations Population Fund, the United Nations Children's Fund, the United States Agency for International Development, and the United Kingdom Department for International Development. I interviewed twenty-six leaders in Peru's civil society (again, some on multiple occasions) who represented organizations with an interest in health reform. These included leaders of associations of health professionals, labor unions, feminist organizations, health-related nongovernmental organizations, Catholic Church representatives, and private health insurers. I combined these interviews with analysis of government policy documents, congressional proceedings, and media reports to determine the politics of the reform process for each of Peru's major health reforms of the 1990s. Examination of the formulation process using these methods allowed me to identify the national and global political dynamics of health sector reform and the ways in which gender and race entered (or did not enter) into the reform agenda.

In the bottom-up analysis presented in the remainder of the book, I used multiple methods to assess the impact of health reforms on gender equity in

Peru, focusing on four poor communities, two urban and two rural. These communities included eight primary-level health centers, six in the urban communities and two in rural ones. (I did not include hospitals because reforms in this sector were too incipient to evaluate at the time that I carried out this research.) Because Peru is over 70 percent urban, I included more urban than rural centers in my sample. The difficulty of reaching the rural health centers and the dispersed populations that they served also led me to limit my rural sample to two health centers. Half of the health centers were CLAS centers, the other half were non-CLAS, PSBT centers.

These communities were all poor, with the urban areas considered poor and the rural areas extremely poor according to government classifications. The urban communities had only obtained water services a few years prior, and some settlements within these communities were still served by water trucks. Roads in these communities were largely unpaved. Most urban residents worked in the informal sector. In the rural areas basic public services were absent altogether, except in the cluster of homes immediately surrounding the health center. Most rural residents engaged in subsistence agriculture.

I employed a number of methods to measure the effects of reforms on gender equity: a survey; observation of health center activities; and interviews with health center staff, community members active in local health administration boards, and leaders of local community organizations. Survey questions measured gender equity in terms of access to services, the distribution of care work, and interfamilial health dynamics. I defined access as economic, geographic, and cultural access, with the redistributive and recognition elements described in chapter 1 in mind. I was also concerned with whether particular gender-based health needs—such as reproductive health care—were served. I asked, for example, whether respondents could pay for health services or medicines, how long it took them to get to the health center, whether health care providers understood their language and health concepts, and whether they felt the health center served their and their communities' health needs and priorities. To measure distribution of care work related to health, questions focused on the amount of time and money invested, and by whom, in both home-based and clinic-based health care. The survey also probed whether there were disparities in access to health care within families, or differential health care treatment within families (i.e., whether boys received more or better health care services than girls).

It was a stratified survey of community residents in the geographic area served by each health center. I piloted the survey in one of the urban communities prior to carrying out the survey in all four. I stratified my sample to include the range of economic variation within each community, with ratios based upon the health center census of each community. In urban areas I roughly determined socioeconomic level before selecting a respondent by observing the construction of their house (brick for better-off residents, adobe or scrap wood for less well off, and straw-mat or plastic-sheeting homes for the worst off). A few residents in each community with telephones were included as the best off. In rural areas, because home construction was almost uniformly of adobe, with an occasional straw or plastic structure, I used distance from the health center as a proxy for economic status. Those residents closer to the health center in the center of the district and thus closer to commerce and government tended to have more access to alternatives to agriculture and perhaps running water or electricity. Distant areas had none of these.

I also sampled each subcommunity or neighborhood served by the health center proportionate to the population it contributed to the geographic area served by the health center as a whole. I sampled men and women proportionately to their actual population in each community. Ten percent of each sample was of single mothers, as this was the percent of single mothers according to district-level 1993 census data (the most recent census at the time). With the aid of assistants, including a Quechua-speaking assistant in rural areas, we conducted the survey by knocking on doors and interviewing residents. Other than some preselection to stratify based on housing type and location, this was random. I administered approximately half of the interviews of the 193 persons interviewed for the survey, and my research assistants administered the other half.

To flesh out the relationship between the health centers and communities, I carried out fifty-nine positional interviews and six group interviews. I interviewed thirteen communal leaders among the four communities, such as leaders of local neighborhood councils, mothers' clubs, communal kitchens, health promoters, and rural militias (*rondas campesinas*). I carried out six group interviews with a selection of these kinds of organizations. I interviewed twenty-eight health professionals—a selection of at least three from each of the eight health centers, including the head doctor, the nurse-midwife, and the person charged with overseeing decisions regarding exoneration (if different from the head doctor). I interviewed twelve local health committee (CLAS) members, three on each board of seven members, at the four centers in my sample that were community-administered. I also interviewed a selection of staff and directors of the regional government health authorities that oversaw the centers, a total of six regional staff from the two regions where the communities were located. These were semistructured interviews, with a schedule of questions for each interview type (community leader, head doctor, etc.). Interview questions asked community leaders to consider whether there were economic, geographic, or cultural barriers that prevented some or all community members from accessing health care. They were asked in particular to think about whether there were different health care issues for women compared to men. In group interviews with women and separately with men, I asked whether their specific health concerns as women or men were addressed. I also asked interviewees what they thought of health center quality and whether the center had good or poor relations with the community and why.

In addition to interviews, I spent hours conducting ethnographic observation, including attending local health committee board meetings, observing health campaigns, participating in health center special events, and observing health center operations from the health center waiting rooms. I also observed and participated in the activities of mothers clubs and communal kitchens in the surrounding neighborhoods.

While the above methods provided me with a detailed picture of the implementation of health reforms in poor communities, and thus a gauge for evaluating their effects on local gender relations, I relied on national statistics and secondary studies to evaluate the effects of reforms to the social security system, which affected better-off Peruvians. I also relied on these secondary forms of data to evaluate more recent reforms to Peru's health system, such as the Seguro Integral de Salud, implemented after my major period of fieldwork in 1998–99.

I made four return trips to Peru after the first major stint of fieldwork to update this research through additional interviews with policy makers and members of health-related organizations in civil society.

references

Abbasi, Kamran. 1999a. "The World Bank and World Health: Changing Sides."
   British Medical Journal 318:865–69.
———. 1999b. "The World Bank and World Health: Under Fire." *British Medical
   Journal* 318:1003–6.
———. 1999c. "The World Bank and World Health: Interview with Richard
   Feachem." *British Medical Journal* 318:1206–8.
Abel, Christopher, and Peter Lloyd-Sherlock. 2000. "Health Policy in Latin America:
   Themes, Trends and Challenges." In Lloyd-Sherlock 2000, 1–20.
Abel-Smith, Brian. 2007. "The Beveridge Report: Its Origins and Outcomes."
   International Social Security Review 45 (1–2): 5–16.
Afshar, Haleh, and Carolyne Dennis, eds. 1992. *Women and Adjustment Policies in
   the Third World.* New York: St. Martin's Press.
Altobelli, Laura C. 1998a. "Comparative Analysis of Primary Health Care Facilities
   with Participation of Civil Society in Venezuela and Peru." Paper prepared
   for the seminar Social Programs, Poverty, and Citizen Participation, State
   and Civil Society Division, Inter-American Development Bank, Cartegena,
   Colombia, March 12–13.
———. 1998b. *Salud, reforma, participación comunitaria e inclusión social: El
   programa de Administración Compartida.* Lima: UNICEF-Peru.
Alvarez, Sonia. 1999. "Advocating Feminisms: The Latin American Feminist NGO
   'Boom.'" *International Feminist Journal of Politics* 2 (1): 181–209.
Amnesty International. 2006. *Perú: Mujeres pobres y excluidas: La negación del
   derecho a la salud materno-infantil.* http://web.amnesty.org/library/index/
   ESLAMR460042006 (accessed July 15, 2006).
Análisis Laboral. 1999. "Análisis del Proyecto de Ley No. 4363/98-CR, Sobre
   SISALUD." 23 (259): xiv–xviii.
Andreassen, Bård A., and Stephen P. Marks, eds. 2006. *Development as a Human
   Right: Legal, Political and Economic Dimensions.* Cambridge, Mass.: Harvard
   School of Public Health, Harvard University Press.
Anthias, Floya, and Nira Yuval-Davis. 1992. *Racialized Boundaries: Race, Nation,
   Gender, Colour and Class and the Anti-racist Struggle.* London: Routledge.
Arenas de Mesa, Alberto, and Veronica Montecinos. 1999. "The Privatization of
   Social Security and Women's Welfare: Gender Effects of the Chilean Reform."
   Latin American Research Review 34 (3): 7–37.
Arretche, Marta. 2004. "Toward a Unified and More Equitable System: Health
   Reform in Brazil." In Kaufman and Nelson 2004, 155–88.
Arróyo Laguna, Juan. 2000. *Salud: La reforma silenciosa.* Lima: Universidad
   Peruana Cayetano Heredia, Facultad de Salud Pública y Administración.

Aslanbeigui, Nahid, and Gale Summerfield. 2001. "Risk, Gender and Development in the 21st Century." *International Journal of Politics, Culture and Society* 15 (1): 7–26.

Babb, Sarah L. 2007. "Embeddedness, Inflation and International Regimes: The IMF in the Early Postwar Period." *American Journal of Sociology* 113 (1): 128–64.

Bachrach, Peter, and Morton S. Baratz. 1962. "Two Faces of Power." *American Political Science Review* 56 (4): 947–52.

Bakker, Isabella, ed. 1994. *The Strategic Silence: Gender and Economic Policy.* London: Zed Books.

———. 2003. "Neoliberal Governance and the Reprivatization of Social Reproduction: Social Provisioning and Shifting Gender Orders." In *Power, Production and Social Reproduction,* edited by Isabella Bakker and Stephen Gill, 66–82. New York: Palgrave Macmillan.

Bakker, Isabella, and Rachel Silvey, eds. 2008. *Beyond States and Markets: The Challenges of Social Reproduction.* New York: Routledge.

Banaszak, Lee Ann, Karen Beckwith, and Dieter Rucht, eds. 2003. *Women's Movements Facing the Reconfigured State.* Cambridge: Cambridge University Press.

Barker, Drucilla K., and Edith Kuiper. 2006. "Feminist Economics and the World Bank: An Introduction." In Kuiper and Barker 2006, 1–10.

Barrett, Deborah, and Amy Ong Tsui. 1999. "Policy as a Symbolic Statement: International Response to National Population Policy." *Social Forces* 78 (1): 213–33.

Barrientos, Armando, and Peter Lloyd-Sherlock. 2002. "Health Insurance Reforms in Latin America: Cream Skimming, Equity and Cost-Containment." In *Social Policy Reform and Market Governance in Latin America,* edited by Louise Haagh and Camilla T. Helgø, 183–99. New York: Palgrave Macmillan.

Barrig, Maruja. 1989. "The Difficult Equilibrium Between Bread and Roses: Women's Organizations and the Transition from Dictatorship to Democracy in Peru." In *The Women's Movement in Latin America: Feminism and the Transition to Democracy,* edited by Jane Jaquette, 114–48. Boston: Unwin Hyman.

———. 1992. "Nos habíamos amado tanto: Crisis del estado y organización feminina." In *La emergencia social en el Perú,* edited by Maruja Barrig, Lidia Elías, and Lisbeth Guillén, 7–17. Lima: ADEC-ATC.

———. 1999. *La persistencia de la memoria: Feminismo y estado en el Perú de los 90.* Lima: Proyecto Sociedad Civil y Gobernabilidad Democrática en los Andes y el Cono Sur, Fundación Ford.

Beall, Jo. 1997. "In Sickness and in Health." In *Searching for Security: Women's Responses to Economic Transformations,* edited by Isa Baud and Ines Smyth, 67–95. London: Routledge.

Bedford, Kate. 2007. "The Imperative of Male Inclusion: How Institutional Context Influences World Bank Gender Policy." *International Feminist Journal of Politics* 9 (3): 289–311.

Benería, Lourdes, and Shelley Feldman, eds. 1992. *Unequal Burden: Economic Crisis, Persistent Poverty and Women's Work.* Boulder: Westview Press.

Benería, Lourdes, and Maria S. Floro. 2006. "Labour Market Informalization, Gender and Social Protection: Reflections on Poor Urban Households in Bolivia and Ecuador." In Razavi and Hassim 2006, 193–216.

Bergeron, Suzanne. 2003. "The Post-Washington Consensus and Economic Representations of Women in the World Bank." *International Feminist Journal of Politics* 5 (3): 397–419.

Berkovitch, Nitza, and Karen Bradley. 1999. "The Globalization of Women's Status: Consensus/Dissensus in the World Polity." *Sociological Perspectives* 42 (3): 481–98.

Berman, Peter. 1995. "Health Sector Reform: Making Health Development Sustainable." In *Health Sector Reform in Developing Countries: Making Health Development Sustainable,* ed. Peter Berman, 13–33. Boston: Harvard University Press.

Bertranou, Fabio M. 2001. "Pension Reform and Gender Gaps in Latin America: What Are the Policy Options?" *World Development* 29 (5): 911–23.

Birkland, Thomas. 1997. *After Disaster: Agenda Setting, Public Policy and Focusing Events.* Washington, D.C.: Georgetown University Press.

Blondet, Cecilia, and Carmen Montero. 1995. *La situación de la mujer en el Perú 1980–1994.* Documento de Trabajo No. 68. Lima: Instituto de Estudios Peruanos.

Bock, Gisela, and Pat Thane, eds. 1991. *Maternity and Gender Policies: Women and the Rise of the European Welfare States, 1880s–1950s.* New York: Routledge.

Bockman, Johanna, and Gil Eyal. 2002. "Eastern Europe as a Laboratory for Economic Knowledge: The Transnational Roots of Neoliberalism." *American Journal of Sociology* 108 (2): 310–52.

Boli, John, and George M. Thomas. 1997. "World Culture in the World Polity: A Century of International Non-governmental Organization." *American Sociological Review* 62 (2): 171–90.

Boloña, Carlos. 1994. *Políticas aracancelerias en el Perú, 1880–1980.* Lima: Instituto de Economía de Libre Mercado.

Bonoli, Giulano, Vic George, and Peter Taylor-Gooby. 2000. *European Welfare Futures.* Cambridge: Polity Press.

Bravo Castillo, Elsi A. S. 1980. "Un enfoque sobre la política de salud en el Perú." In *La salud en el Perú.* Cuaderno No. 28. Lima: Centro Latinoamericano de Trabajo Social.

Bresser Pereira, Luis Carlos, José María Maraval, and Adam Przeworski. 1992. *Economic Reforms in New Democracies: A Social-Democratic Approach.* Cambridge: Cambridge University Press.

Briggs, Charles L., and Clara Mantini-Briggs. 2008. "Why Health Inequalities are Political—and Why LASA Members Should Care." *Latin American Studies Association Forum* 39 (2): 17–21.

Brooks, Sarah M. 2004. "International Financial Institutions and the Diffusion of Foreign Models for Social Security Reform in Latin America." In Weyland 2004, 53–80.

———. 2007. "Globalization and Pension Reform in Latin America." *Latin American Politics and Society* 49 (4): 31–62.

Bunch, Charlotte. 2001. "International Networking for Women's Human Rights." In Edwards and Gaventa 2001, 217–29.

Carbajal, Juan Carlos, and Pedro Francke. 2003. "La seguridad social en salud: Situación y posibilidades." In *La Salud como derecho ciudadano: Perspectivas y propuestas desde América Latina,* coord. Carlos Cáceres, Marcos Cueto, Miguel Ramos, and Sandra Vallenas, 509–25. Lima: Universidad Peruana Cayetano Heredia.

Castiglioni, Rossana. 2001. "The Politics of Retrenchment: The Quandaries of Social Protection Under Military Rule in Chile, 1973–1990." *Latin American Politics and Society* 43 (4): 37–66.

————. 2005. *The Politics of Social Policy Change in Chile and Uruguay: Retrenchment Versus Maintenance, 1973–1998.* New York: Routledge.

Centro de Estudios Sociales y Publicaciones (CESIP) and Movimiento Manuela Ramos. 2005. *Producción legislativa 2001–2005 y equidad de género: Un balance necesario.* Lima: Centro de Estudios Sociales y Publicaciones and Manuela Ramos.

CEPALSTAT. 2008. *Estadísticas de América Latina y el Caribe.* Santiago: Comisión Económica para América Latina y el Caribe. http://websie.eclac.cl/sisgen/ConsultaIntegrada.asp?idAplicacion=6&idTema=151&idioma=e (accessed December 2, 2008).

Cevasco, Gaby. 2004. *25 años de feminismo en el Perú: Historia, confluencias y perspectivas.* Lima: Centro de la Mujer Flora Tristán.

Chacaltana, Juan. 2002. "Social Funds and the Challenge of Social Protection for the Poor in Latin America." Paper presented at Conference on Social Protection, October, Manila.

Chaney, Elsa M. 1979. *Supermadre: Women in Politics in Latin America.* Austin: University of Texas Press.

Chávez, Susana. 2004. *Cuando el fundamentalismo se apodera de las políticas públicas: Políticas de salud sexual y reproductiva en el Perú en el período Julio 2001–Junio 2003.* Lima: Centro de la Mujer Peruana Flora Tristán.

Clark, Mary. 2004. "Reinforcing a Public System: Health Sector Reform in Costa Rica." In Kaufman and Nelson 2004, 189–216.

Collins, Patricia Hill. 1991. *Black Feminist Thought: Knowledge, Consciousness, and the Politics of Empowerment.* New York: Routledge.

El Comercio. 2008. "García promete seguros de salud para dos mil dirigentes y sus familias." December 7. http://www.elcomercio.com.pe (accessed December 7, 2008).

Comité de América Latina y el Caribe para la Defensa de los Derechos de la Mujer (CLADEM). 1999. *Nada personal: Reporte de derechos humanos sobre la aplicación de la anticoncepción quirúrgica en el Perú, 1996–1998.* Lima: CLADEM.

Comité de América Latina y el Caribe para la Defensa de los Derechos de la Mujer (CLADEM), Center for Reproductive Rights (CRLP), and Estudio para la Defensa y los Derechos de la Mujer (DEMUS). 1998. *Derechos sexuales y reproductivos de las mujeres en el Perú.* Reporte Sombra, elaborado para la Décimo Novena Sesión del Comité para la Eliminación de Todas las Formas de Discriminación Contra la Mujer (June).

Conaghan, Catherine M. 1998. "Stars of the Crisis: The Ascent of Economists in Peruvian Public Life." In *The Politics of Expertise in Latin America,* edited by Miguel A. Centeno and Patricio Silva, 142–64. New York: St. Martin's Press.

Contreras, Carlos. 2004. *El aprendizaje del capitalismo: Estudios de historia económica y social del Perú Republicano.* Lima: Instituto de Estudios Peruanos.

Cornia, Giovanni, Richard Jolly, and Frances Stewart, eds. 1987. *Adjustment with a Human Face.* Oxford: Clarendon Press.

Corrêa, Sonia, in collaboration with Rebecca Reichmann. 1994. *Population and Reproductive Rights: Feminist Perspectives from the South.* London: Zed Books in association with Development Alternatives with Women for a New Era.

Cosamalón Aguilar, Jesús A. 2003. "Una visión del cuerpo femenino y de la enfermedad a partir de dos diagnósticos médicos, Lima 1803." *Anuario de Estudios Americanos* 60 (1): 109–38.

Costello, Anthony, Fiona Watson, and David Woodward. 1994. *Human Face or Human Façade? Adjustment and the Health of Mothers and Children.* London: Centre for International Child Health.

Cotler, Julio. 1978. *Clases, estado y nación en el Perú.* Lima: Instituto de Estudios Peruanos.

———. 1995. "Political Parties and the Problems of Democratic Consolidation in Peru." In *Building Democratic Institutions: Party Systems in Latin America,* edited by Scott Mainwaring and Timothy R. Scully, 323–53. Stanford: Stanford University Press.

Council of Europe. 1998. *Gender Mainstreaming: Conceptual Framework, Methodology and Presentation of Good Practices.* Council of Europe EG-S-MS (98) 2 rev.

Craske, Nikki. 1999. *Women and Politics in Latin America.* New Brunswick: Rutgers University Press.

Creese, Andrew. 1998. "In Defence and Pursuit of Equity: A Response." *Social Science and Medicine* 47 (12): 1897–98.

Crenshaw, Kimberlé. 1994. "Mapping the Margins: Intersectionality, Identity Politics and Violence Against Women of Color." In *The Public Nature of Private Violence,* edited by Martha Albertson Fineman and Rixanne Mykitiuk, 93–118. New York: Routledge.

Cruz-Saco, María Amparo, and Carmelo Mesa-Lago, eds. 1998. *Do Options Exist? The Reform of Pension and Health Care Systems in Latin America.* Pittsburgh: University of Pittsburgh Press.

Cúanto, S. A., Richard Webb, and Graciela Fernández Baca. 1991. *Perú en números 1991.* Lima: Cuanto S.A.

Cueto, Marcos. 1992. "Sanitation from Above: Yellow Fever and Foreign Intervention in Peru, 1919–1922." *Hispanic American Historical Review* 72 (1): 1–22.

———, ed. 1994a. *Missionaries of Science: The Rockefeller Foundation and Latin America.* Bloomington: Indiana University Press.

———. 1994b. Introduction to Cueto 1994a, ix–xx.

———. 1994c. "Visions of Science and Development: The Rockefeller Foundation's Latin American Surveys of the 1920s." In Cueto 1994a, 1–22.

———. 1997. *El regreso de las epidemias: Salud y sociedad en el Perú del siglo XX.* Lima: Instituto de Estudios Peruanos.

———. 2001. *Culpa y coraje: Historia de las políticas sobre el VIH/Sida en el Perú.* Lima: Consorcio de Investigación Económica y Social and Facultad de Salud Pública y Administración, Universidad Peruana Cayetano Heredia.

———. 2002. "Social Medicine in the Andes, 1920–50." In *The Politics of the Healthy Life: An International Perspective,* edited by Esteban Rodríguez-Ocaña, 181–96. Sheffield: European Association of the History of Medicine and Health Publications.

———. 2004a. "The Origins of Primary Health Care and Selective Primary Health Care." *American Journal of Public Health* 94 (11): 1864–74.

———. 2004b. "Social Medicine and 'Leprosy' in the Peruvian Amazon." *Americas* 61 (1): 55–80.

———. n.d. "Visiones de medicina y exclusión en los Andes y los Amazonas peruanos en la década de los cuarenta." Universidad Peruana Cayetano Heredia, Lima (unpublished manuscript).

Currie, Dawn H., and Sara E. Wiesenberg. 2003. "Promoting Women's Health-Seeking Behavior: Research and the Empowerment of Women." *Health Care for Women International* 24: 880–99.

Dasso, Elizabeth. 1998. "Nuevas políticas del banco mundial a la sociedad civil." Presentation at "Foro Educativo," November 3, Universidad del Pacífico, Lima.

Davidson, Judith R., and Steve Stein. 1988. "Economic Crisis, Social Polarization and Community Participation in Health Care." In Zschock 1988, 53–77.

Defensoría del Pueblo. 1998. *Anticoncepción quirúrgica voluntaria.* Vol. 1, *Casos investigados por la Defensoría del Pueblo.* Lima: Defensoría del Pueblo.

———. 1999. *La aplicación de la anticoncepción quirúrgica y los derechos reproductivos.* Vol. 2, *Casos investigados por la Defensoría del Pueblo.* Lima: Defensoría del Pueblo.

———. 2000. *Anticoncepción quirúrgica voluntaria.* Vol. 3, *Casos investigados por la Defensoría del Pueblo.* Lima: Defensoría del Pueblo.

———. 2005. *Supervisón de los servicios de planificación familiar.* Vol. 4, *Casos investigados por la Defensoría del Pueblo.* Informe Defensorial 90. Lima: Defensoría del Pueblo.

———. 2007. *Atención de salud para los más pobres: El Seguro Integral de Salud.* Informe Defensorial No. 120. Lima: Defensoría del Pueblo.

de la Cadena, Marisol. 1996. "Las mujeres son más Indias." In *Detrás de la puerta: Hombres y mujeres en el Perú del hoy,* edited by Patricia Ruíz-Bravo, 181–202. Lima: Pontificia Universidad Católica del Perú.

———. 2000. *Indigenous Mestizos: The Politics of Race and Culture in Cuzco, Peru, 1919–1991.* Durham: Duke University Press.

Díaz, Derry. 2006. "EsSalud en la agenda electoral." *Diario La República,* February 22. http://archivo.larepublica.com.pe/index.php?option=com_content&task=view&id=103297&Itemid=30&fecha_edicion=2006-02-22 (accessed July 26, 2006).

Diez Canseco, Javier. 2006. "Recortes a salud y nutrición: ¿"Austeridad"?" *La Primera* 2:498, July 25, 2006. http://www.ednoperu.com/noticia.php?IDnoticia=26119 (accessed July 25, 2006).

Dion, Michelle. 2006. "Women's Welfare and Social Security Reform in Mexico." *Social Politics* 13 (3): 400–426.

Dore, Elizabeth, and Maxine Molyneux, eds. 2000. *Hidden Histories of Gender and the State in Latin America.* Durham: Duke University Press.

Doyal, Lesley. 2000. "Gender Equity in Health: Debates and Dilemmas." *Social Science and Medicine* 51 (6): 931–39.

———. 2002. "Putting Gender into Health and Globalization Debates: New Perspectives and Old Challenges." *Third World Quarterly* 23 (2): 233–50.

Dwyer, Daisy, and Judith Bruce. 1988. *A Home Divided: Women and Income in the Third World.* Stanford: Stanford University Press.

Economic Commission for Latin America and the Caribbean (ECLAC). 2004. *Social Panorama of Latin America.* Santiago: ECLAC.

———. 2005. *Social Panorama of Latin America.* Santiago: ECLAC.

———. 2007. *Social Panorama of Latin America*. Santiago: ECLAC.

———. 2008. *Social Panorama of Latin America*. Santiago: ECLAC.

Edwards, Michael, and John Gaventa, eds. 2001. *Global Citizen Action*. Boulder: Lynne Rienner.

Ehrick, Christine. 2005. *The Shield of the Weak: Feminism and the State in Uruguay, 1903–1933*. Albuquerque: University of New Mexico Press.

Elson, Diane, ed. 1991. *Male Bias in the Development Process*. Manchester: Manchester University Press.

———. 1992a. "From Survival Strategies to Transformation Strategies: Women's Needs and Structural Adjustment." In Benería and Feldman 1992, 26–48.

———. 1992b. "Male Bias in Structural Adjustment." In Afshar and Dennis 1992, 46–68.

Emmerij, Louis. 2005. "How Has the UN Faced up to Development Challenges?" *Forum for Development Studies* 1:21–47.

Encuesta Nacional de Hogares Medición de Niveles de Vida (ENAHO). 1991. Lima: Instituto Nacional de Estadísticas e Informática; Washington, D.C.: World Bank.

———. 1994. Lima: Instituto Nacional de Estadísticas e Informática; Washington, D.C.: World Bank.

Encuesta Nacional de Hogares, Condiciones de Vida y Pobreza (ENAHO). 2000. Lima: Instituto Nacional de Estadísticas e Informática.

———. 2006. Lima: Instituto Nacional de Estadísticas e Informática.

———. 2008. Third trimester. Lima: Instituto Nacional de Estadísticas y Informática.

Esping-Anderson, Gøsta. 1990. *The Three Worlds of Welfare Capitalism*. Princeton: Princeton University Press.

Espinoza Carrillo, Rubén. 2002. "Resumen ejecutivo consultaría en acciones de apoyo al proceso de modernización del subsector público de salud." Internal document, Programa de Fortalecimiento de Servicios de Salud, MINSA-Perú.

EsSalud. 2007. *Memoria Institucional 2006*. Lima: EsSalud.

Evers, Barbara, and Mercedes Juárez. 2002. "Understanding the Links: Globalization, Health Sector Reform, Gender and Reproductive Health." In *Globalization, Health Sector Reform, Gender and Reproductive Health*, 5–52. New York: Ford Foundation.

Ewig, Christina. 1999. "The Strengths and Limits of the NGO Women's Movement Model: Shaping Nicaragua's Democratic Institutions." *Latin American Research Review* 34 (3): 75–102.

———. 2004. "Piecemeal but Innovative: Health Sector Reform in Peru." In Kaufman and Nelson 2004, 217–46.

———. 2006. "Hijacking Global Feminisms: Feminists, the Catholic Church and the Family Planning Debacle in Peru." *Feminist Studies* 32 (2): 632–59.

———. 2008. "Reproduction, Re-reform and the Reconfigured State: Feminists and Neoliberal Health Reforms in Chile." In *Social Reproduction and Global Transformations: From the Everyday to the Global*, edited by Isabella Bakker and Rachel Silvey, 143–58. New York: Routledge.

Ewig, Christina, and Amparo Hernández Bello. 2009. "Gender Equity and Health Sector Reform in Colombia: Mixed State-Market Model Yields Mixed Results." *Social Science and Medicine* 68 (6): 1145–52.

Ewig, Christina, and Stephen J. Kay. 2008. "New Political Legacies and the Politics of Health and Pension Re-reforms in Chile." In *Public and Private Social Policy: Health and Pension Policies in a New Era,* edited by Daniel Béland and Brian Gran, 249–68. Basingstoke: Palgrave Macmillan.

Filgueira, Fernando. 1998. "El nuevo modelo de prestaciones sociales en América Latina: Residualismo y ciudadanía estratificada." In *Ciudadanía y Política Social,* edited by Bryan R. Roberts, 71–116. San José, Costa Rica: FLACSO/SSRC.

Finnemore, Martha. 1993. "International Organizations as Teachers of Norms." *International Organization* 47 (4): 565–99.

———. 1996. "Review: Norms, Culture and World Politics: Insights from Sociology's Institutionalism." *International Organization* 50 (2): 325–47.

Fleury, Sonia, Susana Belmartino, and Enis Baris, eds. 2000. *Reshaping Health Care in Latin America: A Comparative Analysis of Health Care Reform in Argentina, Brazil and Mexico.* Ottawa: International Development Research Center.

Floro, Maria. 1995. "Economic Restructuring, Gender and the Allocation of Time." *World Development* 23 (11): 1913–29.

Floro, Maria, and Hella Hoppe. 2005. *Engendering Policy Coherence for Development: Gender Issues for the Global Policy Agenda in the Year 2005.* Dialogue on Globalization, Occasional Paper no. 17. Berlin: Friedrich-Ebert-Stiftung.

Forget, Evelyn L., Raisa B. Deber, Leslie L. Roos, and Randy Walld. 2005. "Canadian Health Reform: A Gender Analysis." *Feminist Economics* 11 (1): 123–41.

ForoSalud. 2008. *Reporte de la vigilancia ciudadana al seguro integral de salud—sis—en establecimientos de salud de Lima Metropolitana.* Lima: ForoSalud.

Fourcade-Gourinchas, Marion, and Sarah L. Babb. 2002. "The Rebirth of the Liberal Creed: Paths to Neoliberalism in Four Countries." *American Journal of Sociology* 108 (3): 533–79.

Franceschet, Susan. 2003. "'State Feminism' and Women's Movements: The Impact of Chile's Servicio Nacional de la Mujer on Women's Activism." *Latin American Research Review* 38 (1): 9–40.

Francke, Pedro. 1998. *Focalización del gasto público en salud.* Lima: Ministerio de Salud.

Francke, Pedro, Juan Arroyo, and Alfredo Gúzman. 2006. *Políticas de salud 2006–2011.* Lima: Consorcio de Investigación Económica y Social and ForoSalud.

Fraser, Nancy. 1989. *Unruly Practices: Power, Discourse and Gender in Contemporary Social Theory.* Minneapolis: University of Minnesota Press.

———. 1997. *Justice Interruptus: Critical Reflections on the "Postsocialist" Condition.* London: Routledge.

———. 2001. "Recognition Without Ethics?" *Theory, Culture and Society* 18 (2–3): 21–42.

Fraser, Nancy, and Axel Honneth. 2003. *Redistribution or Recognition? A Political-Philosophical Exchange.* New York: Verso.

Friedman, Elisabeth Jay. 2003. "Gendering the Agenda: The Impact of the Transnational Women's Rights Movement at the UN Conferences in the 1990s." *Women's Studies International Forum* 26 (4): 313–31.

Frisancho, Ariel, and Jay Goulden. 2008. "Rights-Based Approaches to Improve People's Health in Peru." *The Lancet* 372:2007–8.

Fukuda-Parr, Sakiko. 2003. "The Human Development Paradigm: Operationalizing Sen's Ideas on Capabilities." *Feminist Economics* 9 (2–3): 301–17.

Fuller, Norma. 2001. "The Social Constitution of Gender Identity Among Peruvian Men." *Men and Masculinities* 3 (3): 316–31.

Gárate Urquizo, Werner, and Rosa Ana Ferrer G. 1994. *En qué trabajan las mujeres: Compendio estadístico 1980–1993.* Lima: ADEC-ATC.

García, María Elena. 2005. *Making Indigenous Citizens: Identity, Development and Multicultural Activism in Peru.* Stanford: Stanford University Press.

García Bedolla, Lisa. 2007. "Intersections of Inequality: Understanding Marginalization and Privilege in the Post-Civil Rights Era." *Politics and Gender* 3 (2): 232–48.

Gargurevich, Gabriel. 2005. "200 Mil niñas empleadas del hogar." *La República,* November 28. http://archivo.larepublica.com.pe/index.php?option=com_content&task=view&id=95836&Itemid=30&fecha_edicion=2005-11-28 (accessed June 8, 2006).

George, Alexander L., and Andrew Bennett. 2005. *Case Studies and Theory Development in the Social Sciences.* Cambridge, Mass.: MIT Press.

George, Alexander L., and Timothy J. McKeown. 1985. "Case Studies and Theories of Organizational Decision Making." *Advances in Information Processing in Organizations* 2:21–58.

George, Susan. 1992. *The Debt Boomerang: How Third World Debt Harms Us All.* Boulder: Westview Press.

Gideon, Jasmine. 2001. "The Politics of Health Reform in Chile: Gender and Participation in Primary Health Care Delivery." Ph.D. diss., University of Manchester.

———. 2006. "Accessing Economic and Social Rights Under Neoliberalism: Gender and Rights in Chile." *Third World Quarterly* 27 (7): 1269–83.

———. 2007. "A Gendered Analysis of Labour Market Informalization and Access to Health in Chile." *Global Social Policy* 7 (1): 75–94.

Giménez, Daniel M. 2005. *Gender, Pensions and Social Citizenship in Latin America.* Santiago de Chile: United Nations, ECLAC, Women and Development Unit.

Gómez Dantés, Octavio. 1999. "Páginas de salud pública." *Salud Pública de México* 41 (4): 356–58.

Gómez Gómez, Elsa. 2002. "Género, equidad y acceso a los servicios de salud: Una aproximación empírica." *Revista Panamericana de Salud Pública* 11:327–34.

Gonzáles-Casanova, Pablo. 1965. "Internal Colonialism and National Development." *Studies in Comparative International Development* 1 (4): 27–37.

González de la Rocha, Mercedes. 1995. "The Urban Family and Poverty in Latin America." *Latin American Perspectives* 22:12–31.

González Rossetti, Alejandra. 2004. "Change Teams and Vested Interests: Social Security Health Reform in Mexico." In Kaufman and Nelson 2004, 65–92.

Gordon, Linda. 1990. *Woman's Body, Woman's Right: Birth Control in America.* Rev. edition. New York: Penguin.

———. 1994. *Pitied but Not Entitled: Single Mothers and the History of Welfare, 1890–1935.* New York: Free Press.

———. 2006. "Internal Colonialism and Gender." In *Haunted by Empire: Geographies of Intimacy in North American History,* edited by Ann Laura Stoler, 427–451. Durham: Duke University Press.

Gough, Ian. 2004. "Welfare Regimes in Development Contexts: A Global and Regional Analysis." In Gough and Wood 2004, 15–48.

Gough, Ian, and Geof Wood, eds. 2004. *Insecurity and Welfare Regimes in Asia, Africa and Latin America: Social Policy in Development Contexts.* Cambridge: Cambridge University Press.

Graham, Carol. 1994. *Safety Nets, Politics and the Poor: Transitions to Market Economies.* Washington, D.C.: Brookings Institution.

———. 1998. *Private Markets for Public Goods: Raising the Stakes in Economic Reform.* Washington, D.C.: Brookings Institution.

Güezmes, Ana. 2000. "Presentación y análisis de la experiencia de la Mesa Tripartita de Seguimiento a la CIPD." In *Al rescate de la utopía: Reflexiones para una agenda feminista del nuevo milenio,* edited by Cecilia Olea Mauleón and Ivonne Macassi León, 199–209. Lima: Centro de la Mujer Peruana Flora Tristán.

Gúzman, Alfredo. 2002. "Para mejorar la salud reproductiva." In *La salud peruana en el siglo XXI,* edited by Juan Arroyo, 185–238. Lima: Consorcio de Investigación Económica y Social, UK Department for International Development and the Policy Project.

Haas, Peter M. 1992. "Introduction: Epistemic Communities and International Policy Coordination." *International Organization* 46 (1): 1–35.

Hacker, Jacob S. 2002. *The Divided Welfare State: The Battle over Public and Private Social Benefits in the United States.* Cambridge: Cambridge University Press.

———. 2004a. "Privatizing Risk Without Privatizing the Welfare State: The Hidden Politics of Social Policy Retrenchment in the United States." *American Political Science Review* 98 (2): 243–60.

———. 2004b. "Review Article: Dismantling the Health Care State? Political Institutions, Public Policies and Comparative Politics of Health Reform." *British Journal of Political Science* 34:1–32.

Haddad, Lawrence, Lynn R. Brown, Andrea Richter, and Lisa Smith. 1995. "The Gender Dimensions of Economic Adjustment Policies: Potential Interactions and Evidence to Date." *World Development* 23 (6): 881–96.

Haddad, Lawrence, John Hoddinott, and Harold Alderman, eds. 1997. *Intrahousehold Resource Allocation in Developing Countries.* Baltimore: Johns Hopkins University Press.

Haggard, Stephen, and Robert Kaufman, eds. 1992. *The Politics of Economic Adjustment.* Princeton: Princeton University Press.

———. 1995. *The Political Economy of Democratic Transitions.* Princeton: Princeton University Press.

———. 2008. *Development, Democracy and Welfare States: Latin America, East Asia and Eastern Europe.* Princeton: Princeton University Press.

Halfon, Saul. 2007. *The Cairo Consensus: Demographic Surveys, Women's Empowerment, and Regime Change in Population Policy.* Lanham: Lexington Books.

Hall, Peter. 1993. "Policy Paradigms, Social Learning and the State: The Case of Economic Policymaking in Britain." *Comparative Politics* 25 (3): 275–96.

———. 2003. "Aligning Ontology and Methodology in Comparative Politics." In *Comparative Historical Analysis in the Social Sciences,* edited by James Mahoney and Dietrich Rueschemeyer, 373–404. Cambridge: Cambridge University Press.

Hancock, Ange-Marie. 2007. "When Multiplication Doesn't Equal Quick Addition: Examining Intersectionality as a Research Paradigm." *Perspectives on Politics* 5 (1): 63–79.

Haney, Lynne A. 2002. *Inventing the Needy: Gender and the Politics of Welfare in Hungary.* Berkeley and Los Angeles: University of California Press.

Hanmer, Lucia. 1994a. *Equity and Gender Issues in Health Care Provision: The 1993 World Bank Development Report and its Implications for Health Service Recipients.* Working Paper Series No. 172. Institute of Social Studies: The Hague-Netherlands.

———. 1994b. *What Happens to Welfare When User Fees Finance Health Care? The Impact Gender on Policy Outcomes; Theory and Evidence from Zimbabwe.* Working Paper Series No. 180. The Hague: Institute of Social Studies.

Hansen, Jakob Kirkemann, and Hans-Otto Sano. 2006. "The Implications and Value Added of a Rights-Based Approach." In *Development as a Human Right: Legal, Political, and Economic Dimensions,* edited by Bård A. Andreassen and Stephen P. Marks, 36–56. Cambridge: Harvard School of Public Health, Harvard University Press.

Hanson, Kara. 2002. "Measuring Up: Gender, Burden of Disease and Priority Setting." In Sen, George, and Östlin 2002, 313–45.

Haq, Mahbab ul. 2003. "The Human Development Paradigm." In *Readings in Human Development: Concepts, Measures and Policies for a Development Paradigm,* edited by Sakiko Fukuda-Parr and A. K. Shiva Kumar, 17–37. New York: Oxford University Press.

Hartmann, Betsy. 1995. *Reproductive Rights and Wrongs: The Global Politics of Population Control.* Rev. ed. Boston: South End Press.

Harvey, David. 2005. *A Brief History of Neoliberalism.* Oxford: Oxford University Press.

Hassim, Shireen, and Shahra Razavi. 2006. "Gender and Social Policy in a Global Context: Uncovering the Gendered Structure of 'the Social.'" In Razavi and Hassim 2006, 1–39.

Havens, A. Eugene, and William L. Flinn. 1970. *Internal Colonialism and Structural Change in Colombia.* New York: Praeger.

Hawkesworth, Mary. 2003. "Congressional Enactments of Race-Gender: Toward a Theory of Race-Gendered Institutions." *American Political Science Review* 97 (4): 529–50.

Hechter, Michael. 1975. *Internal Colonialism: The Celtic Fringe in British National Development, 1536–1966.* Berkeley and Los Angeles: University of California Press.

Hirschmann, Nancy J. 2008. "Mill, Political Economy, and Women's Work." *American Political Science Review* 102 (2): 199–213.

Htun, Mala. 2003. *Sex and the State: Abortion, Divorce, and the Family Under Latin American Dictatorships and Democracies.* Cambridge: Cambridge University Press.

Huber, Evelyne, and John D. Stephens. 2001. *The Development and Crisis of the Welfare State: Parties and Policies in Global Markets.* Chicago: University of Chicago Press.

Hull, Gloria, Patricia Bell Scott, and Barbara Smith. 1982. *All the Women Are White, All the Blacks Are Men, but Some of Us Are Brave: Black Women's Studies.* Old Westbury, N.Y.: Feminist Press.

Instituto Nacional de Estadística e Informática (INEI). 1992. *Perú: Compendio estadístico 1991–1992.* Lima: Instituto Nacional de Estadística e Informática.

———. 1994. *Perú: Mapa de necesidades básicas insatisfechas de los hogares al nivel distrital.* Lima: Instituto Nacional de Estadística e Informática.

———. 1996. *Perú: Compendio estadístico 1995–1996.* Lima: Instituto Nacional de Estadística e Informática.

———. 1999a. *Encuesta nacional de hogares iv trimestre 1999.* Lima: Instituto Nacional de Estadística e Informática. http://www.inei.gob.pe (accessed May 15, 2006).

———. 1999b. *Estimaciones y proyecciones de población 1999.* Lima: Instituto Nacional de Estadística e Informática.

———. 1999c. *Género, equidad y disparidades: Una revisión en la antesala del nuevo milenio.* Lima: Instituto Nacional de Estadística e Informática, Ministerio de la Promoción de la Mujer y el Desarrollo, and Fondo de Población de las Naciones Unidas. http://www1.inei.gob.pe (accessed August 5, 2008).

———. 2001a. *Encuesta nacional de hogares iv trimestre 2001.* Lima: Instituto Nacional de Estadística e Informática. Figures compiled by the INEI at http://www.inei.gob.pe (accessed June 7, 2006).

———. 2001b. *Peru: Estimaciones y proyecciones de población, 1950–2050.* Boletín de Análisis Demográfico No. 35. Lima: Instituto Nacional de Estadística e Informática.

———. 2002. *Perú en cifras.* Censos de población—Estimaciones de población. Lima: Instituto Nacional de Estadística e Informática. http://www.inei.gob.pe (accessed June 7, 2006).

———. 2003–2006. "ENAHO continua 2003–2006: Información socio-demográfica." http://www1.inei.gob.pe/Sisd/index.asp (accessed November 20, 2008).

———. 2004/2005. *Encuesta demográfica y salud familiar.* Lima: Instituto Nacional de Estadística e Informática Figures. Compiled by the INEI at http://iinei. inei.gob.pe/iinei/sisd/index.asp (accessed December 30, 2008).

———. 2005. "Mujeres participan menos en el mercado laboral." Nota de Prensa No. 260. December. Lima: Instituto Nacional de Estadística e Informática.

———. 2006a. "Estadísticas de género: Enero-Feberero-Marzo 2006." Informe Técnico No. 6 (Junio). Lima: Instituto Nacional de Estadística e Informática.

———. 2006b. "Situación del mercado laboral de Lima metropolitana Abril 2006." Informe Técnico No. 5 (Mayo). Lima: Instituto Nacional de Estadística e Informática.

———. 2007a. "Informe técnico: La pobreza en el Perú en el año 2007." Lima: Instituto Nacional de Estadística e Informática.

———. 2007b. *Compendio Estadístico.* http://www1.inei.gob.pe/Sisd/index.asp (accessed January 14, 2009).

Inter-American Development Bank (IDB). 1996. *Apoyo a la reforma en la prestación de servicios sociales.* No. SOC-101. Washington, D.C.: Inter-American Development Bank.

———. 2002. *El sector salud en los proyectos del BID: Una evaluación preliminar.* Nota Técnica de Discusión de Salud. 01:2002. Washington, D.C.: Inter-American Development Bank.

International Conference on Population and Development (ICPD). 1994. *Programme of Action of the International Conference on Population and Development.* Cairo, 1994. Chap. 7, "Reproductive Rights and Reproductive Health." http://www.unfpa.org/icpd/icpd-programme.cfm#ch7.

Jahan, Rounaq. 1995. *The Elusive Agenda: Mainstreaming Women in Development.* London: Zed Books.

Jaramillo, Miguel, and Sandro Parodi. 2004. *El seguro escolar gratuito y el seguro materno infantil: Análisis de su incidencia e impacto sobre el acceso a los servicios de salud y sobre la equidad en el acceso.* Documento de Trabajo 46. Lima: Grupo de Análisis para el Desarrollo.

Johnson, Jaime U. 1998. "Nuevo modelo de seguridad social en salud." *Revista Ideele* (109): 43–46.

Jolly, Richard. 2005. "The UN and Development Thinking and Practice." *Forum for Development Studies* 32 (1): 49–74.

Jones, Nicola, Rosana Vargas, and Eliana Villar. 2007. "Conditional Cash Transfers in Peru: Tackling the Multi-dimensionality of Childhood Poverty and Vulnerability." In *Social Protection Initiatives for Children, Women, and Families: An Analysis of Recent Experiences,* edited by Alberto Minujin and Enrique Delamonica. New York: New School for Social Research and UNICEF.

Kahler, Miles. 1992. "External Influence, Conditionality, and the Politics of Adjustment." In Haggard and Kaufman 1992, 89–136.

Kampwirth, Karen, ed. Forthcoming. *Gender and Populism in Latin America: Passionate Politics.* University Park: Pennsylvania State University Press.

Kaufman, Robert R., and Joan M. Nelson, eds. 2004. *Crucial Needs: Weak Incentives: Social Sector Reform, Democratization and Globalization in Latin America.* Washington, D.C.: Woodrow Wilson Center Press; Baltimore: Johns Hopkins University Press.

Keck, Margaret E., and Kathryn Sikkink. 1998. *Activists Beyond Borders: Advocacy Networks in International Politics.* Ithaca: Cornell University Press.

Kingdon, John. 1984. *Agendas, Alternatives, and Public Policies.* Boston: Little, Brown.

Klarén, Peter Findell. 2000. *Peru: Society and Nationhood in the Andes.* New York: Oxford University Press.

Koivusalo, Meri, and Eeva Ollila. 1997. *Making a Healthy World: Agencies, Actors and Policies in International Health.* London: Zed Books.

Koven, Seth, and Sonya Michel. 1993. *Mothers of the New World: Maternalist Politics and the Origins of the Welfare State.* New York: Routledge.

Kuiper, Edith, and Drucilla K. Barker, eds. 2006. *Feminist Economics and the World Bank: History, Theory and Policy.* New York: Routledge.

Lakshminarayanan, Rama. 2003. *Gender and Health Sector Reform: An Annotated Bibliography.* New York: International Women's Health Coalition.

Lane, Sandra D. 1994. "From Population Control to Reproductive Health: An Emerging Policy Agenda." *Social Science and Medicine* 39 (9): 1303–14.

Larson, Brooke. 2005. "Capturing Indian Bodies, Hearths and Minds: The Gendered Politics of Rural School Reform in Bolivia, 1920s–1940s." In *Natives Making Nation: Gender, Indigeniety and the State in the Andes,* edited by Andrew Canessa, 32–59. Tucson: University of Arizona Press.

Levitt, Barry Steven. 2000. "Continuity and Change in Peru's Political Parties, 1985–2000." Paper presented at the Twenty-first International Congress of the Latin American Studies Association, Miami, March 16–18.

Lind, Amy. 2005. *Gendered Paradoxes: Women's Movements, State Restructuring, and Global Development in Ecuador.* University Park: Pennsylvania State University Press.

———. 2002. "Making Feminist Sense of Neoliberalism: The Institutionalization of Women's Struggles for Survival in Ecuador and Bolivia." *Journal of Developing Societies* 18 (2–3): 228–58.

Lister, Ruth. 1997. "Citizenship: Towards a Feminist Synthesis." *Feminist Review* 57:28–48.

———. 2001. "Towards a Citizens' Welfare State: The 3 + 2 'R's of Welfare Reform." *Theory, Culture and Society* 18 (2–3): 91–111.

Livingston, Steven G. 1992. "The Politics of International Agenda-Setting: Reagan and North–South Relations." *International Studies Quarterly* 36 (3): 313–29.

Lloyd-Sherlock, Peter, ed. 2000. *Healthcare Reform and Poverty in Latin America.* London: Institute of Latin American Studies, University of London.

Locay, Luis. 1988. "Medical Doctors: Determinants of Location." In Zschock 1988, 133–63.

Londoño, Juan Luis, and Julio Frenk. 1997. "Structured Pluralism: Towards an Innovative Model for Health System Reform in Latin America." *Health Policy* 41:1–36.

Long, Carolyn M. 2006. "An Assessment of Efforts to Promote Gender Equality at the World Bank." In Kuiper and Barker 2006, 40–56.

Lukes, Steven. 1974. *Power: A Radical View.* London: Macmillan.

Luna Amancio, Nelly. 2007. "Las postas administradas por la comunidad son más eficientes." *El Comercio,* March 4. http://www.elcomercioperu.com.pe/EdicionImpresa/Html/2007-03-04/ImEcTemaDia0682403.html (accessed June 13, 2007).

Lund, Francie. 2006. "Working People and Access to Social Protection." In Razavi and Hassim 2006, 217–33.

Lycklama à Nijeholt, Geertje, Joke Sweibel, and Virginia Vargas. 1998. "The Global Institutional Framework: The Long March to Beijing." In *Women's Movements and Public Policy in Europe, Latin America, and the Caribbean,* edited by Geertje Lycklama à Nijeholt, Virginia Vargas, and Saskia Wieringa, 25–48. New York: Garland, Inc.

Mackintosh, Maureen, and Paula Tibandebage. 2006. "Gender and Health Sector Reform: Analytical Perspectives on African Experience." In Razavi and Hassim 2006, 237–57.

Madrid, Raul L. 2003. *Retiring the State: The Politics of Pension Privatization in Latin America and Beyond.* Stanford: Stanford University Press.

Madueño, Miguel, Javier Linares, and Alessandra Zurita. 2004. *Instrumento estandarizado de identificación de beneficiarios para programas sociales.* Bethesda, Md.: Partners for Health Reform Project, Abt Associates Inc.

Malloy, James M. 1979. *The Politics of Social Security in Brazil.* Pittsburgh: University of Pittsburgh Press.

Mannarelli, María Emma. 1999. *Limpias y modernas: Género, higiene y cultura en la Lima del novecientos.* Lima: Centro de la Mujer Peruana Flora Tristán.

March, Candida, Ines Smyth, and Maitrayee Mukhopadhyay. 1999. *A Guide to Gender-Analysis Frameworks*. Oxford: Oxfam Great Britain.

Martínez Franzoni, Juliana. 1999. "Poder y alternativas: Las agendas internacionales en las reformas del sector salud en Costa Rica, 1988–1998." *Anuario de Estudios Centroamericanos* 25 (1): 159–82.

———. 2008. "Welfare Regimes in Latin America: Capturing Constellations of Markets, Families, and Policies." *Latin American Politics and Society* 50 (2): 67–100.

Martínez Medina, María Concepción, and Lucía Pérez Fragoso. 2002. *El programa de ampliación de cobertura y el presupuesto federal: Un acercamiento al paquete básico de los servicios de salud desde la perspectiva de género*. Mexico City: Fundar Centro de Análisis e Investigación and Equidad de Género, Ciudadanía, Trabajo y Familia.

Mauceri, Phillip. 1997. "The Transition to 'Democracy' and the Failures of Institution Building." In *The Peruvian Labyrinth: Polity, Society, Economy*, edited by Maxwell A. Cameron and Philip Mauceri, 13–36. University Park: Pennsylvania State University Press.

McCall, Leslie. 2005. "The Complexity of Intersectionality." *Signs* 30 (3): 1771–1800.

McClintock, Anne. 1995. *Imperial Leather: Race, Gender and Sexuality in the Colonial Context*. New York: Routledge.

McClintock, Cynthia. 1999. "Peru: Precarious Regimes, Authoritarian and Democratic." In *Democracy in Developing Countries: Latin America*, 2nd ed., edited by Larry Diamond, Jonathan Hartlyn, Juan J. Linz, and Seymour Martin Lipset, 309–65. Boulder: Lynne Rienner.

McCoy, Terry L., ed. 1974. *The Dynamics of Population Policy in Latin America*. Cambridge: Ballinger.

McNeill, Desmond. 2007. "'Human Development': The Power of the Idea." *Journal of Human Development* 8 (1): 5–22.

McPake, Barbara, Kara Hanson, and Ann Mills. 1993. "Community Financing of Health Care in Africa: An Evaluation of the Bamako Initiative." *Social Science and Medicine* 36 (11): 1383–1405.

Mensch, Barbara. 1993. "Quality of Care: A Neglected Dimension." In *The Health of Women: A Global Perspective*, edited by Marge Koblinsky, Judith Timyan, and Jill Gay, 235–53. Boulder: Westview Press.

Mesa-Lago, Carmelo. 1978. *Social Security in Latin America: Pressure Groups, Stratification, and Inequality*. Pittsburgh: University of Pittsburgh Press.

———. 1989. *Ascent to Bankruptcy: Financing Social Security in Latin America*. Pittsburgh: University of Pittsburgh Press.

———. 1992. *Health Care for the Poor in Latin America and the Caribbean*. Pan American Health Organization Scientific and Technical Publication no. 539. Washington, D.C.: Pan American Health Organization and Inter-American Foundation.

Mesa-Lago, Carmelo, and Katharina Müller. 2002. "The Politics of Pension Reform in Latin America." *Journal of Latin American Studies* 34:687–717.

Mettler, Suzanne. 1998. *Dividing Citizens: Gender and Federalism in New Deal Public Policy*. Ithaca: Cornell University Press.

———. 2002. "Bringing the State Back in to Civic Engagement: Policy Feedback Effects of the G.I. Bill for World War II Veterans." *American Political Science Review* 96 (2): 351–65.

Meyer, John W., John Boli, George M. Thomas, and Francisco Ramírez. 1997. "World Society and the Nation State." *American Journal of Sociology* 103 (1): 144–81.

Ministerio de Economía y Finanzas (MEF). 2000. *Cierre del presupuesto del sector público para 1999.* Lima: Ministerio de Economía y Finanzas. www.mef.gob. pe/dnpp/index1.htm (accessed August 10, 2002).

———. 2001. *Cierre del presupuesto del sector público para 2000.* Lima: Ministerio de Economía y Finanzas. www.mef.gob.pe/dnpp/index1.htm (accessed August 10, 2002).

Ministerio de Promoción de la Mujer y del Desarrollo Humano (PROMUDEH). 1998. "Participación de la mujer en cargos públicos, 1998." Lima: PROMUDEH.

Ministerio de Salud del Perú (MINSA). 1994. "Salud Básica Para Todos." Lima: Ministerio de Salud del Perú.

———. 1996a. *El desafío del cambio de milenio: Un sector salud con equidad, eficiencia y calidad—lineamientos de política de salud 1995–2000.* Lima: Ministerio de Salud del Perú.

———. 1996b. *Segundo censo de infraestructura sanitaria y recursos del sector salud 1996.* Lima: Ministerio de Salud del Perú.

———. 1996c. "Programa de Salud Reproductiva y Planificación Familiar." Lima: Ministerio de Salud del Perú, United Nations Population Fund.

———. 2002. *Propuesta lineamientos de política sectorial para el período 2002–2012 y fundamentos para él plan estratégico sectorial del quinenio Agosto 2001–Julio 2006.* Lima: Ministerio de Salud del Perú.

———. 2005. *Seguro Integral de Salud.* Lima: Ministerio de Salud del Perú. http:// www.sis.minsa.gob.pe (accessed July 25, 2006).

———. 2007. *Plan Nacional Concertado de Salud.* Lima: Ministerio de Salud.

———. 2008. *Cuentas Nacionales de Salud: Perú, 1995–2005.* Lima: Ministerio de Salud del Perú, Oficina General de Planeamiento y Presupuesto and Consorcio de Investigación Económica y Social, Observatorio de Salud.

Ministerio de Salud del Perú (MINSA) and Organización Panamericana de la Salud (OPS). 2003. *Análisis y tendencias en la utilización de servicios de salud: Perú 1985–2002.* Lima: Ministerio de Salud del Perú.

Mogollón, María Esther. 2003. "Peruanas esterilizadas por la fuerza reclaman justicia." Cimac noticias. http://www.cimacnoticias.com/noticias/03mar/ 03030504.html (accessed September 17, 2004).

Mohanty, Chandra. 1991. "Under Western Eyes." In *Third World Women and the Politics of Feminism,* edited by Chandra Mohanty, Ann Russo, and Lourdes Torres, 51–80. Bloomington: Indiana University Press.

Molyneux, Maxine. 2006. "Mothers at the Service of the New Poverty Agenda: Progresa/Oportunidades, Mexico's Conditional Transfer Programme." *Social Policy and Administration* 40 (4): 425–49.

Molyneux, Maxine, and Shahra Razavi, eds. 2002. *Gender Justice, Development, and Rights.* New York: Oxford University Press.

Moraga, Cherríe, and Gloria Anzaldúa, eds. 1981. *This Bridge Called My Back: Writings of Radical Women of Color.* Watertown: Persephone Press.

Murphy, Craig N. 2006. *The United Nations Development Programme: A Better Way?* Cambridge: Cambridge University Press.

Murray, Christopher J. L., and Alan D. Lopez. 1996. *The Global Burden of Disease: A Comprehensive Assessment of Mortality and Disability from Diseases, Injuries, and Risk Factors in 1990 and Projected to 2020*. Boston: Harvard School of Public Health on behalf of the World Health Organization and the World Bank.

Naím, Moisés. 1994. "Latin America: The Second Stage of Reform." *Journal of Democracy* 5 (4): 32–48.

Nanda, Priya. 2002. "Gender Dimensions of User Fees: Implications for Women's Utilization of Health Care." *Reproductive Health Matters* 10 (20): 127–34.

Narayan, Deepa. 1999. *Bonds and Bridges: Social Capital and Poverty*. Poverty Working Paper no. 2167. Washington, D.C.: World Bank. http://info. worldbank.org/etools/docs/library/9747/narayan.pdf.

Nash, Jennifer C. 2008. "Re-thinking Intersectionality." *Feminist Review* 89:1–15.

Nelson, Joan M., ed. 1990. *Economic Crisis and Policy Choice: The Politics of Adjustment in the Third World*. Princeton: Princeton University Press.

———. 1992. "Poverty, Equity and the Politics of Adjustment." In Haggard and Kaufman 1992, 221–69.

———, ed. 1994. *A Precarious Balance*. Vol. 2, *Democracy and Economic Reforms in Latin America*. San Francisco: ICS Press.

———. 1996. "Promoting Policy Reforms: The Twilight of Conditionality." *World Development* 29 (9): 1551–59.

———. 1999. *Reforming Health and Education: The World Bank, the IDB, and Complex Institutional Change*. Policy Essay 26. Washington, D.C.: Overseas Development Council.

———. 2004. "The Politics of Health Sector Reform: Cross-National Comparisons." In Kaufman and Nelson 2004, 23–64.

Nussbaum, Martha. 2000. *Women and Human Development: The Capabilities Approach*. Cambridge: Cambridge University Press.

———. 2003. "Capabilities as Fundamental Entitlements: Sen and Social Justice." *Feminist Economics* 9 (2–3): 33–59.

Nussbaum, Martha, and Jonathan Glover, eds. 1995. *Women, Culture and Development: A Study of Human Capabilities*. Oxford: Clarendon Press.

O'Connor, Julia S. 1996. "From Women in the Welfare State to Gendering Welfare State Regimes." *Current Sociology* 44 (2): 1–124.

O'Connor, Julia S., Ann Shola Orloff, and Sheila Shaver. 1999. *States, Markets, Families: Gender, Liberalism and Social Policy in Australia, Canada, Great Britain and the United States*. Cambridge: Cambridge University Press.

Okin, Susan Moller, et al. 1999. Edited by Joshua Cohen, Matthew Howard, and Martha C. Nussbaum. *Is Multiculturalism Bad for Women?* Princeton: Princeton University Press.

Orenstein, Mitchell A. 2008. *The Transnational Campaign for Social Security Reform*. Princeton: Princeton University Press.

Organización Panamericana de la Salud (OPS) en el Perú. 2002. *Proyecciones de financiamiento de la atención de salud: Perú 2002–2006*. Lima: Organización Panamericana de la Salud.

Orihuela Paredes, Víctor. 1980. "Diagnóstico general de salud." In *La salud en el Perú*, 1–15. Cuaderno No. 28. Lima: Centro Latinoamericano de Trabajo Social.

Orloff, Ann Shola. 1993. "Gender and the Social Rights of Citizenship: The Comparative Analysis of Gender Relations and Welfare States." *American Sociological Review* 58 (3): 303–28.

Pan American Health Organization (PAHO). 1999. "Equidad de género y políticas de reforma del sector salud: Guía para la Preparación de informes." Washington: Pan American Health Organization and World Health Organization.

———. 2002. Special Program for Health Analysis. Regional Core Health Data Initiative; Technical Health Information System. Washington, D.C. http://www.paho.org/English.SHA/CoreData.

———. 2004. *Igualdad de género en salud en las Américas: Marco legal.* Washington, D.C.: Pan American Health Organization.

———. 2005. *Gender, Health, and Development in the Americas: Basic Indicators.* Washington, D.C.: Pan American Health Organization.

———. 2007. Regional Core Health Data Initiative: Technical Health Information System. Health Analysis and Statistics Unit. Washington, D.C. http://www.paho.org/English/SHA/CoreData/Tabulator/newTabulator.htm.

———. 2008. "Health Situation in the Americas: Basic Indicators, 2008." http://devserver.paho.org/hq/index.php?option=com_content&task=view&id=220&Itemid=317 (accessed December 2, 2008).

Parodi, Jorge. 2000. *To Be a Worker: Identity and Politics in Peru.* Chapel Hill: University of North Carolina Press.

ParSalud. 2007. "Evaluación Preliminar del SIS." Working Paper. Lima: Programa de Apoyo a la Reforma del Sector Salud.

Parker, David Stuart. 1998. *The Idea of the Middle Class: White-Collar Workers and Peruvian Society, 1900–1950.* University Park: Pennsylvania State University Press.

Parpart, Jane L., and Marianne H. Marchand, eds. 1995. *Feminism/Postmodernism/Development.* London: Routledge.

Pastor, Manuel, Jr. and Carol Wise. 1999. "The Politics of Second-Generation Reform." *Journal of Democracy* 10 (3): 34–48.

Pérez Fragoso, Lucía C., and María Concepción Martínez Medina. n.d. *El análisis del Programa de Ampliación de Cobertura: Un aporte para la construcción de los presupuestos públicos desde la perspectiva de equidad entre los géneros.* Mexico City: Equidad de Género, Ciudadanía, Trabajo y Familia.

El Peruano: Diario Oficial. 1996. "Carta de intención: Memorándum sobre las políticas económicas y financieras del gobierno del Perú para el período comprendido entre el 1 de Abril de 1996 y el 31 de Diciembre de 1998." Separata Especial. May 11. Lima.

Petchesky, Rosalind Pollack. 1995. "From Population Control to Reproductive Rights: Feminist Fault Lines." *Reproductive Health Matters* 3 (6): 152–61.

———. 2003. *Global Prescriptions: Gendering Health and Human Rights.* London: Zed Books; New York: United Nations Research Institute for Social Development.

Peterson, V. Spike. 2003. *A Critical Rewriting of Global Political Economy: Integrating Reproductive, Productive, and Virtual Economies.* New York: Routledge.

Pierson, Paul. 1993. "When Effect Becomes Cause: Policy Feedback and Political Change." *World Politics* 45 (4): 595–628.

———. 1994. *Dismantling the Welfare State? Reagan, Thatcher and the Politics of Retrenchment.* Cambridge: Cambridge University Press.

———. 2000. "Three Worlds of Welfare State Research." *Comparative Political Studies* 33 (6–7): 791–821.

Phillips, Anne. 2002. "Multiculturalism, Universalism, and the Claims of Democracy." In Molyneux and Razavi 2002, 115–38.

Pollack, Molly E. 2002. *Equidad de género en el sistema de salud Chileno.* Santiago: Economic Commission for Latin America and the Caribbean.

Portocarrero, Gonzalo. 1983. *Ideologías, funciones del estado y políticas económicas, Perú 1900–1980.* Lima: Pontificia Universidad Católica del Perú. Mimeo.

Presser, Harriet B., and Gita Sen. 2000. *Women's Empowerment and Demographic Processes: Moving Beyond Cairo.* New York: Oxford University Press.

Pribble, Jennifer. 2006. "The Politics of Women's Welfare in Chile and Uruguay." *Latin American Research Review* 41 (2): 4–111.

PROMUJER. 1998. *Poder político con perfume de mujer: Las cuotas en el Perú.* Lima: Movimiento Manuela Ramos and Instituto de Estudios Peruanos.

Proyecto Andino de Tecnologías Campesinas (PRATEC). 2002. *Salud y diversidad en la chacra andina.* Lima: PRATEC.

Quadagno, Jill. 1996. *The Color of Welfare: How Racism Undermined the War on Poverty.* New York: Oxford University Press.

Quayum, Seemin. 2002. "Nationalism, Internal Colonialism and the Spatial Imagination: The Geographic Society of La Paz in Turn-of-the-Century Bolivia." In *Studies in the Formation of the Nation-State in Latin America,* edited by James Dunkerley, 275–98. London: Institute of Latin American Studies.

Radcliffe, Sarah A. 1991. "The Role of Gender in Peasant Migration: Conceptual Issues from the Peruvian Andes." *Review of Radical Political Economics* 23 (3–4): 129–47.

———. 1993. "'People Have to Rise Up—Like the Great Women Fighters': The State and Peasant Women in Peru." In *'Viva' Women and Popular Protest in Latin America,* edited by Sarah A. Radcliffe and Sallie Westwood, 197–218. New York: Routledge.

Radcliffe, Sarah, and Sallie Westwood. 1996. *Remaking the Nation: Place, Identity, and Politics in Latin America.* New York: Routledge.

Ramírez, Patricia. 2004. "A Sweeping Health Reform: The Quest for Unification, Coverage and Efficiency in Colombia." In Kaufman and Nelson 2004, 124–54.

Razavi, Shahra. 2007. "The Return to Social Policy and the Persistent Neglect of Unpaid Care." *Development and Change* 38 (3): 377–400.

Razavi, Shahra, and Shireen Hassim, eds. 2006. *Gender and Social Policy in a Global Context: Uncovering the Gendered Structure of "the Social."* Basingstoke: Palgrave Macmillan.

Reeves, Hazel, and Sally Baden. 2000. "Gender and Development: Concepts and Definitions." Brighton: BRIDGE, Institute of Development Studies, University of Sussex.

Remenyi, María Antonia. 1999. *Lineamientos para el diseño de nuevos mecanismos de pago para prestadores públicos.* Lima: Ministerio de Salud del Perú.

Roberts, Kenneth. 1995. "Neoliberalism and the Transformation of Populism in Latin America: The Peruvian Case." *World Politics* 48 (1): 82–116.

Roemer, Milton I. 1964. *La atención médica en América Latina.* Prepared for the Secretary General of the OEA. Washington, D.C.: Unión Panamericana, Secretaría General, Organización de los Estados Americanos.

———. 1969. *The Organization of Medical Care Under Social Security: A Study Based upon the Experience of Eight Countries.* Geneva: International Labour Office.

Rogers, Everett M. 1962. *Diffusion of Innovations.* New York: Free Press of Glencoe.

———. 2003. *Diffusion of Innovations.* 5th ed. New York: Free Press.

Roldan, Martha. 1988. "Renegotiating the Marital Contract: Intrahousehold Patterns, Money Allocation and Women's Subordination Among Domestic Outworkers in Mexico City." In *A Home Divided: Women and Income in the Third World,* edited by Daisy Dwyer and Judith Bruce, 229–47. Stanford: Stanford University Press.

Rosas Lauro, Claudia. 2004. "Madre solo hay una: Ilustración, maternidad y medicina en el Perú del siglo XVIII." *Anuario de Estudios Americanos* 61 (1): 103–38.

Rosemblatt, Karin Alejandra. 2000. *Gendered Compromises: Political Cultures and the State in Chile, 1920–1950.* Chapel Hill: University of North Carolina Press.

Rousseau, Stéphanie. 2006. "Women's Citizenship and Neopopulism: Peru Under the Fujimori Regime." *Latin American Politics and Society* 48 (1): 117–41.

Rueschemeyer, Dietrich, Evelyne Huber Stephens, and John D. Stephens. 1992. *Capitalist Development and Democracy.* Chicago: University of Chicago Press.

Ruger, Jennifer P. 2006. "El rol cambiante del Banco Mundial en la salud global." In *Historia, salud y globalización,* edited by Marcos Cueto and Víctor Zamora, 103–33. Lima: Instituto de Estudios Peruanos and Universidad Peruana Cayetano Heredia.

Saavedra, Jaime. 2000. "La flexibilización el mercado laboral." In *La reforma incompleta: Rescatando los noventa,* vol. 1, edited by Roberto Abusada-Salah, Fritz Du Bois, Eduardo Morón, and José Valderrama, 379–428. Lima: Centro de Investigación de la Universidad del Pacífico and Instituto Peruano de Economía.

Sabhaperu. 2007. *Informe preliminar de medición externa de filtración en la afiliación al SIS en el ámbito del programa de apoyo financiero del comité técnico Belga.* Lima: Sabhaperu Asesoría Tributaria.

Sainsbury, Diane. 1996. *Gender, Equality and Welfare States.* Cambridge: Cambridge University Press.

Schattschneider, Elmer Eric. 1960. *The Semi-sovereign People: A Realist's View of Democracy in America.* New York: Holt, Rinehart and Winston.

Schoenpflug, Karen. 2006. "World Bank Discourse and World Bank Policy in Engendering Development." In Kuiper and Barker 2006, 117–24.

Schoultz, Lars. 1998. *Beneath the United States: A History of US Policy Toward Latin America.* Cambridge: Harvard University Press.

Seguro Integral de Salud (SIS). 2004. *Instructivo de aplicación de la ficha de evaluación económica familiar.* Lima: Seguro Integral de Salud.

Sen, Amartya Kumar. 1989. "Development as Capability Expansion." *Journal of Development Planning* 19:41–58.

———. 2001. *Development as Freedom.* New York: Oxford University Press.

———. 2002. "¿Por qué la equidad en salud?" *Revista Panamericana de Salud Pública* 11:302–9.

Sen, Gita, Asha George, and Piroska Östlin. 2002a. "Engendering Health Equity: A Review of Research and Policy." In Sen, George, and Östlin 2002b, 1–33.

———, eds. 2002b. *Engendering International Health: The Challenge of Equity.* Cambridge: MIT Press.

Sen, Gita, and Caren Grown. 1987. *Development, Crisis, and Alternative Visions: Third World Women's Perspectives.* New York: Monthly Review Press.

Sheahan, John. 1999. *Searching for a Better Society: The Peruvian Economy from 1950.* University Park: Pennsylvania State University Press.

Shepard, Bonnie. 2006. *Running the Obstacle Course to Sexual and Reproductive Health: Lessons from Latin America.* Westport: Praeger.

Shachar, Ayelet. 2000. "On Citizenship and Multicultural Vulnerability." *Political Theory* 28 (1): 64–89.

Simmons, Beth A. 2001. "The International Politics of Harmonization: The Case of Capital Market Regulation." *International Organization* 55 (3): 589–620.

Skocpol, Theda. 1992. *Protecting Soldiers and Mothers: The Political Origins of Social Policy in the United States.* Cambridge: Belknap Press of Harvard University Press.

Smith, Gregory L., George P. Taylor, and Kevin F. Smith. 1985. "Comparative Risks and Costs of Male and Female Sterilization." *American Journal of Public Health* 75 (4): 370–74.

Smith, William C., Carlos H. Acuña, and Eduardo Gamarra, eds. 1994. *Democracy, Markets, and Structural Reform in Latin America.* Coral Gables, Fla.: North-South Center.

Smyth, Ines. 1998. "Gender Analysis of Family Planning: Beyond the 'Feminist vs. Population Control' Debate." In *Feminist Visions of Development: Gender Analysis and Policy,* edited by Cecile Jackson and Ruth Pearson, 217–38. London: Routledge.

Snyder, Margaret. 2006. "Unlikely Godmother: The UN and the Global Women's Movement." In *Global Feminism: Transnational Women's Activism, Organizing, and Human Rights,* edited by Myra Marx Ferree and Aili Tripp, 24–50. New York: New York University Press.

Soederberg, Susanne. 2005. "Recasting Neoliberal Dominance in the Global South? A Critique of the Monterrey Consensus." *Alternatives* 30:325–64.

Sparr, Pamela, ed. 1994. *Mortgaging Women's Lives: Feminist Critiques of Structural Adjustment.* London: Zed Books.

Squires, Judith. 2005. "Is Mainstreaming Transformative? Theorizing Mainstreaming in the Context of Diversity and Deliberation." *Social Politics* 12 (3): 366–88.

Stallings, Barbara. 1992. "International Influence on Economic Policy: Debt, Stabilization and Structural Reform." In Haggard and Kaufman 1992, 41–88.

Standing, Hilary. 1997. "Gender Equity in Health Sector Reform Programmes: A Review." *Health Policy and Planning* 12 (1): 1–18.

———. 1999. "Frameworks for Understanding Gender Inequalities and Health Sector Reform: An Analysis and Review of Policy Issues." Working Paper 99.06 Cambridge, Mass.: Harvard Center for Population and Development Studies.

———. 2000. "Gender Impacts of Health Reforms—The Current State of Policy and Implementation." Paper presented at the ALAMES meeting. Havana, Cuba, July 3–7.

———. 2002. "An Overview of Changing Agendas in Health Sector Reforms." *Reproductive Health Matters* 10 (20): 19–29.

Steinmo, Sven, Kathleen Thelen, and Frank Longstreth, eds. 1992. *Historical Institutionalism in Comparative Analysis.* Cambridge: Cambridge University Press.

Stepan, Nancy. 1981. *Beginnings of Brazilian Science: Oswaldo Cruz, Medical Research and Policy.* New York: Science History Publications.

———. 1991. *The Hour of Eugenics: Race, Gender, and Nation in Latin America.* Ithaca: Cornell University Press.

Stephenson, Marcia. 1999. *Gender and Modernity in Andean Bolivia.* Austin: University of Texas Press.

Stern, Alexandra Minna. 2006. "Yellow Fever Crusade: US Colonialism, Tropical Medicine and the International Politics of Mosquito Control, 1900–1920." In *Medicine at the Border: Disease, Globalization, and Security, 1850 to the Present,* edited by Alison Bashford, 41–59. New York: Palgrave.

Stetson, Dorothy McBride, and Amy Mazur, eds. 1995. *Comparative State Feminism.* Thousand Oaks, Calif.: Sage.

Stiglitz, Joseph E. 1998. "Towards a New Paradigm for Development: Strategies, Policies and Processes." Ninth Raul Prebisch Lecture, delivered at the Palais des Nations, Geneva, October 19, United Nations Conference on Trade and Development.

———. 2002. *Globalization and Its Discontents.* New York: W. W. Norton.

———. 2004. "The Post Washington Consensus Consensus." Initiative for Policy Dialogue Working Paper Series, Task Force on Governance of Globalization, November, Columbia University, New York.

Stoler, Ann Laura. 2002. *Carnal Knowledge and Imperial Power: Race and the Intimate in Colonial Rule.* Berkeley and Los Angeles: University of California Press.

Strange, Susan. 1996. *The Retreat of the State: The Diffusion of Power in the World Economy.* Cambridge: Cambridge University Press.

Stavenhagen, Rodolpho. 1965. "Classes, Colonialism and Acculturation." *Studies in Comparative International Development* 1 (6): 53–77.

Sugiyama, Natasha Borges. 2008a. "Ideology and Networks: The Politics of Social Policy Diffusion in Brazil." *Latin American Research Review* 43 (3): 82–108.

———. 2008b. "Theories of Policy Diffusion: Social Sector Reform in Brazil." *Comparative Political Studies* 41 (2): 193–216.

Superintendencia de Entidades Prestadoras de Salud (SEPS). 2005. *Anuario 2004: Sistema de entidades prestadoras de salud.* Lima: Superintendencia de Entidades Prestadoras de Salud.

Tamayo, Gonzalo, and Pedro Francke. 1997. *Análisis del gasto público en salud.* Seminario Modernización del Sistema de Financiamiento de Salud. Lima: Ministerio de Salud del Perú.

Teichman, Judith. 2001. *The Politics of Freeing Markets in Latin America: Chile, Argentina, and Mexico.* Chapel Hill: University of North Carolina Press.

Theobald, Sally, Rachel Tolhurst, Helen Elsey, and Hilary Standing. 2005. "Engendering the Bureaucracy? Challenges and Opportunities for Mainstreaming Gender in Ministries of Health Under Sector-Wide Approaches." *Health Policy and Planning* 20 (3): 141–49.

Thiedon, Kimberly. 1999. *Análisis situacional de la educación de las niñas en Ayacucho, resumen ejecutivo.* Ayacucho: CARE-Peru, USAID.

Thomas, Duncan. 1997. "Incomes, Expenditures and Health Outcomes: Evidence on Intrahousehold Resources Allocation." In *Intrahousehold Resources Allocation in Developing Countries: Models, Methods, and Policy,* edited by Lawrence Haddad, John Hoddinott, and Harold Alderman, 142–64. Baltimore: Johns Hopkins University Press.

Thorp, Rosemary. 1996. "A Long-Run Perspective on Short-Run Stabilization: The Experience of Peru." In *The Peruvian Economy and Structural Adjustment: Past Present and Future,* edited by Efraín Gonzales de Olarte, 59–75. Miami: North-South Center Press.

Tilly, Charles. 1998. *Durable Inequality.* Berkeley and Los Angeles: University of California Press.

Tinker, Irene, ed. 1990. *Persistent Inequalities: Women and World Development.* New York: Oxford University Press.

Titelman, Daniel. 2000. *Reformas al sistema de salud en Chile: Desafíos pendientes.* No. 104 Serie Financiamiento del Desarrollo. Santiago: Comisión Económica para America Latina y el Caribe, Unidad de Financiamiento para el Desarrollo.

True, Jacqui, and Michael Mintrom. 2001. "Transnational Networks and Policy Diffusion: The Case of Gender Mainstreaming." *International Studies Quarterly* 45:27–57.

Turshen, Meredeth. 1995. "The World Bank Eclipses the World Health Organization." *ACAS Bulletin* 44/45 (Winter/Spring): 25–27.

———. 1999. *Privatizing Health Services in Africa.* New Brunswick: Rutgers University Press.

Tzannatos, Zafiris. 2006. "The World Bank, Development, Adjustment and Gender Equality." In Kuiper and Barker 2006, 13–39.

United Nations (UN). 1962. *The United Nations Development Decade: Proposals for Action.* New York: United Nations.

———. 2002. *Draft Guidelines: A Human Rights Approach to Poverty Reduction Strategies.* New York: United Nations. http://www.unhcr.org/refworld/docid/3f8298544.html.

———. 2005. Millennium Development Indicators, Peru. http://mdgs.un.org/unsd/mdg/Data.aspx (accessed December 30, 2008).

United Nations Children's Fund (UNICEF). 1990. *Revitalizing Primary Health Care/Maternal and Child Health: The Bamako Initiative.* Progress report presented to the UNICEF Executive Board 1990 Session. New York: UNICEF.

United Nations—Department of Economic and Social Affairs (UN-DESA). 1978. *National Experience in the Formulation and Implementation of Population Policy, 1960–1976.* New York: United Nations.

United Nations Development Fund for Women (UNIFEM). 2000. *Progress of the World's Women: UNIFEM Biennial Report.* New York: UNIFEM.

———. 2005. *Violencia doméstica contra las mujeres: Información general, América Latina y el Caribe.* New York: UNIFEM. http://www.unifem.org/attachments/products/ViolenciaDomestica_LAC_spn.pdf.

United Nations Research Institute for Social Development (UNRISD). 2005. *Gender Equality: Striving for Justice in an Unequal World.* New York: UNRISD/United Nations Publications.

UN News Service. 2004. "UN Human Rights Expert Urges Peru, US to Protect Health in Any Trade Deal." http://www.un.org/apps/news/story.asp?NewsID= 11253&Cr=peru&Cr1= (accessed October 18, 2008).

Valverde, Rocio, Victor Salazar, and Robinson Cabello. 2006. *Peru In-Country Monitoring and Evaluation Report on the Implementation of the UNGASS Declaration of Commitment.* International Council of AIDS Service Organizations.

Vargas, Virginia. 1989. *El aporte de la rebeldía de las mujeres.* Lima: Centro de la Mujer Peruana Flora Tristán.

———. 2006. *El movimiento feminista en el horizonte democrático peruano (décadas 1980–1990).* Lima: Centro de la Mujer Peruana Flora Tristán.

———. 2008. *Feminismos en América Latina: Su aporte a la política y a la democracia.* Lima: Programa Democracia y Transformación Global, Centro de la Mujer Flora Tristán, and Universidad Nacional Mayor de San Marcos.

Varillas, Alberto, and Patricia Mostajo. 1990. *La situación poblacional peruana: Balance y perspectivas.* Lima: Instituto Andino de Estudios en Población y Desarrollo.

Vera la Torre, José Carlos. 2003. *Cobertura y financiamiento del seguro integral de salud en el Perú.* Cuaderno de Trabajo No. 2. Lima: ForoSalud and Consorcio de Investigación Económico y Social.

Verdera V., Francisco. 1997. *Seguridad social y pobreza en el Perú, una aproxi-mación.* Documento de Trabajo No. 84. Lima: Instituto de Estudios Peruanos.

Verloo, Mieke. 2005. "Displacement and Empowerment: Reflections on the Concept and Practice of the Council of Europe Approach to Gender Mainstreaming and Gender Equality." *Social Politics* 12 (3): 344–65.

Wade, Peter. 1997. *Race and Ethnicity in Latin America.* London: Pluto Press.

Waitzkin, Howard. 1998. "Is Our Work Dangerous? Should It Be?" *Journal of Health and Social Behavior* 39 (1): 7–17.

Walby, Sylvia. 2001. "From Community to Coalition: The Politics of Recognition as the Handmaiden of the Politics of Equality in an Era of Globalization." *Theory, Culture and Society* 18 (2–3): 113–35.

Wang, Jufen. 2006. "Health Sector Reform in China: Gender Equality and Social Justice." In Razavi and Hassim 2006, 258–77.

Weir, Margaret, and Theda Skocpol. 1985. "State Structures and Possibilities for 'Keynesian' Responses to the Great Depression in Sweden, Britain and the United States." In *Bringing the State Back In,* edited by Peter B. Evans, Dietrich Reuschemeyer, and Theda Skocpol, 107–68. Cambridge: Cambridge University Press.

Weismantel, Mary. 2001. *Cholas and Pishtacos: Stories of Race and Sex in the Andes.* Chicago: University of Chicago Press.

Weldon, S. Laurel. 2006. "The Structure of Intersectionality: A Comparative Politics of Gender." *Politics and Gender* 2 (2): 235–48.

Weyland, Kurt. 1996a. *Democracy Without Equity: Failures of Reform in Brazil.* Pittsburgh: University of Pittsburgh Press.

———. 1996b. "Neopopulism and Neoliberalism in Latin America." *Studies in Comparative International Development* 31:3–31.

———. 2002. *The Politics of Market Reform in Fragile Democracies: Argentina, Brazil, Peru, and Venezuela.* Princeton: Princeton University Press.

———. 2004a. "Assessing Latin American Neoliberalism: Introduction to a Debate." *Latin American Research Review* 39 (3): 143–49.

———, ed. 2004b. *Learning from Foreign Models in Latin American Policy Reform.* Washington: Woodrow Wilson Center Press; Baltimore: Johns Hopkins University Press.

———. 2005. "Theories of Policy Diffusion: Lessons from Latin American Pension Reform." *World Politics* 57:262–95.

———. 2006. *Bounded Rationality and Policy Diffusion: Social Sector Reform in Latin America.* Princeton: Princeton University Press.

Williamson, John. 1990. "What Washington Means by Policy Reform." In *Latin American Adjustment: How Much Has Happened?* edited by John Williamson, 7–20. Washington: Institute for International Economics.

Women's International Network News. 1997. "Women's Eyes on the World Bank: A Global Network to Transform the Bank and to Meet Women's Needs." 23 (1): 14.

World Bank. 1987. *Financing Health Services in Developing Countries: An Agenda for Reform.* Washington, D.C.: World Bank.

———. 1993. *World Development Report 1993: Investing in Health.* Washington, D.C.: World Bank; New York: Oxford University Press.

———. 1999. "Peru: Improving Health Care for the Poor." Report No. 18549-PE, May 28. World Bank, Human Development Department, Bolivia, Paraguay and Peru Country Management Unit, Latin America and the Caribbean Region, Washington, D.C.

World Health Organization (WHO)/Institut Català de Oncologia (ICA) Information Center on HPV and Cervical Cancer. 2007. *Human Papillomavirus and Cervical Cancer: Summary Report, Peru.* http://www.who.Int/hpvcentre (accessed January 14, 2009).

Yamin, Alicia Ely. 2003. *Castillos de arena en el camino hacia la modernidad: Una perspectiva desde los derechos humanos sobre el proceso de reforma del sector salud en el Perú (1990–2000) y sus implicancias en la muerte materna.* Lima: Centro de la Mujer Peruana Flora Tristán.

Yamin, Alicia Ely, and Deborah P. Maine. 1999. "Maternal Mortality as a Human Rights Issue: Measuring Compliance with International Treaty Obligations." *Human Rights Quarterly* 21 (3): 563–607.

Yashar, Deborah J. 1998. "Contesting Citizenship: Indigenous Movements and Democracy in Latin America." *Comparative Politics* 31 (1): 23–42.

Yeates, Nicola. 2001. *Globalization and Social Policy.* London: Sage.

Yoshioka, Hirotoshi. 2006. "A Q-analysis of Census Data: Intra-household Income Allocation and School Attendance in Chiapas, Mexico." *Quality and Quantity* 40: 1061–77.

Yuval-Davis, Nira. 2006. "Intersectionality and Feminist Politics." *European Journal of Women's Studies* 13 (3): 193–209.

Zimmerman, Eduardo A. 1992. "Racial Ideas and Social Reform: Argentina, 1890–1916." *Hispanic American Historical Review* 72 (1): 23–46.

Zinsser, Judith P. 2002. "From Mexico to Copenhagen to Nairobi: The United Nations Decade for Women 1975–1985." *Journal of World History* 13 (1): 139–68.

Zschock, Dieter K., ed. 1988. *Health Care in Peru: Resources and Policy.* Boulder: Westview Press.

Zulawski, Ann. 2000. "Hygiene and 'the Indian Problem': Ethnicity and Medicine in Bolivia, 1910–1920." *Latin American Research Review* 35 (2): 107–29.

———. 2007. *Unequal Cures: Public Health and Political Change in Bolivia, 1900–1950.* Durham: Duke University Press.

Interviews

Aguinaga C., David. Interview by author, July 22, 1998, Lima. Coordinator of Community Participation. CLAS Juan Pablo II.

Aldorodín, Dr. Interview by author, January 25, 1999, Ayacucho. Director, Dirección de Salud Ayacucho.

Altamirano, Hilda. Interview by author, May 13, 1998, Ayacucho. Formerly in charge of evaluating PSBT centers in Ayacucho.

Alviar, Suárez, Tula. Interview by author, February 1, 1999, Ayacucho. Head doctor, CLAS Luricocha.

Amalia, Sra. Interview by author, July 14, 1998, Lima. Coordinator, Vaso de Leche #3, Patria Nueva, CLAS Laura Caller.

Amat y León, Patricia. Interview by author, March 2, 1998, Lima. NGO consortium "Mujer y Ajuste."

Anon. 1. Interview by author, March 3, 1998, Lima. Affiliated with Programa de Salud y Nutrición Básica, MINSA.

Anon. 2. Interview by author, March 10, 1998, Lima. Formerly affiliated with the Inter-ministerial Commission and the national targeted social spending policy plan.

Anon. 3. Interview by author, March 11, 1998, Lima. Member of team that oversaw the overall health sector reform plan.

Anon. 4. Interview by author, March 11, 1998, Lima; March 16, 1998, Lima. Affiliated with the Programa de Salud Básica Para Todos, MINSA.

Anon. 5. Interview by author, April 17, 1998, Lima; April 24, 1998, Lima. Member of team that oversaw overall health sector reform, MINSA.

Anon. 6. Interview by author, August 12, 1998, Lima. Formerly affiliated with the Family Planning Program, MINSA.

Anon. 7. Interview by author, July 23, 1998, Lima. Doctor at CLAS center.

Anon. 8. Interview by author, September 10, 1998, Lima. Consultant to the Program to Strengthen Health Services, MINSA.

Anon. 9. Interview by author. March 2, 1998, Lima. Formerly affiliated with the Programa de Administración Compartida (CLAS), MINSA.

Anon. 10. Interview by author, April 3, 2000, Lima. Affiliated with overall reform process.

Anon. 11. Communication with author, April 8, 1998, Lima. Member of staff, Programa de Administración Compartida (CLAS), MINSA.

Anon. 12. Interview by author, February 23, 1998, Lima. Member of staff, MINSA Department of External Cooperation and the overall reform team.

Anon. 13. Interview by author, November 18, 1998, Lima. Head doctor, PSBT center.

Anon. 14. Interview by author, February 25, 2000, Washington, D.C. Inter-American Development Bank.

Anon. 15. Interview by author, January 19, 1999, Lima. World Bank.

Anon. 16. Interview by author, February 24, 2000, Washington, D.C. Inter-American Development Bank.

Anon. 17. Interview by author, October 8, 1999, Washington, D.C. World Bank.

Anon. 18. Interview by author, April 11, 2000, Lima. Coordinator of Maternal Infant Insurance.

Anon. 19. Interview by author, November 11, 1998, Lima. UNICEF.

Anon. 20. Interview by author, January 15, 1999, Lima. Pan American Health Organization in Peru.

Anon. 21. Interview by author, December 1, 1998, Lima. USAID.

Anon. 22. Interview by author, April 11, 2000, Lima. Affiliated with Maternal Infant Insurance.

Anon. 23. Interview by author, October 7, 1999, Washington, D.C. Pan American Health Organization.

Anon. 24. Interview by author, July 14, 1998, Lima. Social worker, CLAS center.

Anon. 25. Interview by author, February 23, 1999, Ayacucho. Nurse, PSBT center.

Anon. 26. Interview by author, February 23, 1999, Ayacucho. Nurse-midwife, PSBT center.

Anon. 27. Interview by author, August 18, 1998, Lima. Nurse-midwife, CLAS center.

Anon. 28. Interview by author, February 1, 1999, Ayacucho. Nurse-midwife, CLAS center.

Anon. 29. Interview by author, March 9, 1999, Ayacucho. Former nurse-midwife, PSBT Center.

Anon. 30. Interview by author, September 12, 1998, Lima. Head doctor, PSBT Center.

Anon. 31. Interview by author, November 19, 1998, Lima. Social worker, PSBT Center.

Anon. 32. Interview by author, February 11, 1999, Luricocha.

Anon. 33. Interview by author, November 19, 1998, Lima. Nurse-midwife, PSBT Center.

Anon. 34. Interview by author, November 18, 1998, Lima. Nurse-midwife, PSBT Center.

Anon. 35. Interview by author, July 15, 1998, Lima. Doctor, CLAS Center.

Anon. 36. Interview by author, December 3, 1998, Lima. Nurse-midwife, PSBT Center.

Anon. 37. Interview by author, February 23, 1999, Ayacucho. Doctor, PSBT Center.

Anon. 38. Interview by author, May 15, 1998, Ayacucho. Head doctor, PSBT Center.

Anon. 39. Interview by author, April 21, 1998, Lima. Consultant to the Family Planning Program, MINSA.

Anon. 40. Interview by author, February 26, 2000, Washington, D.C. Consultant, Inter-American Development Bank.

Anon. 41. Communication with author, July 2000, Lima. USAID official.

Anon. A1. Interview by author, February 20, 1999, Ayacucho. Person who submitted to surgical sterilization.

Anon. A2. Interview by author with Quechua translation assistance of Madeleine Pariona Oncebay, February 20, 1999, Ayacucho. Person who submitted to surgical sterilization.

Anon. A3. Interview by author with Quechua translation assistance of Madeleine Pariona Oncebay, February 2, 1999, Ayacucho. Person who submitted to surgical sterilization.

Anon. A4. Interview by author with Quechua translation assistance of Madeleine Pariona Oncebay, February 27, 1999, Ayacucho. Person who submitted to surgical sterilization.

Anon. A5. Interview by author with Quechua translation assistance of Madeleine Pariona Oncebay, February 21, 1999, Ayacucho. Person who submitted to surgical sterilization.

Anon. A6. Interview by author, February 27, 1999, Ayacucho. Person who submitted to surgical sterilization.

Arana, María Teresa. Interview by author, June 28, 2005, Lima; June 4, 2007, Lima. Coordinadora Unidad Técnica Funcional de Derechos Humanos, Equidad de Género e Interculturalidad en Salud (at time of first interview).

Arbayza Ramírez, Maura. Interview by author, March 19, 1999, Ayacucho. Coordinator of CLAS for the Dirección de Salud Ayacucho.

Baca Cordova, Elsa. Interview by author, April 24, 1998, Lima. President of the Confederación General de Trabajadores del Perú.

Barboza Merino, Miriam. Interview by author, February 6, 1999. Luricocha, Ayacucho. President, CLAS Luricocha.

Berrocal Perez Palma, Fredy. Interview by author, February 10, 1999. Luricocha, Ayacucho. Vocal, CLAS Luricocha.

Bautista, Luisa. Interview by author, March 18, 1999, Ayacucho. Coordinator of the PSBT for the Dirección de Salud Ayacucho.

Begazo, Hector. Interview by author, January 18, 1999, Lima. General manager, EPS Santa Cruz.

Bendezú, Carlos. Interview by author, March 17, 1998, Lima. Consultant to the Program to Strengthen Health Services, MINSA.

Bermudo Medina, Fredy. Interview by author, February 2, 1999, Ayacucho. Nurse, CLAS Luricocha.

Bottger Bravo, Georgina. Interview by author, November 12, 1998, Lima. Secretaria General del Sindicato Nacional de Enfermeras del IPSS.

Bustamente Castro, Martín. Interview by author, August 27, 1998, Lima. Advisor to Luis Casteñeda Lossio when he was executive president of IPSS.

Cahuana Cordero, Gladys. Interview by author. August 11, 1998, Lima. Secretary of CLAS Laura Caller.

Camacho Gallardo, Carlos. Interview by author, July 23, 1998, Lima. Head doctor, CLAS San Martín de Porres.

Cambria Rosset, Celeste. Interview by author, April 16, 1998, Lima. Programa Salud y Derechos Reproductivos. Centro de la Mujer Peruana Flora Tristán.

Cárdenas, Max. Interview by author, March 16, 1998, Lima. Interview by author, February 12, 1998, Lima. Decano del Colegio Médico and Ex-presidente de la Federación Medica.

Carrasco, Fresia. Interview by author, March 16, 1998, Lima. Equipo Salud, Manuela Ramos.

Casteñeda Lossio, Luis. Interview by author, August 27, 1998, Lima. Former executive president of the Instituto Peruano de Seguridad Social (IPSS).

Castro, Dra. Q. F. Josefa S. Interview by author, April 8, 1998, Lima. Executive director, Pro-Vida.

Chávez, Susana. Interview by author, April 13, 1998, Lima; July 1, 2005, Lima. Programa Repro-Salud, Manuela Ramos (at time of first interview) director of PROMSEX (at time of second interview).

Club de Madres of Vinchos. Group interview by author with the assistance of Madeleine Pariona Oncebay, March 3, 1999, Ayacucho.

Coordinator, Comedor Montenegro, PSBT Cruz de Motupe. Interview by author, January 12, 1999, Lima.

Cuentas Ramirez, Raquel. Interview by author, June 5, 2007, Lima; communication with author, June 27, 2007. Seguro Integral de Salud.

Dador, María Jennie. Communication with author, June 20, 2005; interview by author, June 30, 2005. Formerly of Manuela Ramos.

Degar Romero, Moises. Interview by author, November 17, 1998, Lima. Secretario General de la Federación Gráfica de Lima.

Delgado, Dr. Luis Pro. Interview by author, May 18, 1998, Lima. Director, Dirección de Salud Lima Norte.

Díaz Romero, Ricardo. Interview by author, February 14, 1998, Lima; April 3, 2000, Lima; telephone communication with author, February 19, 2001. Former head of a CLAS health center in Sierra del Pasco; board member, Federación Médica (at time of first interview); director ("Responsibilidad Técnica") of Programa de Administración Compartida, MINSA (at time of second interview).

Dierna, Rosa. Interview by author, June 30, 2005, Lima. Former head of the Pan American Health Organization's Gender Equity and Health Reform project in Peru.

Elisa. Interview by author, July 20, 1998, Lima. President of the health promoters, CLAS/Puesto de Salud San Martín.

Elsa. Interview by author, January 15, 1999, Lima. Health promoter and community kitchen organizer. PSBT C. S. José Carlos Mariátegui.

Fernandez-Castilla, Rogilio. Interview by author, May 6, 1998, Lima. Representative of UNFPA, Peru.

Flecha Zalba, Pedro. Interview by author, January 19, 1999, Lima. Director, EPS Rimac.

Franco Mendoza, Lidia. Interview by author, November 12, 1998, Lima. Secretary, CLAS Juan Pablo II.

Freundt-Thurne, Jaime. Interview by author, April 15, 1998, Lima. Former minister of health.

Gallardo Roncal, Julia Rosa. Interview by author, November 6, 1998, Lima. Treasurer, CLAS Juan Pablo II.

Garavito, Miguel. Interview by author, June 6, 2007, Lima. ParSalud.

García, Uriel. Interview by author, April 16, 1998, Lima. Former minister of health.

Gilman, Josephine B. Interview by author, March 16, 1998, Lima. Executive director of PRISMA.

Gerónimo, Felipe. Interview by author, July 22, 1998, Lima. President, CLAS Juan Pablo II.

Gómez Vargas, Mónica. Interview by author, February 11, 1998, Lima. Director of the Health and Nutrition Program of ADRA/OFASA of Peru.

Gonzales, Diego. Interview by author, April 12, 2000, Lima. Head of health reform team, MINSA.

Gualambo, Antenor. Interview by author. July 19, 1998, Lima. Secretary and former president, CLAS San Martín de Porres.

Guerra García, Roger. Interview by author, September 11, 1998, Lima. Congressional representative, Unión Por el Perú.

Güezmes García, Ana. Interview by author, March 18, 1998, Lima; June 28, 2005, Lima. Coordinator, Programa Salud y Derechos Reproductivos, Centro de la Mujer Peruana Flora Tristán (at time of first interview).

Guillén, Paolo. Interview by author, February 6, 1999, Ayacucho. President Luricocha Self-Defense Committee (Ronderos).

Gutiérrez, Rocio. Interview by author, June 6, 2007, Lima. Coordinadora Área de Salud, Manuela Ramos.

Habich Rospigliosi, Midori de. Interview by author, April 4, 2000. Proyecto 2000 (USAID-funded project in the Ministry of Health of Peru).

Hagei, César. Interview by author, November 18, 1998, Lima. Head doctor, PSBT 10 de Octubre.

Health promoter. Interview by author, August 18, 1998, Lima. Urban CLAS Laura Caller.

Health promoter. Interview by author, February 25, 1999, Ayacucho. Rural PSBT center, Vinchos.

Health promoters of Centro de Salud Mariátegui. Group interview by author, January 15, 1999, Lima.

Health promoters of CLAS Laura Caller. Group interview by author, August 14, 1998, Lima.

Health promoters of CLAS San Martín de Porres. Group interview by author, July 17, 1998, Lima.

Huascaya Medina, Emma Rosana. Interview by author, July 20, 1998, Lima. Treasurer, CLAS San Martín de Porres.

Jara Ortega, Freddy. Interview by author, April 6, 1998, Lima. Federación de Trabajadores en Construcción Civil del Perú.

Jefferson, Luz. Interview by author, April 24, 1998, Lima. Member of national commission appointed by the minister of health to investigate abuses in relation to the family planning program.

Jorge Aguilar, Ulises. Interview with author, January 19, 1999, Lima. Director of Seguro Escolar Gratuito.

Lewis, David. Interview by author, April 30, 1998, Lima. Department for International Development, Great Britain.

Luna Andrade, Fabiola. Interview by author, April 6, 1998, Lima. Director of the Women, Health and Development Program, MINSA.

Male lay midwife. Interview by author, February 22, 1999, Ayacucho. Community of Intay, district of Luricocha.

Manrique, Luis. Interview by author, February 18, 1998, Lima; July 15, 1998, Lima. Formerly affiliated with the national policy on targeting of social spending. Superintendente de la Superintendencia de las Empresas Prestadoras de Salud (at time of second interview).

Mantilla, Julissa. Communication with author, January 20, 1999, Lima. Staff member, Defensoría del Pueblo.

Marín, Mariella. Interview by author, July 16, 1998. Social worker, CLAS San Martín de Porres.

Martínez Padilla, Gretal. Interview by author, July 16, 1998, Lima. Nurse-midwife, CLAS San Martín de Porres.

Maulaui Cahuana, Jeanette. Interview by author, December 11, 1998, Lima. Nurse, PSBT Cruz de Motupe.

Mautino, Walter. Interview by author, July 15, 1998. Treasurer of the Central Neighborhood Council of Laura Caller.

Menchola, Walter. Interview by author, August 28, 1998, Lima. Former manager of health, IPSS.

Miranda Ruíz, Narciso H. Interview by author, July 17, 1998, Lima. Head doctor, CLAS Juan Pablo II.

Morantes, María Elena. Interview by author, June 5, 2007, Lima. Coordinadora Unidad Técnica Funcional de Derechos Humanos, Equidad de Género e Interculturalidad en Salud.

Moreno, Antonio. Interview by author, May 20, 1998, Lima. Director of Communal Participation, Dirección de Salud Lima Norte.

Muñoz, Ismael. Communication with author, March 12, 1998, Lima. Economista, Area de Formación, Instituto Bartolomé de las Casas.

Olea, Cecilia. Interview by author, May 31, 2007, Lima. Centro de la Mujer Peruana Flora Tristán.

Pachas, Juan E. Mauricio. Interview by author, February 17, 1998, Lima. Director of the family planning program, MINSA.

Palomino, Nancy. Communication with author, June 19, 2005, Lima.

Palomino Salazar, Rodrigo. Interview by author, February 10, 1999, Luricocha, Ayacucho. Treasurer, CLAS Luricocha.

Peñaloza, Isaias. Interview by author, February 23, 1998, Lima. Presidente de la Federación Médica.

President Comedor Sagrado Corazon, CLAS JPII. Interview by author, June 13, 1998, Lima.

Rey, Rafael. Interview by author, March 2, 1999, Ayacucho. President of Vinchos Self-Defense Committee (Ronderos).

Rivera Santender, María Adela. Interview by author, March 9, 1998, Lima. Coordinadora del PANSIC, INCAFAM.

Rodríguez, Elcira. Interview by author, July 13, 1998, Lima. Treasurer, CLAS Laura Caller.

Rojas, Marlena. Interview by author, November 18, 1998, Lima. Nurse, PSBT 10 de Octubre.

Rojas Silva, Mimi Lily. Interview by author, July 17, 1998, Lima. Nurse-midwife, CLAS Laura Caller.

Ronderos of Vinchos. Group interview by author with the assistance of Madeleine Pariona Oncebay, March 13, 1999, Ayacucho.

Sánchez Moreno, Francisco. Interview by author, March 10, 1998, Lima. Head of Frente Nacional de Defensa de la Salud y la Seguridad Social and Former Decano of the Colegio Médico of Peru.

Solari Y., Jorge. Interview by author, April 8, 1998, Lima. Capacitación de Medicinas and Director de La Revista, Servicio de Medicinas, Pro-Vida.

Tamayo, Giulia. 1998. Communication with author, April 20, 1998, Lima.

Tejada, David. Interview by author, January 19, 1999, Lima. Former minister of
    health.
Tejada, David, Jr. Interview by author, July 15, 2002, Lima. Former head of the
    Seguro Integral de Salud.
Torres, Raúl. Interview by author, February 25, 1998, Lima; April 12, 2000.
    Director, Comité de Monitoreo de Reforma de Seguridad Social.
Vaso de Leche members of San Martin de Porres, CLAS, Puesto de Salud San Martín
    de Porres. Group interview by author, August 14, 1998, Lima.
Vera del Carpio, Juan José. Interview by author, April 23, 1998, Lima. Director of
    Program of Shared Administration (CLAS), MINSA.
Veyes, Gabriela Angela. Interview by author, December 4, 1998, Lima.
Victoria, Sra. Interview by author. January 12, 1999, Lima. Coordinator of Comedor
    "Tito Condemayta," PSBT center 10 de Octubre.
Vidal, Alvaro. Interview by author, August 17, 1998, Lima. Former president,
    Asociación Médica del IPSS (AMSSOP), and general secretary of the Frente
    Nacional de Defensa de la Salud y la Seguridad Social.
Wicht, Padre Juan Julio. Interview by author, November 13, 1998, Lima.
Yapias Rojas, Edelmira. Interview by author, July 13, 1998, Lima. President, CLAS
    Laura Caller.
Zamora, Victor. Interview by author, July 22, 2002, Lima; interview by author,
    June 29, 2007, Lima. Former regional director of health, San Martín, and
    official at UNFPA in Lima.

index

abortion, 173, 195
absenteeism, health staff, 143
activists, feminist. *See* feminist activists
Acuerdo Político en Salud, 185
Afro-Peruvian, 15, 17
age, health care costs and, 175
agenda-setting, 84
AIDS, 136, 194, 195
alcohol, 4, 7, 134, 136
Alma Alta, 1978 conference at, 69
Amazon, 15, 39
APRA, 48–50
Argentina, 102
Asociación de Empleados del Perú, 50
Asociación Nacional de Médicos del Ministe-
    rio de Salud, 105

Bamako Initiative, 72, 85
Basic Health and Nutrition Program. *See*
    Programa de Salud y Nutrición Básica
basic health care package
    public health system and, 97, 134–37,
        144–46, 208
    social security and private insurers (mini-
        mal plan) and, 107–8, 122, 172–73, 208
Basic Health for All Program. *See* Programa
    de Salud Básica para Todos (PSBT)
Beijing Women's Conference. *See* United
    Nations Fourth World Conference on
    Women
Belaúnde Terry, Fernando, 43–44, 51
Benavides, Oscar, 48–49
Bermúdez, Francisco Morales, 42
Bismarck, 32, 48
Bolivia, 83, 180–81, 210
boomerang pattern, 165
bounded rationality, 62
Brazil, 102
British Department for International Devel-
    opment (DFID), 82
bureaucracy and reform, 63, 78–79, 83
Bustamente Rivero, José L., 50

Cairo accords. *See* International Conference
    on Population and Development (ICPD)
cancer, 134–36
capabilities, human, 74–75
Carbone Campoverde, Fernando, 162–63, 192
CARE, 185
care work
    basic health package and, 137, 144, 207–8
    definition of, 12 n. 11
    health insurance and, 168
    health insurance for community volun-
        teers and, 192, 195
    redistribution and recognition and, 21–22
    Seguro Escolar Gratuito and, 178–79
    waiting times and, 141–43, 144
    See also social reproduction
Catholic Church, 89–90, 149, 157–58
Center for Reproductive Law and Policy, 160
Center for the Defense of Women's Rights.
    See Estudio para la Defensa de los Dere-
    chos de la Mujer
Chile
    as a model of health reform, 24, 83, 106–7
    gender discrimination by private insurers
        in, 170, 174, 210
    gender mainstreaming in, 18
    health decentralization in, 102
    Plan AUGE of, 73, 83, 186
    private interests in, 203
    women's ministry of, 118
chola, 15
Cipriani, Luis, 157
Colegio Médico, 105, 185
Colombia
    health decentralization in, 102
    as a model of health reform, 24, 83, 117,
        187, 210
    social security health coverage in, 17
colonialism, internal, 30–31, 33, 38–40
Comité de América Latina y el Caribe para
    la Defensa de los Derechos de la Mujer
    (CLADEM), 150, 160